Amputation Surgery
and Lower Limb Prosthetics

EDITED BY

G. MURDOCH

MB, ChB, FRCS
Professor of Orthopaedic Surge
University of Dundee

CO-EDITOR

R.G. DONOVAN

AIMBI
Glasgow

GW00601954

FOREWORD BY

E.M. BURGESS

MD
Seattle

BLACKWELL SCIENTIFIC PUBLICATIONS

OXFORD LONDON EDINBURGH
BOSTON PALO ALTO MELBOURNE

© 1988 by
Blackwell Scientific Publications
Editorial offices:
Osney Mead, Oxford OX2 0EL
    (*Orders:* Tel. 0865 240201)
8 John Street, London WC1N 2ES
23 Ainslie Place, Edinburgh EH3 6AJ
3 Cambridge Center, Suite 208, Cambridge,
    Massachusetts 02142, USA
667 Lytton Avenue, Palo Alto,
    California 94301, USA
107 Barry Street, Carlton,
    Victoria 3053, Australia

First published 1988

Set by Scottish Studios and Engravers, Glasgow,
printed by The Alden Press, Oxford, and bound
by Hunter & Foulis, Edinburgh.

DISTRIBUTORS
USA
    Year Book Medical Publishers
    200 North LaSalle Street,
    Chicago, Illinois 60601
    (*Orders:* Tel. 312 726-9733)

Canada
    The C.V. Mosby Company
    5240 Finch Avenue East,
    Scarborough, Ontario
    (*Orders:* Tel. 416-298-1588)

Australia
    Blackwell Scientific Publications
    (Australia) Pty Ltd
    107 Barry Street,
    Carlton, Victoria 3053
    (*Orders:* Tel. [03] 347 0300)

British Library
Cataloguing in Publication Data
Amputation surgery
and lower limb prosthetics.
  1. Amputation
  2. Artificial limbs
I. Murdoch, G.
617'.58059   RD553

ISBN 0-632-01711-2

Contents

CONGENITAL LIMB DEFICIENCY

SPECIAL PROCEDURES IN AMPUTATION SURGERY

PROSTHETIC TECHNOLOGY

PROSTHETIC STANDARDS

Contributors

J.C. ANGEL FRCS, *Consultant Orthopaedic Surgeon, Limb Fitting Centre, Royal National Orthopaedic Hospital, Brockley Hill, Stanmore, Middlesex HA7 4LP*

S.J. ARNOTT MB, ChB(Ed), FRCS, FRCR, *Consultant Radiotherapist, St Bartholomew's Hospital, West Smithfield, London EC1A 7BE*

R.F. BAUMGARTNER MD, *Professor, Westfalische Wilhelms Universitat, Abteilung fur Technische Orthopadie und Rehabilitation, Robert-Koch-Strasse 30, D-4400 Munster, West Germany*

P. BOTTA, *Orthöpadietechniker, H. Botta & Fils, Appareillage Orthopedique, Rue Charles-Neuhaus 23, Biel, Switzerland*

H.U. BÜFF MD, *Associate Professor of Orthopaedics, Department of Dysmelia and Technical Orthopaedics, University of Heidelberg, Schlierbacher Landstrasse 200a, D-6900, Heidelberg, West Germany*

E.M. BURGESS MD, *Principal Investigator, Prosthetics Research Study, Room 409, 1102 Columbia Street, Seattle, Washington 98104, U.S.A.*

D.S. CHILDRESS PhD, *Director, Prosthetics Research Laboratory and Rehabilitation Engineering Program, Northwestern University, 345 East Superior Street, Room 1441, Chicago, Illinois 60611, U.S.A.*

D.N. CONDIE BSc, CEng, MIMechE, *Area Rehabilitation Engineer, Tayside Rehabilitation Engineering Services, Dundee Limb Fitting Centre, 133 Queen Street, Broughty Ferry, Dundee DD5 1AG*

M.E. CONDIE MCSP, *Physiotherapist, National Centre for Training and Education in Prosthetics and Orthotics, University of Strathclyde, Curran Building, 131 St James Road, Glasgow G4 0LS*

R.M. DAVIES PhD, *Professor, Bioengineering Centre, University College London, Roehampton Lane, Roehampton, London SW15 5PR, and Department of Orthopaedics, University of Washington, Seattle, U.S.A.*

xi

H.J.B. DAY MRCS, LRCP, *Senior Medical Officer, Department of Health and Social Security, Artificial Limb and Appliance Centre, Withington Hospital, Cavendish Road, Manchester M20 8LB*

P. DIXON OBE, MA, *Chairman, British Limbless Ex-Servicemen's Association, 185–7 High Road, Chadwell Heath, Essex RM6 6NA*

T.J. DONNELLY MCSP, *Senior Physiotherapist, Prosthetics and Orthotics, Rehabilitation Unit, Southern General Hospital, Glasgow G51 4TF*

B. EBSKOV Dr Med Sc, *Consultant, Department of Orthopaedic Surgery T, Herlev Hospital, DK2730 Herlev, Denmark*

S. FISHMAN PhD, *Professor and Co-ordinator, Department of Prosthetics and Orthotics, Post-graduate Medical School, New York University, 317 East 34th Street, New York, NY 10016, U.S.A.*

D. GARDNER, *Nursing Officer, Dundee Limb Fitting Centre, 133 Queen Street, Broughty Ferry, Dundee DD5 1AG*

R. GILLESPIE MB, ChB, FRCS(Ed), FRCS(C), *Head, Department of Orthopaedic Surgery, The Children's Hospital of Buffalo, 219 Bryant Street, Buffalo, New York, NY 14222, U.S.A.*

S. HEIM, *Orthopaedic Meister, Director, Bundesfachschule fur Orthopadie Technik, Schliepstrasse 8, D-4600 Dortmund 1, West Germany*

J. HUGHES BSc, CEng, FIMechE, *Professor, Director, National Centre for Training and Education in Prosthetics and Orthotics, University of Strathclyde, Curran Building, 131 St James Road, Glasgow G4 0LS*

N.A. JACOBS BSc, MSc, *Deputy Director, National Centre for Training and Education in Prosthetics and Orthotics, University of Strathclyde, Curran Building, 131 St James Road, Glasgow G4 0LS*

K. KAMWENDO, *Occupational Therapist, Department of Occupational Medicine, Örebro Hospital, Örebro, Sweden*

W. KAPHINGST Dipl Ing, *Auf der Pitzes, 3575 Betziedorf, West Germany, formerly of Deutsch Geselschaft fur Technische*

A.N. KEIER MD, *Director, Leningrad Research Institute of Prosthetics, Ministry of Social Security of the RSFSR 117934, 4 Shabolovka Street, Moscow, U.S.S.R.*

R.M. KENEDI, BSc, PhD, ARCST, CEng, FIMechE, MRAes, FHKIE, FRSE, *Foreign Associate of the National Academy of Engineering, U.S.A., and Emeritus Professor, University of Strathclyde, McCance Building, 16 Richmond Street, Glasgow G1 1XG*

B.L. KLASSON PhD, *Vice-president and Head of Research and Development, Een-*

Holmgren Ort AB, Box 60013, 104 01 Stockholm, and Bioengineering Consultant, Department of Orthopaedic Surgery, Karolinska Hospital, Stockholm, Sweden

N.I. KONDRASHIN, Professor, Doctor of Medicine, Director, Central Research Institute of Prosthetics, Ministry of Social Security of the RSFSR, 117934, 4 Shablovka Street, Moscow, U.S.S.R.

O. KRISTINSSON, Director, Össur hf., Box 5288, 125 Reykjavik, Iceland

L.M. KRUGER MD, Chief of Staff, Shriners Hospital for Crippled Children, 516 Carew Street, Springfield, Massachusetts 01104, U.S.A.

D.W. LAMB MB, ChB(Ed), FRCS(Ed), Consultant Orthopaedic Surgeon, Princess Margaret Rose Orthopaedic Hospital, Fairmilehead, Edinburgh EH10 7ED

M. LORD MPhil, Senior Lecturer, Faculty of Engineering, formerly of the Bioengineering Centre, University College London, Roehampton Lane, Roehampton, London SW15 5PR

E. LYQUIST CPO, Principal Prosthetist/Orthotist, The Society and Home for the Disabled in Denmark, Prosthetics and Orthotics Department, Borgervaenget 5, 2100 Copenhagen, Denmark

P.T. McCOLLUM FRCSI, Research Registrar in Surgery, Vascular Laboratory, Ninewells Hospital, Dundee, presently of Department of Surgery, Vascular Laboratory, St James's Hospital, PO Box 580, Dublin 8

A.W. McQUIRK FIBST, Director, Prosthetic Services, J. E. Hanger & Co. Ltd, Roehampton Lane, Roehampton, London SW15 5PL

E.G. MARQUARDT MD, Professor of Orthopaedics, Department of Dysmelia and Technical Orthopaedics, University of Heidelberg, Orthopaedic Hospital, Schlierbacher Landstrasse 200a, D-6900 Heidelberg, West Germany

G. MURDOCH MB, ChB, FRCS, Emeritus Professor of Orthopaedic Surgery, University of Dundee, Dundee, and Dundee Limb Fitting Centre, 133 Queen Street, Broughty Ferry, Dundee DD5 1AG

G. NEFF Dr Med, Oberarzt, Abteilung Technische Orthopadie und Biomechanik, Orthopadische Universitatsklinik und Poliklinik Tubingen, Calwer Strasse 7, 7400 Tubingen 1, West Germany

U. NILSONNE, Dr Med, Orthpedisk Kirugiska Kliniken, Karolinska sjukhuset, 104 01 Stockholm, Sweden

K.E.T. ÖBERG Dr Med Sc, Director, Prosthetic/Orthotic School, Munksjoskolan, Box 1030, S-551 11 Jonkoping, Sweden

J.P. PAUL BSc, PhD, CEng, FIMechE, FBOA, FRSA, FRSE, Professor of Bioengineering, Bioengineering Unit, University of Strathclyde, Wolfson Centre, 106 Rottenrow, Glasgow G5 0NW

H. PFAU Dr, *Orthopadische Werkstatten, Sanitatshaus Heinz Pfau GmbH & Co. KG, Martin-Luther-Strasse 117, 1 Berlin 62, West Germany*

C.H. PRITHAM CPO, *Technical Co-ordinator, Durr-Fillauer Inc., Orthopedic Division, 2710 Amnicola Highway, Chattanooga, Tennessee 37406, U.S.A.*

E. RAMSAY MCSP, *Superintendent Physiotherapist, Dundee Limb Fitting Centre, 133 Queen Street, Broughty Ferry, Dundee DD5 1AG*

R.G. REDHEAD MBBS, PhD, *Senior Medical Officer, Department of Health and Social Security, Limb Fitting Centre, Roehampton Lane, Roehampton, London SW15 5PR*

G. ROBERTSON OBE, FHA, *13 Lockharton Crescent, Edinburgh EH14 1AX, formerly Administrator, Scottish Home and Health Department, Edinburgh*

A.V. ROZHKOV Dr, *Leningrad Research Institute of Prosthetics, Ministry of Social Security of the RSFSR, 117934, 4 Shablovka Street, Moscow, U.S.S.R.*

M. SALEH MB, ChB, MSc(Bioeng), FRCS(Eng) FRCS(Ed), *Senior Lecturer and Honorary Consultant, Northern General Hospital, Harriers Road, Sheffield S5 7AU*

S. SAWAMURA MD, *Director, Hyogo Rehabilitation Center, 1070 Akebono-cho, Tarumi-ku, Kobe 673, Japan*

J.T. SCALES OBE, FRCS, CIMechE, *Professor of Biomedical Engineering, Institute of Orthopaedics, University of London, Royal National Orthopaedic Hospital, Brockley Hill, Stanmore, Middlesex HA7 4LP*

H. SCHMIDL, *Professor of Orthopaedics, Istituto Nazionale per l'Assicurazione, Contro gli Infortuni sul Lavoro, Vigorso di Budrio, 40054 Bologna, Italy*

O.Y. SHATILOV, *Doctor of Medicine, Head of Division of Clinical Problems in Prosthetics, Leningrad Research Institute of Prosthetics, Ministry of Social Security of the RSFSR, 11793, 4 Shabolovka Street, Moscow, U.S.S.R.*

B.V. SHISHKIN Med Sc Cand, *Senior Researcher, Central Research Institute of Prosthetics, Ministry of Social Security of the RSFSR, 117934, 4 Shabolovka Street, Moscow, U.S.S.R.*

J.J. SHORTER MIIM, MBIM, *Technical Director, Chas. A. Blatchford & Sons Ltd, Research and Development Unit, Unit 6, Sherrington Way, Basingstoke, Hampshire RG22 4LU*

A. SMITH DipCOT, *Senior Occupational Therapist, Dundee Limb Fitting Centre, 133 Queen Street, Broughty Ferry, Dundee DD5 1AG*

S.E. SOLOMONIDIS BSc, ARCST, CEng, MIMechE, *Lecturer, Bioengineering Unit, University of Strathclyde, Wolfson Centre, 106 Rottenrow, Glasgow G4 0NW*

V.A. SPENCE PhD, *Principal Physicist, Vascular Laboratory, Ninewells Hospital, Dundee DD1 9SY*

W.D. SPENCE MSc, *Prosthetist Orthotist, Bio-Engineering Unit, University of Strathclyde, Wolfson Centre, 106 Rottenrow, Glasgow G4 0NW*

J. STEEN JENSEN, MD, PhD, *Department of Orthopaedics, Rigshospitalet, University of Copenhagen, DK2100 Copenhagen, Denmark*

C.P.U. STEWART MD, D Med Rehab, *Associate Specialist (Prosthetics and Orthotics), Dundee Limb Fitting Centre, 133 Queen Street, Broughty Ferry, Dundee DD5 1AG*

M.L. STILLS CO, *Assistant Professor and Instructor in Orthopedics, The University of Texas, Health Science Centre at Dallas, Southwestern Medical School, 5323 Harry Hines Boulevard, Dallas, Texas 75235, U.S.A.*

A.J.G. SWANSON MB, ChB, FRCS, *Consultant Orthopaedic Surgeon, Caird Block, Dundee Royal Infirmary, DD1 9ND*

J.S. TAYLOR FBIST, *Chief Prosthetist, National Centre for Training and Education in Prosthetics and Orthotics, University of Strathclyde, Curran Building, 131 St James Road, Glasgow G4 0LS*

I.M. TROUP MB, ChB, D Med Rehab, *Formerly Medical Rehabilitation Consultant, Dundee Limb Fitting Centre, 133 Queen Street, Broughty Ferry, Dundee DD5 1AG. Home address: 3 Bonspiel Gardens, Camphill Road, Broughty Ferry, Dundee, Scotland*

R.L. VAN VORHIS MS, *Prosthetics Research Laboratory and Rehabilitation Engineering Program, Northwestern University, 345 East Superior Street, Room 1441, Chicago, Illinois 60611, U.S.A.*

W.F. WALKER DSc, FRCS, FRCSE, *Professor, Vascular Laboratory, Ninewells Hospital, Dundee DD1 9SY*

M. WALL *Orthopaedic Consultant, Samariterhemmets Sjukhus, Box 609, 751 25 Uppsala, Sweden*

A.B. WILSON Jr BSME, *Associate Professor of Prosthetics/Orthotics, Department of Orthopaedics and Rehabilitation, Rehabilitation Research and Training, University of Virginia Medical Center, Box 159, Charlottesville, Virginia 22908, U.S.A.*

M.S. ZAHEDI BSc, PhD, *Chas. A. Blatchford & Sons Ltd, Sherrington Way, Basingstoke, Hampshire, RG22 4LL*

Foreword

This publication documents an excellent and timely educational event. Not only does it present a comprehensive summary of current state-of-the art practice and research, it additionally outlines the challenge of future needs. Few areas of health services are experiencing as great a change as is now under way in prosthetics and orthotics. This volume brings together the wisdom and experience of many world-wide leaders in amputation surgery and in prosthetic rehabilitation. Appropriately, all disciplines directly responsible for team service are included. This unified approach is a cardinal requisite for holistic care. Without it amputee management falls short of what it can and should achieve.

The dynamic nature of amputation surgery is refreshingly reported. Current concepts of level determination, wound healing, functional assessment and the reconstructive nature of limb ablation are emphasized. Advances in prosthetic technology, in particular automated fabrication of mobility aids, highlights research reports.

It is a delight and an inspiration to read and study these monographs. Professor George Murdoch and his staff have again demonstrated their ability to organize a comprehensive, powerful conference. ISPO sponsorship underlies this effort. Those of us who were privileged to attend and the many others who can now read the papers should use these data to extend the quality of care. Each contributor and especially the internationally recognized and respected Dundee host participants deserve our gratitude. Wide readership is assured.

E. M. Burgess

Preface

Over a number of years, conferences in the field of rehabilitation engineering, and particularly on amputation surgery, prosthetics and orthotics, have been held in Dundee. The meetings have traditionally involved the foremost world authorities as principal speakers. The first publication in the field of amputation surgery and prosthetics was *Prosthetic and Orthotic Practice* published in 1970. Since that time there have been many requests to convene another conference on the same subjects and to produce another publication. Accordingly, in July, 1985, a conference was held on Amputation Surgery and Prosthetics of the Lower Limb, and this volume is the resultant. The book is not simply a compendium of the proceedings of a conference randomly organized. Indeed the conference was structured so that it would be reflected in this volume and ensure the publication of the papers presented by these acknowledged authorities in their allotted fields in an orderly and comprehensive way. As before, the influence of the clinic team has been emphasized because of its importance in effecting a comprehensive and successful rehabilitation of the patient. It is hoped that the integration of information on amputation surgery and biomechanics, prosthetic prescription and fabrication, rehabilitation and management will increase understanding of the complexity of delivering patient care in this field.

George Murdoch

Acknowledgements

I wish straightaway to acknowledge the extent of sponsorship in the production of this volume. Without it the cost would have been beyond the resources of some members of the clinic team. The principal sponsor is the International Society for Prosthetics and Orthotics, a society comprising individual professionals representing all the disciplines involved in the rehabilitation of the amputee. The British Limbless Ex-Servicemen's Association representing the consumer has, as always, supported this effort in education and training. Finally the commercial suppliers of prostheses and prosthetic components have responded in an enlightened way by contributing handsomely; they are Otto Bock Limited and the British manufacturers Messrs Chas. A. Blatchford & Sons Ltd, Messrs J. E. Hanger & Co. Ltd, and Messrs Hugh Steeper Ltd.

Next I wish to recognize the contribution of the authors. As world authorities they have provided us with a unique body of knowledge derived from their extensive experience and research. All gave of their valuable time and it is to be hoped that they in turn gained from contact with their colleagues. Certainly their readers will have a rewarding experience to the ultimate benefit of their patients.

The staff of Dundee Limb Fitting Centre and their colleagues in Kings Cross Hospital, Ninewells Hospital and Dundee Royal Infirmary have contributed by their unfailing enthusiasm and high competence expressed day by day in their clinical practice. I am pleased we have been able to record that experience which is a tribute in itself. Tayside Health Board and the University of Dundee have always supported our efforts and did not fail us on this occasion.

Special thanks are due to a number of colleagues but the contribution of some requires special mention, namely Dr Ian Troup for the contribution he made to the welfare of our patients over so many years; and to David Condie for our many fruitful years of collaboration and his help in formulating the conference and thus the contents of this volume.

I wish to make a very special acknowledgement of the considerable contribution made by Ron Donovan, my colleague of more than 30 years' standing for the painstaking work he has done as co-editor in handling the material emanating from so many disciplines and language sources. His experience and meticulous attention to detail have been invaluable.

I must reserve my final thanks and acknowledgement to Jean Whyte, my secretary, who has been responsible for all the real work of organizing the material, maintaining a day-to-day update to the files and of course all the typing involved, but most of all for her quick and lively intelligence and good humour.

While an acknowledgement of fruitful collaboration with our publishers represented by Nigel Palmer and his staff is something of a formality, I like to think it has gone beyond that. Certainly I have appreciated the understanding, encouragement and tolerance displayed and my hope is that our combined efforts will go some way to helping the clinic team in its efforts towards better clinical practice.

GENERAL PRINCIPLES

1

Trends in Lower Extremity Amputation (Denmark, 1978–1983)

B. EBSKOV

Introduction

In the past it has generally not been possible to identify trends in lower extremity amputation because nationwide surveys have not been accessible. With the Danish Amputation Register (DAR), however, it is feasible to record, year by year, the total number of amputations (Ebskov 1977). This chapter aims to present the results of a nationwide study of Danish lower extremity amputations during the period 1978–1983.

Material and methods

Since the mid-seventies the Danish National Patient Register (NPR) has recorded all admissions to hospitals dealing with physical problems. Among other data the recordings comprise dates of admission and discharge, diagnoses according to the International Classification of Diseases (ICD), the date and code of operations performed, and, of course, personal data on each individual patient, including age, sex, and habitat. Initially the NPR did not record data from all hospitals, and the recordings were not invariably exact. By 1978, however, the problems had been eliminated, and the material thereafter was considered fully reliable. Since that year the DAR has had access to the NPR and has extracted pertinent data on all significant amputations on a yearly basis. The present material comprises all amputations from the transmetatarsal level proximally during 1978–1983. Based upon the ICD diagnoses the patients were sorted into ten aetiological groups, i.e. 01, arteriosclerosis; 02, diabetes mellitus; 03, trauma; 04, benign tumours; 05, malignant tumours; 06, congenital deformity; 07, congenital amputation; 08, infection (NB: *not* infected gangrene); 09, intractable pseudarthrosis; and 10, miscellaneous (e.g. Buerger disease).

Results

Table 1.1 shows the total number of amputations year by year as well as the

3

Table 1.1 Lower extremity amputations in Denmark, 1978–1983.

Year	Total	01 Arterio-sclerosis (%)	02 Diabetes mellitus (%)	03 Trauma (%)	05 Tumour (%)	06 Congenital deformity (%)	08 Infection (%)	09 Pseud-arthrosis (%)	10 Miscellaneous (%)
1978	1838	61.0	26.6	3.4	2.2	0.1	2.9	0.1	2.9
1979	1969	59.6	27.6	4.6	2.0	0.5	2.1	0.1	3.4
1980	2168	61.1	27.4	4.0	1.5	0.3	2.2	0.1	3.6
1981	2125	61.0	27.1	4.0	2.1	0.2	2.8	0.1	4.4
1982	2165	61.9	24.8	3.7	1.5	0.5	3.3	0	4.4
1983	2200	64.1	23.2	3.5	1.8	0.2	3.1	0	4.1

percentage representation of the ten aetiological groups related to the individual year's total. The annual totals are plotted in Figs 1.1 and 1.2. Apparently the trend is upward, and assessed by the chi-square method the increase is significant ($p <$ 0.001). The majority of amputations were found in aetiological groups 01 and 02, these causal conditions being responsible for more than 85% overall (Fig. 1.3). Whereas these totals are largely unchanged over the years, the relative share of arteriosclerosis seems to be increasing, while the share of diabetes mellitus seems to be decreasing. However, in the material so far available the changes are not statistically significant. The tendencies seen are further demonstrated in Fig. 1.4, which includes aetiology group 03 as well. Trauma seems to be a very constant cause of amputation, accounting for roughly 4% every year.

Fig. 1.5 shows the relative share of the aetiological groups: malignant tumour, congenital deformity, infection, and pseudarthrosis. Each of these groups is represented somewhere between 0 and 3% with no apparent change in either direction. During the period in question no lower extremity amputations were performed for benign tumour, and no congenital amputations were recorded.

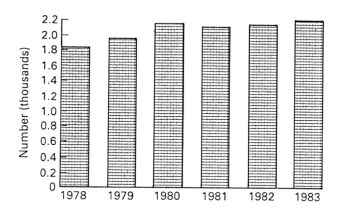

Fig. 1.1 Total number of lower extremity amputations from the transmetatarsal level proximally, 1978–1983.

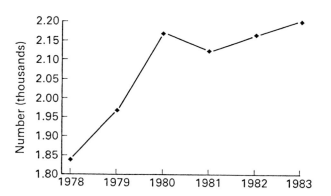

Fig. 1.2 The trend regarding an increase in amputations is demonstrated. It is statistically significant by the chi-square method ($p < 0.001$).

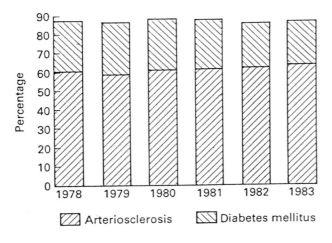

Fig. 1.3 The combined share of arteriosclerotic and diabetic gangrene consistently accounts for more than 85% of all lower extremity amputations.

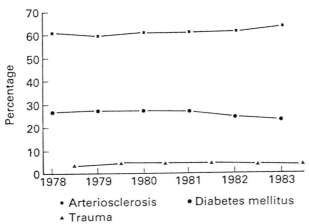

Fig. 1.4 Trends in amputation for arteriosclerotic and diabetic gangrene as well as trauma. The changes within each aetiology are not statistically significant.

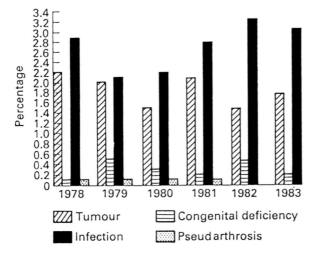

Fig. 1.5 Comparison of amputations for malignant tumour, congenital deformity, infection, and intractable pseudarthrosis as a percentage of the total.

Discussion

The only statistically significant trend being the increase in the total number of amputations, it seems relevant to consider possible explanations of this phenomenon. For a number of years the older age groups in Denmark have constituted an ever-increasing percentage of the total population. Since arteriosclerosis is the predominant aetiology leading to lower extremity amputation, it seemed reasonable to assume a connection with the increasing number of amputations. In a previous study (not published) no connection was demonstrated between the increase in the number of citizens over 69 years of age and the incidence of lower extremity amputation, as assessed nationwide, county by county. Furthermore, the age groups in question have, for the period studied, shown no increase in any way close to the percentage increase in total number of amputations from 1978 to 1983 (17.8%), or to the increase of arteriosclerotic amputees (19.3%).

Theoretically the upward trend might be explained by a change in indications for amputation. According to available information no such change has taken place. Is it possible then that the 'significant' increasing trend might in fact be non-existent? From previous studies (Ebskov & Josephsen 1980), it is known that the incidence of ipsilateral reamputation following a 'first lower extremity amputation' is very high during the first half-year after original surgery, and in particular in the first three months; in contrast ipsilateral reamputation after that period of time is very rare. This fact was interpreted as the unintended result of an increasingly conservative policy of preservation of limb length, or in other words a too optimistic interpretation of tissue viability. On the other hand, contralateral amputation shows an ever-increasing incidence year after year during the four-year observation period. The material analysed was collected by the DAR, using questionnaires returned from the surgical departments participating in the project. In this way information on the side amputated (right/left) was obtained, as well as details of any earlier amputation(s), and this information was updated by new reports in the case of later amputation. The information on eventual cause of death was furnished in the reports, and later confirmed and supplemented by comparison with the National Person Register, which records personal data, including death. The National Patient Register, on the other hand, records operations (i.e. amputations), not persons, and also the operation codes do not contain information on laterality. Consequently the increasing number of amputations does not necessarily mean a correspondingly increasing number of amputees, but an increasing number of patients with ipsilateral reamputation as well as contralateral amputation.

Based upon these observations a study is being planned, whereby amputees subject to more than one amputation may be isolated. This is easily accomplished by sorting the material derived from the 'personal number', which is recorded for all patients. Once located it is possible to obtain from the relevant surgical departments the discharge notes on the persons in question, thereby accessing the missing details, including laterality.

Acknowledgement

The present study was generously supported by a grant from the Krista and Viggo Petersen Foundation, to which the author is deeply grateful.

References

Ebskov B. (1977) Fruhergebnisse des Danischen Amputationsregisters — ein nationales Registrierungs-system. *Orthopädische Praxis* **13** 430–433.

Ebskov B. & Josephsen P. (1980) Incidence of reamputation and death after gangrene of the lower extremity. *Prosthetics and Orthotics International* **4**, 77–80.

2

Recommendations for the Objective Determination of the Level of Limb Viability

V.A. SPENCE, P.T. McCOLLUM & W.F. WALKER

Introduction

In 1971 Romano and Burgess suggested that most amputations for peripheral vascular disease will heal at the below-knee level. This statement was reinforced by Murdoch in 1975, who declared that 'there is ample evidence that more knees can be saved than a decade ago'. Despite these firm convictions, there remains a disappointingly high rate of above-knee amputations (AKAs) in relation to below-knee amputations (BKAs) (Barnes *et al.* 1976, Finch *et al.* 1980, Porter *et al.* 1981), although there has been a shift in emphasis towards preservation of the knee joint (Thompson *et al.* 1974). It is quite feasible to achieve BKA to AKA ratios of 3:1 or better with excellent healing rates (Malone *et al.* 1981, McCollum *et al.* 1984), but this degree of success is limited to a few specialized centres. There are many good reasons for this. In the first instance, amputation services are generally not centralized, resulting in relatively low amputation numbers in individual hospitals and a consequent lack of experience. Secondly, few surgeons have recourse to ancillary methods to aid in the selection of the precise level of amputation.

It is clear that there are two questions to be considered: (a) will a distal (e.g. part-foot) amputation heal, and (b), if not, can the knee joint be preserved? Determination of the level of foot viability is quite a different problem, and it is important to stress that criteria used in the assessment of below-knee level viability do not necessarily apply to the foot.

Clinical assessment

Whilst much criticism can be made against the use of clinical judgement alone in the selection of amputation level, good results can be obtained by an experienced amputation surgeon (Romano & Burgess 1971, Robinson 1972, Burgess & Matsen 1981). In some patients, however, assessment of the level of limb viability will not be obvious on clinical inspection, even by the most experienced surgeon, and additional objective tests will be required to supplement clinical judgement. Such information will be of particular importance in those patients in whom preservation

9

of the knee joint might require a specifically designed skin-flap other than the long posterior flap.

Ancillary methods

A wide variety of potentially useful investigations is available to the amputating surgeon (Table 2.1), but many of the techniques listed are not in general use, mainly because they do not fulfil the exacting demands which are necessary for a method to be clinically useful; simplicity, reliability and reproducibility are essential characteristics. The aim of this chapter is to investigate the claims made for methods in common use, and to recommend particular techniques if they provide reliable objective information.

Table 2.1 Ancillary methods used to aid the selection of optimum amputation level.

Arteriography	Thermography
Plethysmography	Laser Doppler flowmetry
Doppler ultrasound	Fluorescein flowmetry
Radioisotope clearance	Photoplethysmography
Tissue Po_2/pH	Radioactive microspheres
Transcutaneous Po_2	Electromagnetic flowmetry

Systolic pressure measurements

The commonest investigation currently used in vascular laboratories is the measurement of Doppler systolic pressures. However, the significance of simple pressure measurements in the choice of amputation level is controversial. Several workers have found that ankle, below-knee or thigh pressure studies may be of value in predicting the outcome of BKA procedures (Dean *et al.* 1975, Cooperman *et al.* 1977, Pollack & Ernst 1980, Barnes *et al.* 1981, Creaney *et al.* 1981) although there is some disparity between the various recommended lower limits of pressure consistent with healing of a wound. Also, many diabetics have apparently high limb pressures because of rigid-walled arteries, rendering the investigation of doubtful significance in these patients (Lee *et al.* 1979). In addition, some BKAs will heal in spite of low ankle or below-knee pressures. This was emphasized by Lepantalo *et al.* (1982), who commented on the variability of outcome in BKAs performed on patients with calf pressures between 35 and 65 mmHg. Thigh pressure measurements may well have the most useful predictive value (Dean *et al.* 1975), and the authors have recently confirmed that a thigh pressure value of greater than 50 mmHg is a good indicator of potential below-knee viability. Plethysmographic pressure studies also have deficiencies, and techniques such as the mercury strain gauge become inaccurate and difficult to interpret at the low levels of arterial inflow that exist in critical ischaemia (Burgess & Matsen 1981). Measurement of big toe systolic pressure will give a good indication of flow resistance in the foot, but such a measurement is impractical in critically ischaemic limbs where distal gangrene or a low flow/pressure situation is common. Ankle pressures are also a poor guide to foot viability (Nicholas *et al.* 1982), and a high pressure does not guarantee healing (Raines *et al.* 1976).

This lack of correlation between healing of a distal amputation and the arterial systolic inflow pressure to the foot highlights the importance of measuring microcirculatory parameters when assessing the viability of a particular area of skin. The disordered capillary bed in the foot of diabetic patients, where microvascular stasis and ischaemia may coexist with a normal ankle pressure, is a good example of this problem. It is also clear that autoregulatory mechanisms and dependency can maintain perfusion in severely ischaemic, non-diabetic feet with low pressures.

Summary:
1 Below-knee amputation is worth attempting if the thigh pressure is greater than 50 mmHg.
2 Below-knee amputations can heal in the presence of very low ankle pressures.
3 Ankle pressures are of little value in determining the outcome of distal amputations.
4 Toe pressures may provide an index of viability for the foot, if they can be measured.

Skin blood flow measurement

A quantitative measurement of blood flow in the nutrient capillary loops of the skin can be calculated from the clearance of a biologically inert radioactive tracer, as first described by Kety in 1949. This technique has been developed and modified by others (Bohr 1967, Sejrsen 1967, Carr *et al.* 1977, Moore *et al.* 1981, Stockel *et al.* 1981), and at present the freely diffusible inert gas xenon-133 (^{133}Xe) is the most frequently used isotope. The problem with xenon is that it is highly fat-soluble and so the clearance from the skin is complicated by the dermal and subcuticular fat content. However, good results have been obtained with this tracer, and indeed the results obtained by Malone *et al.* (1981), where amputation level was selected on the basis of blood flow criteria, have not been bettered. The minimum blood flow, below which healing would not take place, was 2.0 ml/100 g/min. This contrasts with the experience of Holloway and Burgess (1978), who found that 'flows of 1.0 ml/100 g/min or below are to be viewed as borderline' and that no definite level of blood flow could be identified below which healing could not take place.

The authors' past experience, using xenon-133 as a tracer, was also disappointing, and indeed the clearance technique was dismissed as an unreliable method for determining skin viability. Later, it was discovered that a stable solution of ^{125}I-4-iodoantipyrine (^{125}I-4-IAP) gave a highly reproducible monoexponential clearance from colonic tissue (Forrester *et al.* 1980) and that the washout was unaffected by tissue fat content. Using this tracer for skin blood flow measurements (McCollum *et al.* 1985a), the authors have recently shown that it provides a monoexponential clearance in nearly every patient, and that the criteria laid down by Malone *et al.* (1981) seem justified. However, the authors are unsure of Malone's methodology, because it is quite clear that xenon-133 underestimates tissue blood flow, especially in ischaemic skin. Evidence for this has been obtained from recent work where a mixture of ^{125}I-4-IAP and ^{133}Xe was injected intradermally and their relative clearances monitored and plotted simultaneously. Results from one site on a severely ischaemic limb are illustrated in Fig. 2.1: ^{125}I-4-IAP clearance is significantly faster than that of ^{133}Xe. This disparity is probably due to the diffusion of ^{133}Xe into fat, which is accentuated in a tissue with a very reduced blood supply because of the increased time available for diffusion.

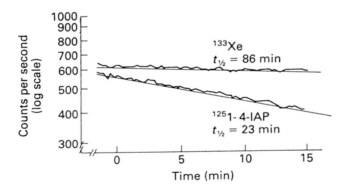

Fig. 2.1 Simultaneous washout of ^{125}I-4-iodoantipyrine and xenon-133 following an intradermal injection of a combination of the two isotopes. The calculated blood flows from the two washouts are significantly different, which demonstrates the inability of ^{133}Xe clearance to reflect accurately skin blood flow in a low-flow situation.

Using ^{125}I-4-IAP as a tracer, it is found that there is a significant blood flow gradient at the below-knee level. The medial skin has a better supply than the lateral, and this gradient is especially significant in a limb of marginal below-knee viability (McCollum *et al.* 1985a). It is therefore extremely important that at least two, and preferably three, blood flow measurements are made around the below-knee level before reliable predictions can be made as to healing potential. If these three measurements are available, then a mean blood flow of 2.5 ml/100 g/min or greater will be consistent with viability at the below-knee level. However, a specifically designed below-knee flap may be required if the measurements which made up the mean blood flow value are significantly skewed, especially if one measurement (generally the lateral) is less than 1.5 ml/100 g/min.

Similar skin blood flow measurements made on the foot are, unfortunately, not indicative of healing potential (McCollum *et al.* 1985b). Indeed, a blood flow measurement as high as 10–15 ml/100 g/min at a particular skin site on the foot is meaningless, and this highlights the principal inadequacy of the clearance technique — spot measurements are not necessarily indicative of regional blood flow characteristics. This problem applies particularly to the ischaemic foot, where microvascular blood flow patterns are dominated by flow through non-nutritional thoroughfare channels such that patches of ischaemia can co-exist with areas of normal perfusion.

Summary:

1 Multiple skin blood flow measurements can provide a good index of tissue viability at the below-knee level.

2 Above-knee amputation should be performed if the mean below-knee skin blood flow is less than 2.5 ml/100 g/min.

3 Skin blood flows in the foot are not indicative of regional tissue viability.

Transcutaneous oxygen measurements

The measurement of tissue oxygen tension in the skin of ischaemic limbs was first described in 1950 by Montgomery and Horwitz, but although reliable modern polarographic microelectrodes have been developed (Spence & Walker 1976), the direct measurement of oxygen tension in the skin is, in general, too difficult to be of practical use at present. However, the development of a transcutaneous oxygen electrode for monitoring neonatal arterial oxygen tension, first described by Huch et al. in 1969, renewed interest in the measurement of oxygen transport to the skin. Despite the simplicity of use of transcutaneous oxygen ($TcPo_2$) monitoring, the interpretation of such measurements in adult skin is difficult (Spence & McCollum 1985). Variables such as the arterial oxygen tension, transmural pressure, local oxygen availability, skin thickness, and local skin blood flow all contribute to the measured $TcPo_2$. In normal skin, many of these variables are counteracted by the maximum vasodilatory response produced under the electrode by its heater, leading to $TcPo_2$ values just below the arterial oxygen tension. However, in ischaemic skin, $TcPo_2$ measurements are not necessarily indicative of the local oxygen exhange rate but are more likely to be related to the underlying perfusion pressure.

Despite these reservations, several workers have found $TcPo_2$ studies to be useful in the assessment of the ischaemic limb (Matsen et al. 1980, Eickoff & Engell 1981, Clyne et al. 1982, Mustapha et al. 1983), and more recently a number of studies have proposed the method as a valuable adjunct to choosing the optimum level of amputation (Burgess et al. 1982, Franzeck et al. 1982, Dowd et al. 1983, Ratcliff et al. 1984). Although there is a general agreement that $TcPo_2$ measurements greater than 35 mmHg are consistent with healing, most studies have been unable to define a lower limit of $TcPo_2$ below which healing will not take place. This is further complicated by the fact that healing can sometimes occur at a $TcPo_2$ value of zero (Katsamouris et al. 1984).

One possible means of improving the discriminating ability of the TcPo$_2$ method for tissue viability studies might be achieved by monitoring the TcPo$_2$ changes induced by oxygen inhalation. The reasoning behind this dynamic evaluation of the tissue oxygen exchange rate stems from previous experimental work (Spence & Walker 1984a) which showed that the tissue oxygen tension may be maintained in ischaemic skin, but that the response to oxygen breathing was impaired. In critically ischaemic skin, the oxygen inhalation response was reduced or absent. The authors have recently reported on preliminary findings using a TcPo$_2$ electrode on ischaemic skin (Spence & McCollum 1985) and have shown that the lack of response to oxygen breathing was indeed a much better predictor of wound healing than the actual TcPo$_2$ value, breathing air. Other experimental work reflects the value of oxygen inhalation-induced changes in the evaluation of the ischaemic limb (Harward *et al.* 1985).

Summary:
1 A TcPo$_2$ value of 35 mmHg or more is associated with viable skin.
2 A TcPo$_2$ value of less than 35 mmHg does not always denote non-viable tissue.
3 A skin-flap may be viable despite a zero TcPo$_2$ reading.
4 Oxygen inhalation-induced changes can improve the sensitivity and specificity of the TcPo$_2$ method; severe impairment of the response to oxygen indicates critical ischaemia.

Infrared thermography

Infrared thermography has been used in the assessment of peripheral vascular disease for some 20 years (Branemark *et al.* 1967, Winsor 1971, McLoughlin & Rawsthorne 1973, Henderson & Hackett 1978), and indeed was suggested as a possible means of selecting amputation level by Lloyd-Williams in 1964. However, despite the obvious potential of the method, results have, until recently, been disappointing. There are two main reasons for this. In the first instance, the quality of most thermographic images has been relatively poor in terms of their spatial resolution. Thermograms have not been easy to quantify, and this has led to subjective and qualitative interpretations with consequent shortcomings. Secondly, the relationship between thermography and the underlying blood flow is poorly understood.

Recently, high-resolution digital thermographic systems became commercially available, and when linked to a microcomputer the output from these systems can be quantified. It is now possible to obtain an accurately calibrated thermal map of the limb such that the level of viability can be ascertained in an ischaemic leg. This level of viability is defined by specific isothermal criteria which are directly related to the underlying skin blood flow (Spence & Walker 1984b), and this evidence has supported previous studies which have recommended thermography as a useful adjunct to amputation level selection (Spence *et al.* 1981).

The great advantage of thermographic mapping of skin lies in the ability to assess whole skin areas. This contrasts with the principal difficulty of point source measurements which have to assume a regional homogeneity of flow around the measurement site. Such an assumption is not always valid, and the authors have recently demonstrated circumferential skin blood flow differences in the lower leg which are especially significant in the critically ischaemic leg (McCollum *et al.* 1985a). The ability to show this gradient is one of the assets of thermography, and can be used to help in the design of specific skin-flaps (Fig. 2.2a). However, the calibration of a thermographic image remains subjective and this means that the gradient which outlines the level of limb viability may be misrepresented by a few vital centimetres either way. Fig. 2.2b & c illustrate this difficulty, which may be overcome by measuring the skin blood flow concurrently at one or two points on the gradient.

Whereas thermographic gradients around the knee joint can reliably be used to demonstrate skin viability, such a simple relationship between flow and temperature does not exist in the ischaemic foot. The existence of a significant thermal gradient in the foot may indeed be indicative of the level of viability, but such gradients are rarely straightforward, being often quite different on the plantar and dorsal aspects of the same foot. Furthermore, similar gradients may exist in perfectly normal feet, depending upon the tone of the abundant thermoregulatory arteriovenous shunts. These shunts also contribute to the problem of foot hyperthermia, which is a common feature of the chronically ischaemic limb (Fig. 2.2d). The mechanism of dilated arteriovenous channels in ischaemic skin allows large volumes of blood to be held in the superficial venous plexuses, and this explains the phenomenon of inadequate foot perfusion in the presence of a larger than normal volume blood flow.

Summary:
1 The optimum level of amputation around the knee joint can be reliably predicted by thermographic mapping. However, measurement of blood flow in at least one spot on the gradient greatly enhances the specificity of the method.
2 Thermographic mapping is ideally suited to the delineation of specific skin-flaps.
3 Thermographic patterns of ischaemic feet are extremely complicated and do not, at present, add much objectivity to clinical assessment.

Skin fluorescence

The use of skin fluorescence to outline viable tissue has been recommended by several studies (Lange & Boyd 1942, Myers *et al.* 1971, Lawrence *et al.* 1980). A small quantity of fluorescein is injected intravenously, and this quickly diffuses across perfused capillary beds into the interstitial space. Ischaemic tissues will have little or no uptake of fluorescein, and when examined under ultraviolet light the demarcation between areas of viable and non-viable skin can be determined by the degree of fluorescence present. Using this method, recent studies have indicated

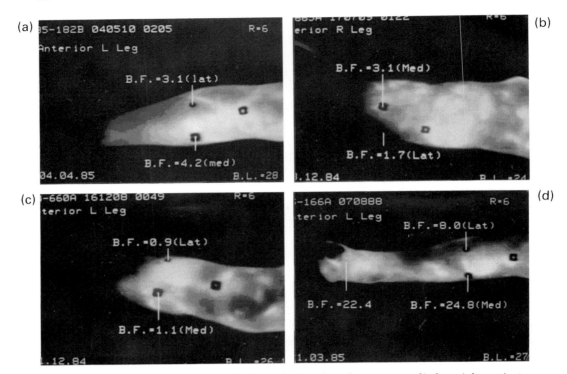

Fig. 2.2 Black and white reproductions of high-resolution colour thermograms of ischaemic legs prior to amputation. The black level (BL) and temperature range (R) calibrate the temperature scale of each image. The tibial tuberosity is identifiable (○) and blood flow values are superimposed on each image at two points 10 cm distal to the tibial tuberosity and at 3 cm medial and lateral to the anterior tibial border. (a) An example of a significant transverse thermal gradient around the level of limb viability with a marked hyperthermia just below the knee on the medial aspect, reflecting superficial arterial collaterals. (b) An example of a critically ischaemic limb with a blood flow value (lateral) less than 2.0 ml/100 g/min. The thermographic outline of the level of viability corresponds perfectly with the skin blood flow measurements and a medially skewed flap was recommended. (c) An example of a lack of correlation between the thermographic delineation of the level of viability and the skin blood flow measurements, which are clearly not consistent with below-knee healing. The black level is probably set too low on this image, and an above-knee amputation was recommended on the basis of the skin blood flow values. (d) A thermogram of the limb of a patient with gangrene of the big toe. There is hyperthermia of the foot and an excellent skin blood flow at the site of measurement. The hyperthermia extends up the medial aspect of the leg in the line of the saphenous vein, reflecting the warmer venous blood.

that the level of amputation can be reliably predicted (McFarland & Lawrence 1982, Tanzer & Horne 1982). Like thermography, it has the potential for outlining skin-flaps, but has been limited by purely qualitative interpretations, although it is probable that the objective methodology developed by Silverman and Wagner (1983) will impart the same degree of objectivity which thermography has recently gained. Of all the investigations available, skin fluorescence is the only method, apart from angiography, which can have potentially fatal side-effects (Buchanan & Levine 1982).

Other methods

Several alternative investigative techniques have been proposed, and have generally been found wanting in terms of reliability and usefulness as methods of assessing tissue viability. There have been reports on muscle pH (Young *et al.* 1978), radioactive microspheres (Fee *et al.* 1977), photoplethysmography and non-invasive electromagnetic flowmeter studies (Lee *et al.* 1979) and laser Doppler measurements (Holloway & Burgess 1983). Of these, laser Doppler has perhaps the most exciting potential, but as yet the method has been unable to give sufficiently quantitative data for accurate assessment of tissue viability in a limb. Its ability to measure changes in skin blood flow is well recognized, and indeed it provides one of the few currently available techniques which may truly be said to assess the microcirculation.

Conclusion

In the description of the various methods used for amputation level selection emphasis has been placed on the assessment of skin viability, by whatever means, as the most important criterion. This is certainly so for amputations at the below-knee level (Young *et al.* 1978), but it is not true for part-foot amputations, where skin blood flow differs anatomically and functionally. A good BKA with early mobilization is surely preferable to multiple 'conservative' procedures on an ischaemic foot, which often result ultimately in a higher amputation, and certainly contribute to increased patient morbidity (McCollough 1972). The exception is the ischaemic diabetic foot without proximal arterial disease, in which a local procedure is more likely to be successful (Gibbons *et al.* 1979, Ger 1984).

Of the methods described, thermography and fluorescein angiography have the potential to outline skin-flaps; however, skin fluorescence has the disadvantage of being invasive, and while thermography is non-invasive it requires an initial capital expenditure, although this cost is quickly offset by the salvage of only a few extra BKAs. Assessment of skin blood flow using radioisotopes has now become the standard by which other criteria are compared (Malone *et al.* 1981). The main disadvantage of this method is its inability to assess the whole limb, even with multiple measurements, a problem which is also true of skin perfusion pressure. Thus, there is a logic in using one of these measurements in conjuction with thermography of skin fluorescence to assess the critically ischaemic limb.

References

Barnes R. W., Shanik G. D. & Slaymaker E. E. (1976) An index of healing in below-knee amputation: leg blood pressure by Doppler ultrasound. *Surgery* **79**, 13–20.

Barnes R. W., Thornhill B., Nix L., Rittgers E. & Turley G. (1981) Prediction of amputation wound healing. *Archives of Surgery* **116**, 80–83.

Bohr H. (1967) Measurement of the blood flow in the skin with radioactive xenon. *Scandinavian Journal of Clinical and Laboratory Investigations* **19**, (suppl. 99), 60–61.

Branemark P. I., Fagerberg S. E., Langer L. & Save-Soderbergh J. (1967) Infrared thermography in diabetes mellitus. *Diabetologia* **3**, 529–532.

Buchanan R. T. & Levine N. S. (1982) Blood pressure drop as a result of fluorescein injection. *Plastic and Reconstructive Surgery* **70**, 363–368.

Burgess E. M. & Matsen F. A. (1981) Determining amputation level in peripheral vascular disease. *Journal of Bone and Joint Surgery* **63A**, 1493–1497.

Burgess E. M., Matsen F. A., Wyss C. R. & Simmons C. W. (1982) Segmental transcutaneous measurements of Po_2 in patients requiring below-the-knee amputation for peripheral vascular insufficiency. *Journal of Bone and Joint Surgery* **64A**, 378–382.

Carr M. J. T., Crooks J. A., Griffiths P. A. & Hopkinson B. R. (1977) Capillary blood flow in ischaemic limbs before and after surgery assessed by subcuticular injection of xenon-133. *American Journal of Surgery* **133**, 584–586.

Clyne C. A. C., Ryan J., Webster J. H. H. & Chant A. D. B. (1982) Oxygen tension of the skin of ischaemic legs. *American Journal of Surgery* **143**, 315–318.

Cooperman M., Clark M. & Evans W. E. (1977) Use of Doppler ultrasound in the selection of patients for below-knee amputation. *Review of Surgery* **34**, 362–363.

Creaney M. G., Chattopadhaya D. K., Ward A. S. & Morris-Jones W. (1981) Doppler ultrasound in the assessment of amputation level. *Journal of the Royal College of Surgeons of Edinburgh* **26**, 278–281.

Dean R. H., Yao J. S. T., Thompson R. G. & Bergan J. J. (1975) Predictive value of ultrasonically derived arterial pressure in determination of amputation level. *American Surgeon* **41**, 731–737.

Dowd G. S. E., Linge K. & Bentley G. (1983) Measurement of transcutaneous oxygen pressure in normal and ischaemic skin. *Journal of Bone and Joint Surgery,* **65B**, 79–83.

Eickhoff J. H. & Engell H. C. (1981) Transcutaneous oxygen tension ($TcPo_2$) measurements on the foot in normal subjects and in patients with peripheral arterial disease admitted for vascular surgery. *Scandinavian Journal of Clinical and Laboratory Investigation* **41**, 743–748.

Fee H. J., Friedman B. H. & Siegel M. E. (1977) The selection of an amputation level with radioactive microspheres. *Surgery, Gynecology and Obstetrics* **144**, 89–90.

Finch D. R. A., MacDougal M., Tibbs D. J. & Morris P. J. (1980) Amputation for vascular disease: the experience of a peripheral vascular unit. *British Journal of Surgery* **67**, 233–237.

Forrester D. W., Spence V. A. & Walker W. F. (1980) The measurement of colonic mucosal–submucosal blood flow in man. *Journal of Physiology* **299**, 1–11.

Franzeck U.K., Talke P., Bernstein E. F., Golbranson F. L. & Fronek A. (1982) Transcutaneous Po_2 measurements in health and peripheral arterial occlusive disease. *Surgery* **91**, 156–163.

Ger R. (1984) Newer concepts in the surgical management of lesions of the foot in the patient with diabetes. *Surgery, Gynecology and Obstetrics* **158**, 213–215.

Gibbons G. W., Wheelock F. C. Jr, Siembieda C., Hoar C. S. Jr, Rowbotham J. L. & Persson A. B. (1979) Non-invasive prediction of amputation level in diabetic patients. *Archives of Surgery,* **114**, 1253–1257.

Harward T. R. S., Volny J., Goldbranson F. L., Fronek A. & Bernstein E. F. (1985) Oxygen inhalation-induced transcutaneous Po_2 changes as a predictor of amputation level. *Journal of Vascular Surgery,* **2**, 220–227.

Henderson H. P. & Hackett M. E. J. (1978) The value of thermography in peripheral vascular disease. *Angiology* **29**, 65–75.

Holloway G. A. Jr & Burgess E. M. (1978) Cutaneous blood flow and its relation to healing of below knee amputation. *Surgery, Gynecology and Obstetrics* **146**, 750–756.

Holloway G. A. & Burgess E. M. (1983). Preliminary experiences with laser Doppler velocimetry for the determination of amputation levels. *Prosthetics and Orthotics International* **7**, 63–66.

Huch, A., Huch R. & Lubbers D. W. (1969) Quantitative polarographische sauerstoffdruckmessung auf der Kopfhaut des Neugeborenen. *Archive Gynaekologie* **207**, 443–451.

Katsamouris A., Brewster D. C., Megerman J., Cina C., Darling R. C. & Abbott W. M. (1984) Transcutaneous oxygen tension in selection of amputation level. *American Journal of Surgery* **147**, 510–517.

Kety S. S. (1949) Measurement of regional circulation by local clearance of radioactive sodium. *American Heart Journal* **38**, 321–327.

Lange K. & Boyd L. J. (1942) Use of fluorescein to determine adequacy of circulation. *Medical Clinics of North America* **26**, 943–952.

Lawrence P. F., McFarland D. C., Seeger J. M. & Lowry S. F. (1980) Evaluation of extremity ischaemia by skin fluorescence. *Surgical Forum* **31**, 349–351.

Lee B. Y., Trainor F. S., Kavner D., McCann W. J & Madden J. L. (1979) Non-invasive haemodynamic evaluation in selection of amputation level. *Surgery, Gynecology and Obstetrics* **149**, 241–244.

Lepantalo M. J. A. Haajanen J., Lindfors O., Paavolainen P. & Scheinin T. M. (1982) Predictive value of pre-operative segmental blood pressure measurements in below-knee amputations. *Acta Chirugia Scandinavica* **148**, 581–584.

Lloyd-Williams K. (1964) Pictorial heat scanning. *Physics and Medical Biology* **9**, 433–456.

McCollough N. C. III (1972) The dysvascular amputee. *Orthopedic Clinics of North America* **3**, 287–301.

McCollum P. T., Spence V. A., Walker W. F., Swanson A. J. G., Turner M. S. & Murdoch G. (1984) Experience in the healing rate of lower limb amputations. *Journal of the Royal College of Surgeons of Edinburgh* **29**, 358–362.

McCollum P. T., Spence V. A. & Walker W. F. (1985a) Circumferential skin blood flow measurements in the ischaemic limb. *British Journal of Surgery* **72**, 310–312.

McCollum P. T., Spence V. A., Walker W. F., Murdoch G., Swanson A. J. G. & Turner M. S. (1985b) Antipyrine clearance from the skin of the foot and the lower leg in critical ischaemia: clinical implications. In *Practical Aspects of Skin Blood Flow Measurement* (eds Spence V. A. & Sheldon C. D.), pp. 47–51. BES.

McFarland D. C. & Lawrence P. F. (1982) Skin fluorescence, a method to predict amputation site healing. *Journal of Surgical Research* **32**, 410–415.

McLoughlin G. A. & Rawsthorne G. B. (1973) Thermography in the diagnosis of occlusive vascular disease of the lower limb. *British Journal of Surgery* **60**, 655–656.

Malone J. M., Leal J. M., Moore W. S., Henry R. E., Daly M. J., Patton D. D. & Childers S. J. (1981) The 'gold standard' for amputation level selection: xenon-133 clearance. *Journal of Surgical Research* **30**, 449–455.

Matsen F. A. III, Wyss C. R., Pedegana L. R., Krugmire R. B., Simmons C. W., King R. V. & Burgess E. M. (1980) Transcutaneous oxygen tension measurement in peripheral vascular disease. *Surgery, Gynecology and Obstetrics* **150**, 525–528.

Montgomery H. & Horwitz O. (1950) Oxygen tension of tissues by the polarographic method. Introduction; oxygen tension and blood flow of the skin of human extremities. *Journal of Clinical Investigation* **29**, 1120–1130.

Moore W. S., Henry R. E., Malone J. M., Daly M. J., Patton D. & Childers S. J. (1981) Prospective use of xenon-133 clearance for amputation level selection. *Archives of Surgery* **116**, 86–88.

Murdoch G. (1975) Below-knee amputation and its use in vascular disease and the elderly. 'Immediate' prosthetic fitting and early walking. *Recent Advances in Orthopaedics* **2**, 152–172.

Mustapha N. M., Redhead R. G., Jain S. K. & Wielogorski J. W. J. (1983) Transcutaneous partial oxygen pressure assessment of the ischaemic lower limb. *Surgery, Gynecology and Obstetrics* **156**, 582–584.

Myers M. B., Brock D. & Cohn I. Jr (1971) Prevention of skin slough after radical mastectomy by the use of a vital dye to delineate devascularised skin. *Annals of Surgery* **173**, 920–924.

Nicholas G. G., Myers J. L. & DeMuth W. E. Jr (1982) The role of vascular laboratory criteria in the selection of patients for lower extremity amputation. *Annals of Surgery* **195**, 469–473.

Pollack S. B. & Ernst C. B. (1980) Use of Doppler pressure measurements in predicting success in amputation of the leg. *American Journal of Surgery* **139**, 303–306.

Porter J. M., Baur G. M. & Taylor L. M. Jr (1981) Lower-extremity amputations for ischaemia. *Archives of Surgery* **116**, 89–92.

Raines J. K., Darling R. C., Buth J., Brewster D. C. & Austen W. G. (1976) Vascular laboratory criteria for the management of peripheral vascular disease of the lower extremities. *Surgery* **79** 21–29.

Ratcliff D. A., Clyne C. A. C., Chant A. D. B. & Webster J. H. H. (1984) Prediction of amputation wound healing: the role of transcutaneous PO_2 assessment *British Journal of Surgery* **71**, 219–222.

Robinson K. P. (1972) Long posterior flap myoplastic below-knee amputation in ischaemic disease. Review of experience in 1967–71. *Lancet* **1**, 193–195.

Romano R. L. & Burgess E. M. (1971) Level selection in lower extremity amputations. *Clinical Orthopaedics and Related Research* **74**, 177–184.

Sejrsen P. (1967) Cutaneous blood flow in man studied by freely diffusible radioactive indicators. *Scandinavian Journal of Clinical Laboratory Investigation* (Suppl. **99**), 52–59.

Silverman D. & Wagner F. W. Jr (1983) Prediction of leg viability and amputation level by fluorescein uptake. *Prosthetics and Orthotics International* **7**, 69–71.

Spence V. A. & McCollum P. T. (1985) Evaluation of the ischaemic limb by transcutaneous oxymetry. In *Diagnostic Techniques and Assessment Procedures in Vascular Surgery,* (ed. Greenhalgh R. M.), pp. 331–341. London: Grune & Stratton.

Spence V. A. & Walker W. F. (1976) Measurement of oxygen tension in human skin. *Medical and Biological Engineering* **14**, 159–165.

Spence V. A. & Walker W. F. (1984a) Tissue oxygen tension in normal and ischaemic human skin. *Cardiovascular Research* **18**, 140–144.

Spence V. A. & Walker W. F. (1984b) The relationship between temperature isotherms and skin blood flow in the ischaemic limb. *Journal of Surgical Research* **36**, 278–281.

Spence V. A., Walker W. F., Troup I. M. & Murdoch G. (1981) Amputation of the ischaemic limb: selection of the optimum site by thermography. *Angiology* **32**, 155–169.

Stockel M., Jorgensen J. P., Jorgensen A., Brochner-Mortensen J. & Emneus H. (1981) Radioisotope washout technique as a routine method for selection of amputation level. *Acta Orthopaedica Scandinavica* **52**, 405–408.

Tanzer T. L. & Horne J. G. (1982) The assessment of skin viability using fluorescein angiography prior to amputation. *Journal of Bone and Joint Surgery* **64A**, 880–882.

Thompson R. G., Keagy R. D., Compere C. L. & Meyer P. R. (1974) Amputation and rehabilitation for severe foot ischaemia. *Surgical Clinics of North America* **54**, 137–154.

Winsor T. (1971) Vascular aspects of thermography. *Journal of Cardiovascular Surgery* **12**, 379–388.

Young A. E., Henderson B. A. & Couch N. P. (1978) Muscle perfusion and the healing of below-knee amputations. *Surgery, Gynecology and Obstetrics* **146**, 533–534.

3

Pre-operative and Post-operative Care: Stump Environment

I.M. TROUP

Introduction

This chapter endeavours to cover pre-operative and post-operative care, including stump environment, albeit in an abbreviated form.

The decisions relating to levels (Spence *et al.* 1981) and limiting factors, although primarily based on surgical factors, should properly involve the opinion of the consultant in prosthetics during the pre-operative period. Essentially, amputee care can be divided into four areas of primary importance:

1 Pre-operative care.
2 Surgery.
3 Post-operative care.
4 Prosthetic management.

All are critical areas and are interactive — excellent surgery followed by poor post-operative care, including stump environment, may well result in an outcome which is less than desirable.

Pre-operative care

It is important to optimize the patient's general condition. Inevitably this involves careful comprehensive assessment, including biochemical and bacteriological analyses. Blood chemistry is frequently disturbed by disease or trauma, and a recorded baseline is useful in continuing care. In particular, one should be aware of the undiagnosed diabetic, the condition only becoming obvious some time after surgery (McCollum *et al.* 1984). This is relevant inasmuch as the management of the patient with vascular disease varies; thus the atherosclerotic patient and the diabetic patient with small vessel disease require different approaches.

Recent work has indicated the importance of blood viscosity in the avascular patient (Bailey *et al.* 1979, Bouhoutsos *et al.* 1974, Yates *et al.* 1979). Blood transfusion, given pre-operatively because of low haemoglobin levels, may simply increase the blood viscosity, thus decreasing the flow. Therefore, it may be wise, if clinically valid, to delay transfusion until the post-operative period.

The patient is frequently confused, but the possible cause must be considered carefully. A toxic confusional state due to infection is indeed the likeliest cause, but a long history of pain and its relief may mean that the confusional state is drug-induced. Certainly amputation cures the toxic confusional state quite dramatically, and the need for pain-relieving drugs is reduced, but drug monitoring is still essential, since drug-induced confusion undoubtedly complicates the clinical picture. At this stage counselling is of extreme importance. The patient must see a solution to his problem — he must be told the likely steps in his recovery in some detail. Fear of the unknown is a major difficulty and need not occur. It may be that the confusional state delays adequate counselling, but nevertheless it must take place, if need be later. At this stage some mention must be made of the phantom limb which the patient will inevitably experience and the possibility of associated pain which should gradually disappear.

Two drugs should be given to cover the surgical event and the immediate post-operative period — penicillin and *Minihep. Penicillin guards against the possibility of *Clostridium welchii* infection, and should the patient be sensitive to penicillin erythromycin is the drug of choice. Neither of these drugs will necessarily cover a pre-existing infection already identified bacteriologically. In that case it is necessary to give a second antibiotic specific to the infection. Minihep should be given to minimize the risk of deep venous thrombosis.

All of these areas of pre-operative care should involve both the surgeon and the prosthetic consultant, the latter being concerned particularly with patient counselling since he will probably be responsible for continuing post-operative care.

Post-operative care

An immediate responsibility in post-operative care is the control of pain. This presents in varying degrees. The avascular patient has, in all probability, suffered chronic pain for long periods, so that surgery when required, often urgently, paradoxically comes as a relief, and post-operative pain is minimized. On the other hand, surgery carried out after due deliberation as part of a planned programme of events, and also surgery following trauma, can produce a greater degree of post-operative pain. A variety of drugs may be used — from cyclomorphine to the simpler forms of analgesia — and preferably should be given on demand and not by the clock.

It is vitally important to control pain, but it is equally important to minimize the use of drugs. Very often one finds that simple drugs like mefenamic acid and paracetamol effectively control post-operative pain after the first 48 hours. Continued heavy sedation can do nothing but harm, interfering with the patient's ability to increase activity towards final mobilization. Activity itself reduces the level of pain, particularly when directed at early active movement of the stump.

*Sodium heparin.

General post-surgical care continues. Vacuum drainage of the wound is necessary to avoid the formation of a haematoma. This can be discontinued after 48–72 hours, and bacteriological examination of the drainage fluid is always a prudent measure. If stump problems do arise due to infection then the organism and its sensitivity are already known. Minihep is continued for five days, and this, along with early mobilization, ensures that deep venous thrombosis rarely occurs. Penicillin, at first parenterally and later orally, is continued for the first seven days. The value of prophylaxis against infection can only be realized if one has seen, and attempted to manage, a *Clostridium welchii* septicaemia.

Biochemical monitoring should be maintained. It may be that at this stage diabetes can be confirmed by plasma glucose levels and glucose tolerance testing. The known diabetic requires special care — the absence of an infected foot and the increasing post-operative activity and general well-being cause marked changes in plasma glucose levels, thus altering the need for insulin and oral hypoglycaemic drugs. Frequently insulin is required at the time of surgery, but it is possible to change to oral hypoglycaemic drugs during the post-operative phase, which, of course, is a much better solution for the patient.

Whilst blood transfusion may have been contraindicated in the pre-operative phase, it may now become necessary. Even a moderate drop in haemoglobin level induces tiredness and lethargy, which interfere with the patient's rehabilitation.

Concurrent and complicating problems require management. Some 75% of all primary amputees present with a concurrent problem. This may be another manifestation of vascular disease or simply defective vision or hearing — both of importance in rehabilitation, especially to the therapist. Complicating problems may be associated with the stump — ischaemia, infection, or non-viability. The elderly person with a minor myocardial infarction will require little, if any, treatment, and similarly the chronic bronchitic suffering an acute exacerbation of chest infection is readily controlled, although such a complication is fortunately rare, probably due to the use of spinal anaesthesia.

It is during the post-operative phase that the remainder of the clinic team becomes increasingly involved — the nurse, physiotherapist, occupational therapist, social worker, engineer, and finally the prosthetist. Truly a team of specialists, thus raising the question of the correct environment for all their activities. It is suggested that a small unit specializing in amputee care, concerned in both in-patient and out-patient situations, with staff thoroughly versed in the specialty, is ideal. The best encouragement an amputee can get in the early post-operative phase is to see another amputee walking out of the hospital following completion of his treatment. Experience suggests that a 40-bedded unit per million population is required, comprising 50% of the beds providing full nursing care, 25% partial nursing care, and 25% hostel accommodation. This formula would seem to meet the needs of most western European countries.

Stump environment is a subject of considerable debate. Essentially it is a question of creating a comfortable and effective interface between a newly fashioned stump and its environment. This can be dictated by convention or by rather more studied methods. The management is bound to be heavily influenced by the nature of ischaemic tissue, but similar issues will also apply to tissues damaged by trauma or other disease. The pressure applied to the skin and the blood flow required to maintain nutrition are absolutes and have to be satisfied. There are several methods in use in providing a stump – environment interface.

1 A free stump.
2 A soft dressing.
3 A rigid dressing and a rigid dressing with mobility ('immediate post-operative fitting').
4 Controlled environment treatment.

1 Free stump

If no dressing is applied then the inevitable response to surgical trauma operates — oedema forms with possible diminution of vascular supply. Moreover, lack of protection results in pain. This is not the management of choice, although it may perforce be employed following above-knee amputation.

2 Soft dressing

Soft dressings protect the wound and apply varying degrees of pressure. How much pressure and how it can be controlled is a difficult problem. Certainly too much pressure will devitalize tissues to the extent that survival is doubtful. Conventional stump bandaging can create a detrimental environment. Isherwood *et al.* (1975) have demonstrated in a very clear way that even experienced bandagers can inadvertently create pressures as high as 130 mmHg. Such pressures are certainly lethal to skin survival.

3 Rigid dressing

Rigid dressings (Fig. 3.1) in the form of a plaster of Paris cast have been advocated by Burgess *et al.* (1969) and exposed to evaluation by Mooney *et al.* (1971), a study which demonstrated an advantage over soft dressings. Experience strongly suggests that pain is diminished, and of course the stump is protected and casual inspection of the wound is prevented. The patient is free to move and can start walking training using such aids as the pneumatic post-amputation mobility (PPAM) aid (Redhead 1983). The application of a rigid cast does require some skill, but this is readily acquired. Muscle 'setting' can be practised within the cast without danger to distal muscle sutures. Certainly the cast has a fixed volume, but stump volume reduction can be overcome to some extent by using a distal end-cap which expands as the stump reduces, provided sufficient distal pressure is applied to the dressing in its initial application. The technique advocated by Burgess, the use of Spandex

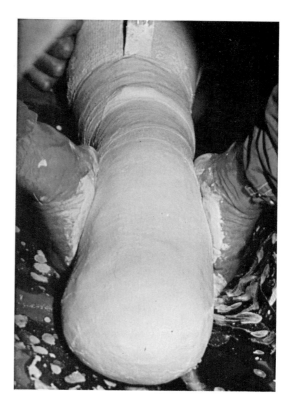

Fig. 3.1 Rigid dressing.

socks and elasticated plaster of Paris (Burgess *et al.* 1969), is easily learned, and correctly applied produces an excellent interface. It can be used equally well in through-knee and Syme levels.

The application of a rigid cast also permits so-called immediate post-operative fitting (Burgess *et al.* 1967). 'So-called' because it is rarely used nowadays in the immediate post-operative period, application being delayed until the seventh to tenth day. In both through-knee and Syme amputations, patients are fitted with pylon prostheses (Figs 3.2 & 3.3) from the seventh to tenth day and continue weight-bearing throughout until delivery and check-out of the definitive prosthesis. The use of this technique at above-knee levels is technically just possible, but it is not recommended because of the difficulty in maintaining satisfactory suspension to ensure an adequate stump – socket interface.

4 Controlled environment treatment

This method of stump environment (Fig. 3.4) was developed by Redhead and Snowdon (1978). It was the first attempt to create an environment which was precise, controllable, and therefore sensible. The stump, enclosed in a plastic Sterishield with a distal air inlet and a proximal, internal, pleated, partial seal, is

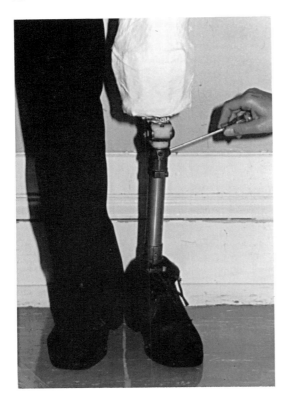

Fig. 3.2 Immediate post-operative fitting for through-knee level.

subjected to controllable pressure, cycled between low and high pressure levels, with a controlled temperature, and a dressing of sterile air, thus avoiding any extraneous environmental problems. No skills are demanded and no dressing of any kind is employed. The system can be varied as the clinical situation demands and, provided staff are appropriately trained, presents no operating problem. The stump is visible throughout and active movements can be carried out within 24 hours of surgery. There are undoubtedly some limitations placed upon the patient by virtue of the machine and the air supply hose, but generally it is an acceptable form of environment which promotes lymphatic and venous return, reducing oedema and improving the peripheral circulation, and by virtue of this enhancing the healing process (Troup 1980).

Whatever environment is used, the intention is to obtain rapid healing of the stump and to promote an optimum situation which will allow early casting and limb-fitting. Throughout all amputee care it is essential to know and understand the patient's needs. One must respect his aspirations, understand his difficulties, and promote his general well-being.

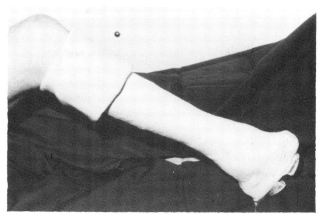

Fig. 3.3 Immediate post-operative fitting for Syme level.

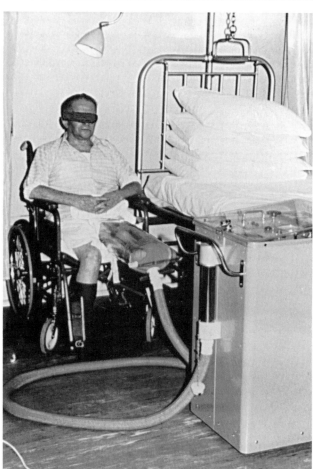

Fig. 3.4 Controlled environment treatment.

References

Bailey M. J., Johnston C. L. W., Yates C. J. P., Somerville P. G. & Dormandy J. A. (1979) Pre-operative haemoglobin as predictor of outcome of diabetic amputations. *Lancet* **July**, 168–170.

Bouhoutsos J., Morris T., Chavatzas D. & Martin P. (1974) The influence of haemoglobin and platelet levels on the results of arterial surgery. *British Journal of Surgery* **61**, 984–986.

Burgess E. M., Traub J. E. & Wilson A. B. (1967) Immediate post-surgical prosthetics in the management of lower extremity amputees. Publication for the *Prosthetics and Sensory Aids Service*, Veterans Administration, Washington.

Burgess E. M., Romano R. L. & Zettl J. H. (1969) The management of lower extremity amputations. Publication for the *Prosthetics and Sensory Aids Service*, Veterans Administration, Washington.

Isherwood P. A., Robertson J. C. & Rossi A. (1975) Pressure measurements beneath below-knee stump bandages. Elastic bandaging, the Puddifoot dressing and a pneumatic bandaging technique compared. *British Journal of Surgery* **62**, 982–986.

McCollum P. T., Spence V. A., Walker W. F., Swanson A. J. G., Turner M. S. & Murdoch G. (1984) Experience in the healing rate of lower limb amputations. *Journal of the Royal College of Surgeons of Edinburgh*, 358–362.

Mooney V., Harvey J. P., McBride E. & Snelson R. (1971) Comparison of post-operative stump management: plaster versus soft dressings. *Journal of Bone and Joint Surgery* **53A**, 241–249.

Redhead R. G. (1983) The early rehabilitation of lower limb amputees using a pneumatic walking aid. *Prosthetics and Orthotics International* **7**, 88–90.

Redhead R. G. & Snowdon C. (1978) A new approach to the management of wounds of the extremities: controlled environment treatment and its derivatives. *Prosthetics and Orthotics International* **2**, 148–156.

Spence V. A., Walker W. F., Troup I. M. & Murdoch G. (1981) Amputation of the ischeamic limb: selection of the optimum site by thermography. *Angiology* **32(3)**, 155–169.

Troup I. M. (1980) Controlled environment treatment. *Prosthetics and Orthotics International* **4**, 15–28.

Yates C. J. P., Berent A., Andrews V. & Dormandy J. A. (1979). Increase in leg blood flow by normovolaemic haemodilution in intermittent claudication. *Lancet*, **July**, 166–168.

4

Prosthetic Fitting: General Concepts

C.H. PRITHAM

The act of fitting a prosthesis is the quintessential element of the prosthetist's role. It sets him apart from all other members of the clinic team, and it demands of him and the patient the greatest measure of co-operation and interaction. Accordingly, it is proposed that the subject of prosthetic fitting be treated in an abstract manner, with the hope of identifying topics of interest and thereby providing the groundwork for discussion.

Measurement and casting

Once a patient has been assessed for his needs and capabilities, and a prescription has been formulated, the act of fitting begins. The process is initiated by a session in which the prosthetist obtains a more detailed set of facts about the patient. The measurements taken are of two types. One type is used to obtain components of appropriate size and assemble them in the correct configuration. The other set of measurements is used in the production of a three-dimensional positive model for fabrication of the desired socket. The information necessary for the production of this positive model is obtained by taking a negative model or cast of an appropriate portion of the patient's involved limb. To date, the best and most universally applicable material for this has been proven to be plaster of Paris bandage, which is readily available, inexpensive, and requires no special environment. Moreover, the process can hardly be said to be capital-intensive, for it most frequently requires little more than a pail. The skills necessary are readily taught and an experienced prosthetist can achieve results that are quite satisfactorily reproducible.

Aside from the data recorded in some physical form or another, the prosthetist acquires another set of information during the measurement and casting process. As the prosthetist makes the necessary measurements and marks relevant reference points, he gains a sense of feel that permits evaluation of such factors as tissue compressibility, pressure tolerance, skin mobility, and range of motion. Most of these factors cannot be measured or recorded in any meaningful fashion at present, but they are of the greatest aid to the prosthetist during the act of modifying the positive model. It is for this reason that most authorities insist that the prosthetist who measures the patient modifies the positive model, and the modification should be accomplished within 24 hours of obtaining the cast.

Over the years a number of elaborations on the basic fitting techniques have been described. Fundamentally, these have been intended to simplify the modification process and to obviate the need for these last two requirements. Methods using felt or clay to produce relief areas, and techniques using positive or negative pressure to compress and mould soft tissue, have all been reported. While doubtlessly of great aid to their developers, these various methods have never gained widespread popularity.

Cognizance must also be taken of the various schemes put forth to supplant the reliance on plaster of Paris bandages. The most elaborate of these schemes involves the utilization of CAD–CAM technology. This approach may be possible, but it must be viewed with a healthy scepticism, due to its apparent lack of relevance to the way prosthetics is practised in the real world, and also due to the economic constraints. It is altogether possible that a prosthetist may become so involved with the act of coping with the computer that he looks upon the presence of the patient as an unwelcome distraction.

However the positive model is obtained, its shape must be modified from the anatomical in accordance with certain principles. These principles vary with amputation level and the functions to be provided by the socket. Moreover, they must be applied with due regard to the condition and shape of the patient's extremity. Two fundamental principles are common to all sockets: pressure is applied by a socket in proportion to the ability of the tissue to sustain the load, and the socket must bear a certain relationship in volume to the volume of the limb segment enclosed.

From the modified positive model, a socket is produced. This socket may be either the actual socket used in the prosthesis, or it may be a check socket. This latter course of action is becoming increasingly popular in the U.S.A. A variety of reasons account for this increase in popularity, but fundamental to it is the availability of transparent sheet thermoplastics and the technology to form sockets readily and inexpensively.

Check socket

Utilization of a check socket potentially leads to a better fit for a variety of reasons.
1 Since the check socket is disposable and must be replaced, the prosthetist has less emotional investment in it, is more likely to evaluate it objectively, and is thus more likely to refine the fit that 'last little bit'.
2 Fitted in a static situation in the first instance prior to dynamic alignment, the check socket provides both participants with the opportunity to focus on the fit without the distracting eagerness to take the first step.
3 The check socket promotes communication between the prosthetist and patient because both can see and talk about the same thing. In many respects a check

socket is of considerably more psychological value to a patient than it is to an experienced prosthetist.

4 The advantage of transparency is obvious.

5 The ability to produce successive check sockets quickly and inexpensively promotes innovation and change. This fact as much as anything underlies the development of contoured adducted trochanteric-controlled alignment method (CAT-CAM) fitting techniques for the AK amputee as pioneered in the United States.

Check sockets have a number of other implications that perhaps deserve comment. A check socket isolates the element of fit, and separates it from the actual physical structure of the socket to be used in the final prosthesis. With an accurate fit thus assured, the actual socket can be made as thin as is consistent with the loads imposed upon it. If a check socket is used in the assembly of a prototype prosthesis for the performance of dynamic alignment, a prosthesis can be subsequently fabricated with structural materials strategically located for maximum strength and mimimum weight. This idea is embodied in the TPJ system of Een-Holmgren, Sweden.* A prosthetist can concentrate on the production of such prototype prostheses and leave the manufacture of the actual prosthesis to someone else, since all the information necessary is embodied in the prototype prosthesis. This allows a prosthetist to devote his time to his patients and makes central fabrication much more efficient.

Socket function

As alluded to above, the socket provides at least two functions. Primarily it provides for fit (safe and comfortable transmission of forces to and from the patient and the control of soft tissue volume), and secondarily it acts as a structural element. Theoretically at least, it is possible to assign these separate functions to different portions of the socket. Interaction between the patient and the prosthesis is carried out by the inner surface. It is this function of a socket that people are referring to when they use the word interface in place of the word socket. The interface can be imagined as being infinitely thin or something akin to a coat of varnish. Everything peripheral to the interface, the socket wall, fulfils the role of load-bearing element. Ideally, the wall should be no thicker than is absolutely necessary for structural integrity. In many instances walls are made thicker than necessary to allow space for modifying the fit of the interface by expanding it outwards into the wall; that is, by grinding away material. Conversely, pads or filler may be added to alter the interface in the opposite direction. This concept suggests that it is possible to combine materials synergistically so as to provide a degree of function that neither of them alone is capable of providing. This explains the preference that many amputees profess for such 'old-fashioned' forms of construction as leather

*Information from: Viktor Begat & Co. AB, Grevturegatan 75, S–114 38 Stockholm, Sweden.

socket with steel frames. It also underlies the success of such designs as the flexible above-knee socket of Kristinsson (1983) and of the Sauter below-elbow prosthesis with silicone elastomer suction socket (1975). Prosthetists need to utilize new materials and fabrication techniques to exploit this design principle and others, such as the concepts that Murphy (1971) and Bennett (1971) have identified.

Alignment

Once a satisfactory socket or socket analogue is obtained, alignment proceeds. The temporarily assembled prosthesis that is initially presented to the patient is said to have been been bench-aligned. That is, the prosthesis has been assembled in accordance with the recorded measurements of the patient and the principles of biomechanics known to govern the behaviour of that class of prosthesis. The initial stages of static and dynamic alignment may well proceed quite rapidly, since an experienced prosthetist can frequently refine the basic alignment to his satisfaction in short order. The subsequent stage in the alignment procedure is more problematic. During this stage, as the amputee walks the prosthetist asks a number of questions intended to gain information about the patient's subjective impression of the prosthesis. Every prosthetist has a series of stereotype questions which he uses and to which he expects fairly predictable responses. Unfortunately not all amputees are so well-versed, and their comments may be more confusing than illuminating. The amputee may have difficulty interpreting what he is feeling. His responses may confuse the prosthetist, and it may take a fairly long time to establish what he really means. Worse yet, the prosthetist may think he is hearing the desired response when something quite different is intended.

Over the years it has been proposed that the resources of the gait laboratory or alignment units adjustable by the ambulating patient be used to facilitate the process. None of these techniques has so far had any influence. In the U.S.A. the use of videotape equipment to provide the patient and prosthetist with another viewpoint has gained some popularity. However, utilization of this equipment, despite such refinements as freeze frame and slow motion, still depends on visual observation and communication between the two participants.

Finishing and delivery

Once the alignment process has been completed, and comfort and function assured, the prosthesis is finished providing for the third element in the triad, cosmesis. The provision of cosmesis is one fraught with frustration and confusion. The uninitiated patient's expectation is that the prosthesis will be indistinguishable from his sound side. Clearly this expectation is rarely if ever met, and the patient's ability to pass unidentified as an amputee depends more on his own ability and patience in practising his gait. In providing cosmesis the prosthetist must contend with a number of factors which limit his ability to create a truly realistic facsimile. In fact, what he does more often than not is to achieve a result that conforms to a set of generally held precepts that dictate what a prosthesis should look like. The word 'cosmetic' is used when it would be more accurate to use the word 'aesthetic'.

The process of fitting culminates in delivery of the prosthesis. At this time, the last-minute adjustments take place and the patient is instructed about such matters as building up wearing tolerance. Aside from a clinic visit for follow-up and evaluation, it is quite likely that the patient will have to be seen at least once more for minor adjustments.

This then is the sequence of events involved in the fitting of a prosthesis. Attention has been purposely focused on the act of providing the prosthesis. This is, of course, not the only element involved. Equally important is the process by which it is decided what a patient is to receive and the ones involved in follow-up, assessment, and training. Also ignored is the fabrication of the device which is so inextricably bound up in the act of fitting. The author's purpose has been to concentrate strictly on the act of fitting and the interaction between prosthetist and patient. This role is seen to be crucial and will continue to be so despite the efforts of developers to supplant or augment it by various mechanical or electronic means.

References

Bennett L. (1971) Transferring load to flesh. Part II. Analysis of compressive stress. *Bulletin of Prosthetic Research* **10–16**, 45–63.

Kristinsson O. (1983) Flexible above-knee socket made from low density polyethylene, suspended by a weight transmitting frame. *Orthotics and Prosthetics* **37(2)**, 25–27.

Murphy E. F. (1971) Transferring load to flesh. Part I. Concepts. *Bulletin of Prosthetics Research* **10–16**, 38–44.

Sauter W. (1975) Flexible suction sockets for short below-elbow amputees. *Orthopaedic Prostheses* **9(3)**, 19–22.

BELOW-KNEE AMPUTATION

5

Surgery, Including Levels, Alternative Techniques, Growth Period

E.M. BURGESS

Introduction

Prior to and during World War II, above-knee amputation held centre stage in surgical interest. This emphasis also applied to lower limb prosthetics. Above-knee suction socket suspension and the development of a whole family of prosthetic knees epitomized this era. Since that time, slowly at first, and then at an accelerated rate, emphasis has shifted to the lower leg level. Several factors are responsible for the below-knee amputation being today by far the most frequently performed major level in the lower limb. The first of these resulted from a realization of the critical importance of the knee in stance and gait. People function reasonably well with a hip arthrodesed in the proper position. The same is true of ankle arthrodesis. On the other hand, fusion of the knee, functioning as it does between the two long lever arms of the femur and tibia, critically compromises limb function. Mechanical knee function replacement proved to be, and continues to be, an elusive engineering challenge, even using hydraulic, pneumatic, electrical, and ingenious mechanical systems. The overriding need to retain, when possible, a functional knee has placed increased emphasis on below-knee amputation techniques. The second factor contributing to the increasing numbers of below-knee amputations relates to the ischaemic limb. Improved below-knee surgical techniques and better knowledge of limb viability have challenged the surgeon to perform below-knee amputation rather than accepting the above-knee level often considered to be required for wound healing.

Objectives of surgery

Surgeons carrying out below-knee amputation should first understand that this is not inconsequential surgery: it offers a significant technical challenge. Most general surgical texts, even those recently published, are inadequate as amputation reference guides. The surgeon must have a good knowledge of the anatomy and functional characteristics of cross-sectional structures, so that his surgery will result in an end-organ capable of utilizing the excellent new family of beautiful and well-engineered below-knee prostheses. He must be innovative, particularly in the presence of trauma, including burns, and must also be aware of the scope of prosthetic substitution. He must create a residual limb that with the aid of a prosthesis can achieve useful function.

Skin management

A healthy, pressure-tolerant skin envelope must be the goal. This can be achieved by using well-understood plastic and reconstructive skin management when the skin available for closure is healthy, sensible, mobile, and well-nourished. Position of the skin incision or incisions is of secondary importance, because the total-contact socket environment anticipates tissue–interface contact no matter where the incisions lie.

A less than satisfactory skin envelope does not, however, preclude a good functioning below-knee amputation. The degree of compromise will vary depending on the type of skin trauma present — from those which heal with minimal scarring to massive burns with split-skin or full-thickness skin graft coverage. Skin, including grafted skin, when properly programmed can adapt to accommodate pressure. The need for skin grafting does not necessarily change the amputation level.

In peripheral vascular disease, skin management is especially critical. With low viability, slow-healing skin must be handled with particular care to avoid isolation from blood and nerve supply and unnecessary surgical trauma.

Surgical procedures

The nature of below-knee cross-sectional anatomy eliminates the need for subcutaneous sutures. This is especially the case when myofascial approximation is performed. Muscles and tendons make up the largest proportion of the cross-sectional area. These musculotendinous structures have been, and continue to be, largely neglected by many surgeons. The need for distal muscle stabilization is absolutely necessary if full potential is to be achieved.

For some years the author has performed and advocated myodesis: suture of severed muscles to the distal tibia. Many of these residual limbs functioned beautifully, and active, voluntary, and involuntary muscle contractions resulted. Complications included occasional necrosis of the distal tibia around the drill sites and slow healing in cases of peripheral vascular disease. The subcutaneous medial tibial surface does not lend itself well to effective myodesis. Myoplasty, however, can be carried out. This is a particularly effective technique when using the posterior flap closure.

Myoplasty in conjunction with tibiofibular synostosis, the Ertl procedure (1949), is also effective. Some degree of muscle stabilization can be accomplished in almost every instance if the surgeon is aware of its importance and addresses it technically.

Severed blood vessels and nerves are treated in the same way as with other levels of amputation. Gentle traction and high circular ligation of nerves with sharp section is preferred. Some surgeons have revived the technique of nerve stump cauterization, and a few are crushing the nerve ends below the suture. They suggest that such management diminishes local neuroma tenderness and phantom sensations. The author knows of no statistical verification.

Bone management is straightforward in that bone ends should be very carefully tailored to eliminate local pressure problems. The open medullary cavities, especially of the tibia, should be sealed off either by soft tissue, as with a myofascial flap, or by osteoperiosteal coverage, as with the Ertl procedure. The need for good haemostasis and meticulous skin closure is self-evident.

There has been renewed interest in tibiofibular synostosis, but this procedure is not recommended in the presence of peripheral vascular disease. These fragile ischaemic tissues frequently will not tolerate the added trauma of surgical manipulation. With ischaemic tissues, healing, rather than achieving high performance levels, is the primary goal. In general the below-knee amputation for ischaemia is short, which further discourages the use of the Ertl technique.

For those cases in which tissue viability is adequate, particularly in amputation resulting from trauma, there is a real and important place for synostosis surgery. When carefully performed it need not result in significant additional loss of length, and while the healing time following surgery and rehabilitation is slower than with so-called conventional techniques, the resulting residual limb is strong and non-tender. The degree of end-bearing it permits further enhances its value.

Not only should the well-performed below-knee amputation permit total interface contact, whenever possible some end-bearing capacity should be incorporated into this diaphyseal level. This goal can be particularly well accomplished using the posterior flap technique.

Summary

Below-knee amputation is statistically the single most important level in the lower limb. Great advances have been made in below-knee amputation surgery over the last two decades. The time has come when the available techniques should be critically reviewed in the light of modern principles of plastic and reconstructive surgery with the goal of further improving and innovating this very important operation. When it is performed thoughtfully, and when tissue conservation is combined with rigid-dressing post-surgical management, the below-knee amputation can be a major factor in improved mobility.

Reference

Ertl J. (1949) Uber Amputationsstumpf. *Chirurgie* **20**, 218.

Further reading

Burgess E. M. & Matson F. A. (1981) Determination of amputation levels in periperhal vascular disease. *Journal of Bone and Joint Surgery* **63**, 1493–1497.

Spence V. A., McCollum P. T., Walker W. F. & Murdoch G. (1984) Assessment of tissue viability in relation to the selection of amputation level. *Prosthetics and Orthotics International* **8**, 67–75.

6

Biomechanics and Prosthetic Practice

J. HUGHES & J.S. TAYLOR

Introduction

It is now almost quarter of a century since Radcliffe and Foort (1961) described in great detail the design philosophy and the practical application of the patellar tendon-bearing (PTB) below-knee prosthesis. The description itself represented the culmination of an activity extending over several years and involving many people in an attempt to distil all that was then best in the current 'state of the art' of below-knee prosthetics. Twenty-five years later the prosthesis described, with its solid ankle cushion heel (SACH) foot, its reinforced fibreglass construction, and its cuff suspension must now be considered as the 'conventional' prosthesis for this level. This biomechanical basis of the design has proved sound in application and, by simple extension, provides an understanding of the basis of recent variants.

Biomechanics

Basic considerations

The design of any prosthesis is approached in the same basic way. The prosthesis is required to provide support, to permit or facilitate progression and to give an appearance of normality — the various elements of which are often referred to as 'cosmesis'. The first stage in the design process is to identify the parts of the stump which may provide the support function, determine the mode of progression, and then study the force effects which result. This will determine the design specification.

The most important part of the prosthesis, to most amputees, is the socket. Without a comfortable and functional socket the prosthesis cannot be considered successful. The socket is the interface between the patient and the prosthesis across which must be transmitted the forces due to support and progression. Unfortunately in most prostheses, the socket is applying force to tissue which is not particularly well suited to load-bearing, or indeed developed for that purpose, as is, for example, the sole of the foot. The most important factor in providing effective force application, while affording maximum comfort, is to avoid excessive pressure. Pressure is directly proportional to the force applied and indirectly proportional to the area of application. One obvious way to reduce pressure is to reduce the forces applied to the minimum; the other is to increase the area over which the force is applied. In principle, it would seem to be a simple matter to reduce pressure by increasing the contact areas. In practice, it is more difficult because the relative firmness and softness of the tissues involved is not uniform. A second factor which must be considered is that some areas tolerate pressure quite well, while other areas are relatively sensitive to pressure. The aim, therefore, is to distribute the load as widely as possible over pressure-tolerant tissue. Both of these factors can be accommodated by appropriate design of the contours and shape of the socket.

Consider a stump which is essentially circular in cross-section encased in a socket which accurately matches the periphery of the stump. If the stump were of uniform firmness the stump–socket pressure would also be uniform when load was applied. In Fig. 6.1a, which shows the cross-section of the stump, the areas indicated by the letter 'F' are relatively firm, while softer areas are indicated by the letter 'S'. If the socket were shaped to match the stump accurately, the pressure on the stump would not be evenly distributed. The firm areas, designated by 'F', would take relatively more of the load, while the soft areas, designated by 'S', would take relatively less. A more even distribution of pressure would be obtained by purposely modifying the socket by making reliefs in the socket over the firm areas and bulging the socket inward over the soft area (Fig. 6.1b). This same strategy, i.e. using reliefs and inward contours in the socket, can be used to compensate for the different pressure tolerance of the various areas of the stump. In this case the purpose is different. Instead of producing an even distribution of pressure, the objective is to produce a selective loading of the tissues so that more of the weight will be supported by the pressure-tolerant areas and less weight will remain on the pressure-sensitive areas.

Fig. 6.1c shows the schematic diagram of a theoretical stump of uniform firmness, encased in a socket. The socket has reliefs over the pressure-sensitive

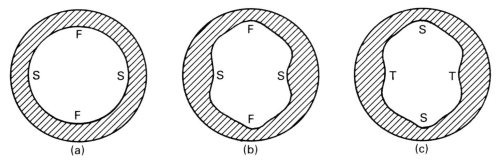

Fig. 6.1 Schematic cross-section. (a) Relative tissue stiffness: F, firm; S, soft. (b) Socket modified to equalize load pressure. (c) Differing stump tissue: S, pressure-sensitive; T, pressure-tolerant. Socket modified to redistribute load selectively.

areas which are designated by 'S', and inward contours over the pressure-tolerant areas, which are designated by 'T'. The inward bulges over the pressure-tolerant areas will cause the tissues in these locations to sustain a relatively larger portion of the load, leaving a smaller part of the load to be borne by the sensitive areas. The reliefs in the socket will assist further in reducing the pressure on the sensitive areas.

The PTB socket

The general statement may be made that disability and energy cost are increased the greater the number of joints which are lost. This is not a linear relationship. The most important joint to retain in the lower limb amputee is the knee joint. The normal knee joint functions over a wide range of angles. It is controlled and actuated by powerful muscle groups and plays an important part in 'smoothing' the path of progression, in absorbing shock, and in reducing the energy cost of walking. It is vital, where possible, to save this joint. The difference in loss of function from below-knee to above-knee amputation is very great.

The patellar tendon-bearing (PTB) prosthesis for the below-knee amputee (Radcliffe & Foort 1961) is designed to permit the amputee to retain the full function of the knee joint which is, after all, more or less intact. This means that the socket must be designed to transmit all the forces which are involved in such a way that the joint is relatively unrestricted.

The first stage in the design of the socket is to identify the supporting areas. In this prosthesis the major part of this function is provided by the patellar tendon area — a tough tendinous structure with skin and underlying tissue adapted to kneeling — and by the medial flare of the tibia. By studying the walking pattern of the amputee, the forces which must occur between the socket and the stump if the amputee walks in a relatively normal way may then be identified. Figs 6.2a & b show, respectively, the force patterns produced in the plane of progression and the plane at right angles to this. The aim is to transmit these forces to the stump, keeping pressures as low as possible, while avoiding load on pressure-sensitive areas.

The next stage in using this information to produce a functional and comfortable socket is for the prosthetist to examine the stump and by palpation identify the firmness and softness of the tissues in different areas. He will also identify those areas which are pressure-tolerant and those which are sensitive. He then covers the stump with a thin sock on which he marks with an indelible pencil important features of the particular stump — sensitive areas, neuroma, skeletal landmarks, etc. A plaster of Paris wrap cast of the stump is applied over this sock — identifying the patellar tendon and the popliteal areas with the fingers during the 'setting up' of the wrap cast. Using this female cast a male model of the stump is then poured, which bears the marks of the indelible pencil previously made on the sock. A socket produced exactly to the dimensions of this cast, however, would not be

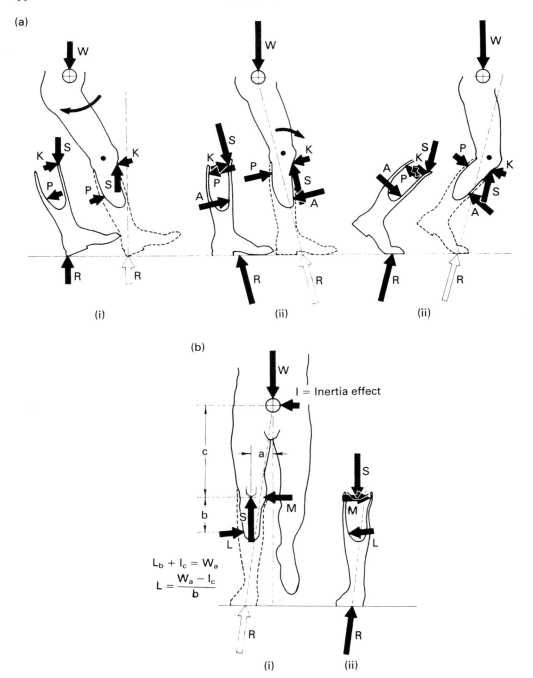

Fig. 6.2 (a) Anteroposterior force diagram, PTB prosthesis (i) heel contact; (ii) shock absorption; (iii) push-off. (b) Mediolateral force diagram, PTB prosthesis: (i) forces on the amputee; (ii) forces on the prosthesis.

'modified' with build-ups and reliefs to apply selectively load on tolerant and sensitive areas or allow for the differing tissue stiffness in different parts of the stump. The cast must be 'modified' or 'rectified' by the prosthetist — adding plaster for reliefs, and removing plaster for build-ups, in the appropriate areas (Fig. 6.3). The socket laminated on this model will apply load to the stump in a predetermined way, providing function and comfort.

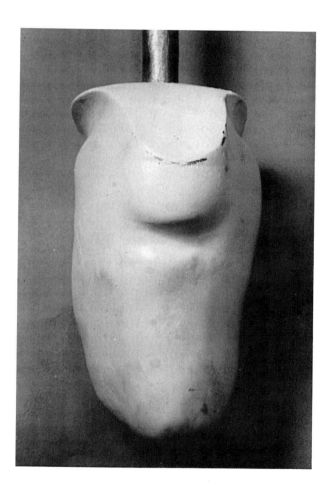

Fig. 6.3 Rectified PTB plaster cast.

Suspension considerations

The original PTB design described two basic suspension variants. The first and preferred system used a cuff which passed round the knee above the femoral condyles and was attached by two tabs to the proximal part of the prosthesis. The cuff-suspension was said to have two functions: it suspended the prosthesis on the stump during the swing phase, and during stance it acted as a check against hyperextension of the knee joint. The second suspension system was used, for example, for very short stumps, lack of muscle control and joint instability, and employed a thigh corset and metal side joints. Both these solutions resist the distraction forces during the swing phase in the same way. The most significant difference, in biomechanical terms, is in the potential for the accommodation of the lateral stabilizing forces. From Fig. 6.2b it was seen that a medially directed force on the distal lateral aspect of the stump, and a laterally directed force on the proximal medial aspect, were necessary to provide lateral stabilization during stance. The closer these forces are together, as in short stumps, the greater their magnitude to provide the stabilizing moment required. It is known that these forces may be reduced by lateral displacement of the foot to alter the inertia effects. With very short stumps it may still not be possible by this means to reduce the forces to a tolerable level and, consequently, side irons and a thigh corset would be used to increase substantially the lever arm between medial and lateral stabilizing forces with a consequent reduction in the magnitude of the forces.

Variants which employ supracondylar or patellar suspension have as their primary objective the efficient resistance to distraction during the swing phase with minimal 'pistoning', achieved in a cosmetic way with no unsightly protuberances to damage clothing. It must be recognized that their other biomechanical effect is extremely significant. The supracondylar 'wings' not only provide suspension, they also permit the application of mediolateral force and consequently, by extending the lever arm as described above, permit the fitting of extremely short stumps, virtually eliminating the justification for side joints and corset.

SACH foot

Biomechanically, the SACH foot, which was designed to be incorporated in the PTB prosthesis, provides a stable base at heel-strike, the flat sloping plantar surface of the keel being combined with a facility to roll forward over the foot on the curved support surface of the keel. The SACH foot achieves this using a simple, strong, maintenance-free, and relatively inexpensive, construction. It is apparent that the SACH foot has not been universally adopted for use in this prosthesis. In the authors' view, this and the problems which have been encountered are almost invariably due to design faults, changes introduced to the original concept, or to the use of poor materials.

Prosthetic considerations

Prior to the introduction of the PTB prosthesis, the application of biomechanical principles was largely intuitive, based on clinical experience and trial and error. After 25 years' accumulation of knowledge and experience of the PTB, combined with the overwhelming advantage of this prosthesis, it is strange to find such a high percentage of below-knee amputees still wearing the older thigh corset types of device.

The development of the PTB prosthesis has made it possible to transmit all the weight-bearing loads through the stump comfortably and with the maximum stability required without the need for thigh support. The close fit of the socket leaves little room for error and, therefore, the whole procedure must be well controlled by the prosthetist. The common practice of sending plaster casts to a distant place to be modified, as was the standard procedure with some conventional limbs, can only result in poor fittings and may well account for the high percentage of thigh corset below-knee limbs still in use.

The great diversity of practice and resulting variable quality of the end product has been the reason for all the attempts made to produce models by means other than human hands, none of which has been wholly successful. The current research using computers and associated equipment to produce stump images may be the way of the future (Hughes & Jacobs 1985). The socket produced by whatever means over the modified cast should produce the desired stump/prosthesis interface. The success of this process will determine whether the leg will be comfortable under load-bearing and during all conditions of use, or else the patient will suffer discomfort and perhaps breakdown of stump tissues.

By spreading the load over as large an area as possible, the pressures are greatly reduced. This is the guiding principle of cast modification. It is unfortunate that the total area of the stump cannot be used. Areas such as the head of the fibula, crest of the tibia, distal end of the stump, and sometimes areas with split skin grafting, have to be avoided. The remaining areas can tolerate pressure, to a greater or lesser degree, providing there are no unusual circumstances (Fig. 6.4). The areas of maximum load-bearing potential must be identified and used. Forces are applied to the stump in various predetermined directions, and the correct transmission of these forces will determine whether or not interface problems will occur. The final factor is the alignment of the foot in relation to the socket. If this is not correct, then it does not matter how well the socket fits. Malalignment can produce intolerable pressures and can result in localized breakdown of the tissue of the stump.

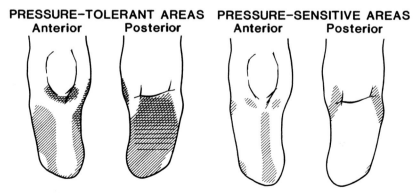

PRESSURE–TOLERANT AREAS **PRESSURE–SENSITIVE AREAS**
Anterior   Posterior   Anterior   Posterior

Fig. 6.4 Pressure-tolerant and pressure-sensitive areas.

Therefore, presented with the ideal stump and a prosthetist who can interpret the stump properly and carry out the correct modification, the below-knee amputee can be easily rehabilitated. However, in practice a large number of problems continue to occur. Problems which are said to arise from the use of the PTB are oedema, breakdown of the stump, and gross shrinkage. Oedema is usually present in the primary stump, but with good fitting should soon be eliminated. The same applies to shrinkage. The rate at which shrinkage occurs should reduce as the stump matures and should be minimal, if it takes place at all, after 9–12 months.

The fault most commonly encountered with the PTB socket is an excessively tight fit proximally. If the bulge into the popliteal area of the stump is made too large this can affect circulation, causing oedema and, eventually, deterioration and breakdown of the distal tissues of the stump. Pressure is necessary in the popliteal area to balance the posteriorly directed force applied by contact of the socket and patellar tendon, but should not be excessive.

It is sometimes seen that the posterior brim of the socket is carried high up into the popliteal area, with grooves made medially and laterally for the hamstring tendons. This can also cause constriction and abrasions both during walking and while in a sitting position. The posterior brim can be kept fairly high and made parallel to the floor, provided it is flared properly and use is made of the posteromedial and posterior structures of the tibial condyles and their tendinous structures (Fig. 6.5). The bulge into the posterior portion of the stump can then be reduced. The same applies to the patellar tendon area; a common error is to cut the indentation too deep and too narrow during cast modification. This produces a bar in the socket which is too long and narrow. This, in turn, produces severe localized pressures on the tendon, breakdown of the overlying tissue, and, in some cases, bursae and cysts develop. These problems can be overcome by using all the area around the inferior border and medial and lateral edges of the patella to spread the load and reduce the pressure on the tendon.

Oedema can also be caused by fitting too tightly at mid-stump level. This is usually a result of modifying the cast too severely in order to provide mediolateral stability. The most common fault is to push in too hard on the lateral side along the shaft of the remaining fibula.

Mediolateral stability is best provided for by placing the foot in the correct position under the socket, using the medial and lateral surfaces of the knee joint, and fitting closely on either side of the crest of the tibia to form a wedge shape. The fibula is usually fairly mobile, and if excessive pressure is applied to it severe pain can be produced by pinching of nerve and tissue between it and the tibia. The head of the fibula must also be relieved of pressure. Contact there with the socket wall can cause pain and breakdown. Pressure on the peroneal nerve, which passes around the neck of the fibula, must be avoided.

If the contact at the end of the stump is too heavy, breakdown of the skin may occur. Breakdown can also be caused by too tight a fit at the mid-portion of the socket, causing traction of the skin. Space between stump and socket may cause

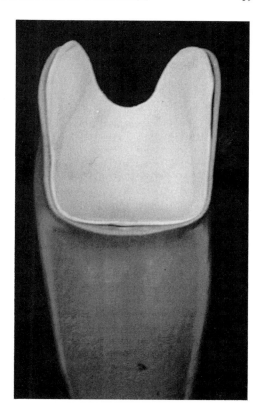

Fig. 6.5 Posterior brim of socket.

swelling and excessive sweating and blistering. These complications can be largely eliminated by ensuring that there is a good fit between stump and socket.

Many changes have taken place since the introduction of the PTB, including sockets without liners and prostheses made of thermoplastic materials, such as polypropylene. The most significant, however, has been the change in the amount of rectification applied to the cast. The model which appears in the PTB manual (Radcliffe & Foort 1961) shows figures of ⅜'' depth of plaster removed from the area below the medial flare and ¼'' deep on the lateral side of the tibia, ¼''–⅜'' removed along the shaft of the fibula, and a large bulge made into the popliteal area. These figures can be reduced by well over 50%. The same applies to the extent of build-ups to the sensitive areas. These have also been reduced by up to 50% from the early days, and the build-up which was deemed necessary along the entire length of the tibial crest has been dispensed with; only the distal tip need be increased.

The indentation into the patellar tendon has been reshaped entirely: it is less deep and curves up and around the patella using all the area available. To overcome many of the problems which occurred during the early years of the PTB, many variants of the standard version were introduced:

The KBM (*Kondylen Bettung Münster*) socket which extended over the knee on the medial and lateral sides (Lyquist 1970).

The PTS (*prothèse tibiale supra-condylienne*) socket which enclosed the whole of the patella and the medial and lateral epicondyles of the femur.

The air cushion socket (Wilson *et al.* 1968) designed to deal with tender distal ends of stumps.

The Dundee socket (Murdoch 1964, 1968), a pressure casting system using a sealed container and water pressure, was very successful and taught more about cast modification than was realized at the time. This technique produced socket volumes far in excess of the then standard versions, and the sockets, without modification except for the addition of a PT bar, were comfortable. Stumps treated in this manner did not atrophy at such an alarming rate as previously. It was from this experience that the extent of modification was gradually reduced to that seen today.

So far as the authors' unit is concerned, the standard PTB socket is now rarely prescribed. The troublesome cuff strap suspension has given way to supracondylar and suprapatellar suspending prostheses; in other words, the so-called PTB variants have become standard. They are found to be especially beneficial for the older amputee because they give far greater stability. If properly fitted, there is less constriction around the area formerly occupied by a tight-fitting strap. Less piston movement is possible, and consequently the leg feels lighter with the stump in constant contact with the socket. Modification has been reduced to a minimum as a result of lower mediolateral loads required to provide stability because of the increase in length of the socket. Atrophy has also been greatly reduced, and in patients with vascular disease all this must be beneficial.

The quality of socket fit, the quality of the prosthetic foot, and the positioning of these two in relation to each other, are crucial factors in below-knee prosthetic provision. It is the duty of the operating surgeon to produce a satisfactory organ for locomotion. Unfortunately, the end product is very often less than adequate for the purpose, and needless pain and expense are the consequence when all that is required is education and communication. In many cases it is found that the cut end of the tibia has not been rounded sufficiently at the anterior aspect during amputation. This can be a source of great irritation, irrespective of allowance being made in the modified cast. If the socket fit is tight, then traction of the skin during load-bearing over this sharp area of bone can make limb-wearing almost unbearable. It is also sometimes found that the fibula has been left longer than the tibia. This can be a difficult problem to overcome in a socket. It is much better if the fibula is 1–2 cm shorter than the tibia.

Excessive weight can be a problem with some methods of production, but is something which is easily overcome by using the right materials, even with conventional methods of construction. It is possible to make prostheses of less than 1 kg while maintaining strengths well above the Philadelphia standard (ISPO 1978).

There are many new interesting methods of construction which may enhance the lot of the below-knee amputee in the future and also improve the service in general, such as the use of thermoplastic materials and carbon fibre. Component parts and methods of construction are secondary, however, to having involved with the amputee a team of people who understand their business and who are willing to listen to each other's point of view. Contact between the units sending the amputees for prosthetic treatment and the prosthetic fitting units is often non-existent and, at worse, may consist of the standard departmental form requesting limb fitting; nothing more. The quality of the components and material available has kept pace with new technology. Great advances have been made in the education of prosthetist/orthotists; this should not be wasted by lack of communication.

References

Hughes J. & Jacobs N. J. (eds) (1985) CAD/CAM — computer aided design and manufacture. *Prosthetics and Orthotics International* 9, 1–47.

International Society for Prosthetics and Orthotics (1978) Standards for lower limb prostheses: report of a conference, 1977. Philadelphia: ISPO.

Lyquist E. (1970) Recent variants of the PTB prosthesis (PTB, KBM and air-cushion sockets). In *Prosthetic and Orthotic Practice* (ed. Murdoch G.), pp.79–88. London: Edward Arnold.

Murdoch G. (1964) The 'Dundee' socket — a total contact socket for the below-knee amputation. *Health Bulletin* 22(4), 70–71.

Murdoch G. (1968) The 'Dundee' socket for the below-knee amputation. *Prosthetics International* 3 (4–5), 15–21.

Radcliffe C. W. & Foort J. (1961) The patellar-tendon-bearing below-knee prosthesis. Biomechanics Laboratory, University of California, Berkeley.

Wilson L. A., Lyquist E. & Radcliffe C. W. (1968) Air-cushion socket for patellar-tendon-bearing below-knee prosthesis. Technical Report 55, Department of Medicine and Surgery, Veterans Administration, Washington, D.C.

7

Ankle–Foot Devices

D.N. CONDIE

Introduction

Virtually every patient who suffers a lower limb amputation will require an ankle–foot mechanism as a component of their prosthetic replacement. It is perhaps surprising therefore that there has been so little apparent change in the design of ankle–foot devices currently in widespread use since this topic was last reviewed in Dundee in 1969 (Condie 1970). Two explanations may be postulated for this observation: either the contemporary designs are entirely satisfactory or, alternatively, the challenge of overcoming their limitations is so severe that it has daunted even the most talented prosthetic designers. In this chapter the evidence in support of each of these theories will be examined.

The biomechanical functions of the ankle joint

The axis of motion of the ankle joint lies horizontally and perpendicular to the line of progression. Its motions are under the control of ten muscles, of which three are capable of exerting an upward movement upon the foot and are collectively referred to as the *dorsiflexors*. The remaining seven, which are responsible for producing a downward movement, are referred to as the *plantarflexors*. The action of these two muscle groups during normal level walking has been frequently described and may be summarized as follows:

1 *Heel contact to foot-flat*

A *shock absorption* phase during which the external plantarflexing moment resulting from the ground reaction force is resisted by the action of the dorsiflexors, resulting in a controlled movement of the ankle from its initial plantigrade attitude to a position of approximately 15° plantarflexion at foot-flat.

2 *Foot-flat to mid-stance*

A period of active dorsiflexion follows as the body pivots over the ankle joint, during which contraction of the dorsiflexors is required to overcome the plantarflexion moment resulting from the ground reaction.

3 Mid-stance to heel-off

From mid-stance the centre of gravity of the body moves forward with the plantarflexors acting to resist the external dorsiflexion moment and control the resulting rate of dorsiflexion.

4 Heel-off to toe-off

The direction of ankle motion reverses abruptly as the plantarflexors contract and lift the body onto the forefoot prior to swing.

5 Swing phase

During the swing phase the foot is held slightly dorsiflexed with the dorsiflexors acting to overcome the gravitational and inertia forces.

Thus the muscular activity during the stance phase may be summarized as comprising for each group of muscles (plantarflexors and dorsiflexors) a period of eccentric activity which may be regarded as involving the absorption of energy followed by a period of contraction during which energy is produced in order to overcome the external force actions on the body.

The nature of the energy exchanges occurring at the ankle joint was analysed by Bresler and Berry (1950), who highlighted the principal problem which faces designers who would attempt to replace the function of the ankle joint using *passive* designs of mechanisms. While the net energy output during the dorsiflexion phase is minimal, the very significant net output of energy occurring during the plantarflexion phase associated with push-off cannot possibly be simulated by a passive design of system, no matter how effective the energy storage mechanism may be. This analysis, which has provided the design criteria for most contemporary designs of ankle–foot device, does not take account of the changing situation that arises when walking up or down slopes. In the natural ankle joint, changes in the slope of the walking surface are readily accommodated by a shift in the neutral position of the joint with associated adjustments in muscle phasing. Equally, changes in shoe design, particularly heel height, are instantly accommodated with barely conscious adjustments in ankle function.

It is now possible to consider how prosthetic designers have responded to the challenge of replacing the functions of the ankle joint.

The conventional uniaxial ankle–foot

The traditional uniaxial prosthetic ankle–foot comprises essentially a standard foot blank, in wood or plastic, attached to the leg by a simple horizontally placed ankle bolt rotating in plain bushes. The construction of the joint may vary in the choice of bearing material and the means of mounting. The resisting and restoring moments necessary to simulate ankle flexion are obtained by the use of a compressible plantarflexion bumper located posteriorly and a rather stiff dorsiflexion bumper located anteriorly, designed to permit the required degree of motion under the anticipated external loading. A toe break is normally provided by means of a further rubber bumper placed between the foot and toe sections. Correctly fitted, which includes the selection of bumpers of appropriate stiffness, this design of foot is generally capable of providing an acceptable simulation of the normal ankle functions, the sole exception being the inability of the device to provide active plantarflexion during the terminal swing phase. This design of ankle–foot is intended for level walking conditions only and will normally be assembled for use with one single height of shoe heel. Problems with device failure resulting from the wear of mechanical parts and work hardening of the rubber bumpers encouraged the development of a new design of prosthetic ankle–foot some years ago in the U.S.A.

The SACH foot

The solid ankle jointed foot developed by the University of California (1957) has revolutionized prosthetic practice, providing the first viable alternative to the traditional uniaxial design. This foot, which has no moving parts, achieves its function by means of the wedge of cushioning material inserted in the region of the heel, which replaces the function of the heel bumper in the earlier designs, and the rigid internal keel, which controls the transfer of body weight from mid-stance until toe-off, replacing the normally occurring dorsiflexion and plantarflexion. In spite of the apparent simplicity of this design many problems were encountered initially by would-be users due to their failure to adhere to the correct procedures when selecting and fitting the foot. This problem has been aggravated on occasions by the failure of manufacturers to provide a sufficient range of feet with heel cushions matched to the full range of prosthetic users. The advantages claimed for this design of foot relate to its superior durability and the suggestion that it permits a smoother, more natural ankle–foot action. Disadvantages not already mentioned are common to the uniaxial foot and relate to its passive design.

Since the appearance of the SACH foot more than 20 years ago a considerable debate has been waged between practitioners who still favour the traditional uniaxial design and proponents of the new 'rubber foot'. In the U.K. this debate has resulted in an informal consensus which favours the use of the SACH foot for most below-knee prostheses but which prefers the use of the uniaxial foot on above-knee prostheses. This attitude is justified by the view that the action of the uniaxial foot provides greater knee stability immediately following heel contact.

This controversy has recently been refuelled by the appearance of several comparative biomechanical studies of amputees wearing both types of feet. First Doan and Holt (1983) and then Goh *et al.* (1984) have published detailed analyses of the differences encountered in the resulting gait patterns. Similar findings are reported by both groups; however, the Strathclyde report is of greater interest since the information published also includes kinetic data. Analysis of the kinetic data does appear to confirm the view expressed by practitioners that with the SACH foot the period from heel-strike until foot-flat is almost twice as long as with the uniaxial foot, which more closely resembles the timing of normal ankle motion. For patients fitted with a SACH foot this deviation is associated with an increase in the degree of knee flexion required to achieve foot-flat. It is postulated that this manoeuvre could be perilous for an elderly or frail above-knee amputee.

The analysis of the ground-to-foot vector data demonstrates clearly the smoother transition from heel contact to toe-off which has long been claimed by SACH foot users. Surprisingly, in spite of these clear differences, no significant deviations were identified in the pattern of the moments occurring at the proximal joints for either foot design. The Strathclyde team also commented on the difficulties encountered in obtaining the correct stiffness characteristics for both designs of feet, highlighting the importance of proper selection, fitting, and alignment of any prosthetic foot.

The biomechanical function of the subtalar joint

The discussions of ankle–foot design have so far been confined to devices which are designed to replace the function of the ankle joint alone. Substantial evidence exists, however, to demonstrate the importance of the movements which occur in the more distal joints of the foot in enabling normal function. Certainly the most important of these joints is the subtalar joint.

The axis of motion at the subtalar joint has been demonstrated to lie obliquely from a point laterally on the calcaneus to a point anteriorly on the neck of the talus. The movements obtainable at this joint may be described as comprising in one direction plantarflexion/inversion/internal rotation (usually referred to as supination) and in the other direction dorsiflexion/eversion/external rotation (termed pronation). These movements are under the control of the same ten muscles which control plantarflexion and dorsiflexion.

Doubts surrounding the function of this joint during walking were dispelled by the publication of the excellent study by Levens *et al.* (1948) at the University of California, which described the relationship between subtalar motion and the transverse rotation of the whole leg. Stated briefly, during the swing phase and the first 15% of the stance phase, while the pelvis is rotating internally, the foot moves into a pronated position. This action, which occurs in conjunction with external rotation at the hip, enables the foot to maintain its attitude in relation to the direction of progression. During the remainder of the stance phase, as pelvic rotation reverses, the foot moves into a supinated position, combining with internal rotation of the hip to eliminate slippage between the foot and the ground.

The significance of this feature of subtalar function when considering prosthetic design has long been questioned. Many practitioners have pointed to the soft tissue interface between stump and socket as an alternative site for the absorption of these motions. No scientific studies have been performed to clarify this issue; however, it is possible to offer an informal view based on clinical experience. Certainly for those patients who exhibit a full normal range of hip rotation, the absence of subtalar motion would appear to be of little significance. In contrast, a single experience with a below-knee amputee with marked limitation of hip rotation has demonstrated the disastrous effect of the resulting torsional forces which were thus transmitted across the socket interface. It is suggested therefore that the inclusion of a mechanism within the ankle–foot to permit controlled internal/ external rotation should be regarded as a compensation for abnormal hip function rather than as a replacement for normal subtalar function.

It remains therefore to examine the other important function of the subtalar joint, that relating to adjustments in the attitude of the foot required by sidehill slopes. Reference has already been made to the inversion/eversion element of supination and pronation. If motion at the subtalar joint takes place in conjunction with compensatory ankle dorsiflexion and plantarflexion movements, it will therefore be possible to produce pure foot inversion and eversion. If these movements and adjustments can be co-ordinated with the ankle joint motions necessary for normal walking they will provide a fully effective mechanism for coping with a sidehill situation.

It is now possible to examine how prosthetic designers have approached the task of replacing the function of the subtalar joint during walking.

Multiaxial designs of prosthetic feet

The wave of prosthetic design activity which followed the institution of the U.S. Artificial Limb Program in 1945 resulted in the development of a large number of multifunctional ankle–foot assemblies, none of which achieved any significant success. Worthy of mention, however, is the experimental torque absorber designed at the University of California, experience with which provided the basic design data which have been employed in many subsequent developments in this area. Three later designs of multiaxial foot–ankle which have emerged have reached the stage of commercial supply.

The *Teufel Telasto* ankle–foot assembly is essentially a modification of the standard uniaxial foot by the addition of a rubber bushing within the housing of the ankle joint which permits a mild degree of inversion and eversion.

The *Greissinger* foot–ankle assembly features a wood ankle section and a moulded rubber block recessed into a plastic foot. The foot and ankle section are joined by a U-bolt and yoke-type assembly which permits controlled plantar/ dorsiflexion, inversion/eversion, and transverse rotation. This device is in widespread use in continental Europe, although little or no scientific evidence exists to support this practice. A limited biomechanical study of patients using this foot (Spiers 1982) yielded inconclusive biomechanical evidence; however, the younger, more active patients reportedly favoured the 'greater freedom' afforded by this design.

The *Trautman* foot–ankle assembly designed in the U.S.A. consists of a wood ankle section mounted on a moulded plastic base, a wood foot with rubber ankle fairing, and a rubber ankle block. Two cables are located along the mid-sagittal line, the anterior cable securing the entire assembly and the posterior permitting adjustment of the plantar/dorsiflexion attitude of the foot. This design also permits inversion/eversion and transverse rotation.

Statistics of the scale of use of these multiaxial joints are not available; however it is probably safe to state that they have scarcely dented a market dominated internationally by the SACH foot and standard uniaxial designs.

More recently there has been an upsurge in interest in multiaxial ankle–foot devices, with several additional devices making an appearance. Most prosthetic practitioners will be familiar with the extended history of the *Mauch hydraulic foot–ankle* development. A preliminary clinical evaluation of the latest version of this system was reported (Sowell 1981), and several features of the design are worthy of description. Four rubber washers embodied in the housing of the unit are positioned and shaped such that they pemit 10% of inversion but strongly resist eversion. This arrangement is designed to permit a straddled gait or for the downhill foot on sloping ground. Two rubber bumpers interposed between the piston rod and the inside of the shank section provide torsion resistance to transverse rotations. The most revolutionary feature of this design however relates to the use of a hydraulic unit to control the plantarflexion/dorsiflexion characteristics of the foot. This ingenious unit contains a gravity-controlled element which automatically adjusts the 'neutral' position of the ankle joint to accommodate uphill and downhill surfaces. This same mechanism will also accommodate different heights of heel. A further feature of the design of the hydraulic unit utilizes a weight-controlled port which functions to free the foot to adopt any position from 10° of dorsiflexion to 20° of plantarflexion when the leg is unloaded. This feature allows the wearer to adopt a more natural leg and foot position when seated.

The conclusion to the evaluation of the system reported that the study 'had revealed' that the system does simulate the anatomical ankle functions for an ambitious range of indoor and outdoor activities; however, the evaluation techniques employed were totally subjective and nothing further has been heard regarding this development.

A new 'oldie' has recently joined the commercial product range with the appearance of the *McKendrick foot and ankle joint*. Initial inspection of this device suggests that it is a hybrid embodying a front bumper, as in uniaxial designs, a heel cushion and a keel drawn from the SACH foot design, and a 'memory block' and steel retaining tendon similar to the Trautman design. Sales literature states that the mechanism provides a full range of ankle–foot motion; however, no technical specification is available, nor any report of clinical experience.

Perhaps the most ambitious recent development in the field of multifunctional ankle–foot design is the *Multiflex ankle–foot* (Fig. 7.1) which has been produced as part of the Blatchford Endolite system. This mechanism is immediately reminiscent of the Metalastik unit developed at Roehampton many years ago; however, the Blatchford designers have employed modern materials and manufacturing methods to overcome the weight and wear problems which condemned that earlier unit.

The essential components of the Multiflex ankle–foot are the moulded plastic foot with its carbon-fibre box construction keel and a metal ankle assembly which houses the controlling mechanism and provides a means of attachment for the shin tube. The primary control of ankle motions is obtained by the deflection of a rubber ball and stem assembly located in the ankle housing. Secondary resistance to dorsiflexion is provided by a 'snubber O ring' located below the ball which acts against a stop on the housing. The combination of controlling elements described

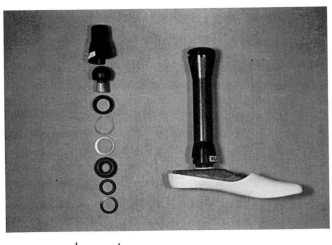

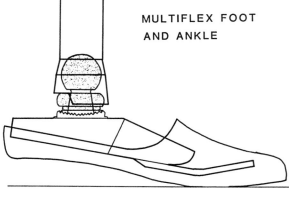

MULTIFLEX FOOT
AND ANKLE

Fig. 7.1 Blatchford Multiflex ankle–foot.

provides a full range of dorsiflexion/plantarflexion controlled inversion/eversion and some rotation or torque absorption. A range of balls and snubber rings is available, colour-coded to provide a range of stiffness characteristics designed to match the full range of prosthetic activity levels. The foot is secured to the ankle assembly by a single bolt, and adjustment to accommodate a 40 mm variation in heel height is available through the curved serrated design of the matching surfaces on the foot and the ankle assembly. The developers report that more than 2500 of these feet are in service in the U.K. and Europe; however, no scientific or clinical data are available with which to judge their performance.

In 1966 the U.S. Veterans Administration published the results of a laboratory study of two multifunctional ankle joints (Greissinger and Trautman) where the range of motion produced by the application of the normally encountered maximum external moments were compared with the corresponding natural ankle movements. These results are probably of little significance, since they take no account of the changes in the external loading pattern which might be expected as a result of the normal joint structure and its controlling mechanism. It is interesting, however, to compare these results with data provided by the developers of the Multiflex ankle (Table 7.1). Not surprisingly, the Multiflex data compare rather closely with both the normal and the previous experimental data, with the exception of eversion where the motion obtained is significantly smaller than the normal movement. It should be repeated, however, that the normal data used to carry out these comparisons were obtained from non-amputees walking on level surfaces, whereas the most significant advantage of multifunctional ankle joints is likely to be the ability to accommodate side-sloping surfaces. Regrettably, experimentally derived data for this situation do not appear to be available.

Table 7.1 Comparison of the functional properties of a range of multiaxial prosthetic feet.

Motion	Normal max loads (ft/lb)	Rotation (degrees)			
		Normal	Trautman	Greissinger	Multiflex
Plantarflexion	18.0	18	8.5	15.0	9.5–13.5
Dorsiflexion	80.0	10	4.5	12.5	Max. 10
Eversion	2.0	6	4.0	0.5	0.6–1.7
Inversion	15.0	6	18.0	4.5	4.5–8.0
Internal	6.0	9	12.0	7.0	3.0–9.0
External	6.0	8	12.0	7.0	3.0–9.0

The almost total lack of scientifically obtained information regarding experience with multifunctional ankle–foot devices makes it impossible to reach any concrete conclusions regarding the merit of these designs. It is to be hoped that the work already reported on the uniaxial and SACH foot function will be extended in the future to include these aspects of foot design.

Conclusion

The available clinical evidence regarding the acceptability of the most commonly used ankle–foot devices suggests that the majority of patients can be treated successfully with these devices. There appears, however, to be a strongly held view amongst prosthetists and designers that reliable multifunctional devices are required if it is to be possible to satisfy fully the aspirations of the younger, more active patients. Whether the new generation of these devices will succeed in filling this need will require some time to evaluate. The final lasting problem of ankle–foot design relates to the inability to current designs to simulate push-off. Once again the clinical and experimental evidence suggests that this is not a serious handicap for the majority of amputees; however, it is significant that the recent development of the *Seattle* foot is designed specifically to utilize more effectively the stored and released gravitational energy in an attempt to respond to the needs of the physically active lower-limb amputee. Further information on this development is eagerly awaited.

References

Bresler B. & Berry F. R. (1950) Energy characteristics of normal and prosthetic ankle joints. University of California, Berkeley, Series II, Issue 12.

Condie D. N. (1970) Ankle–foot mechanisms. In *Prosthetic and Orthotic Practice* (ed. Murdoch G.), pp. 89–103. London: Edward Arnold.

Doan N. E. & Holt L. E. (1983) A comparison of the SACH and single axis foot in the gait of unilateral below-knee amputees. *Prosthetics and Orthotics International* 7, 31–36.

Goh J. C. H., Solomonidis S. E., Spence W. D. & Paul J. P. (1984) Biomechanical evaluation of SACH and uniaxial feet. *Prosthetics and Orthotics International* 8, 147–154.

Levens A. S., Inman V. T. & Blosser J. A. (1948) Transverse rotation of the segments of the lower extremity in locomotion. *Journal of Bone and Joint Surgery* 30A, 859–872.

Sowell T. T. (1981) A preliminary clinical evaluation of the Mauch hydraulic foot–ankle system. *Prosthetics and Orthotics International* 5, 87–91.

Spiers R. W. (1982) A biomechanical assessment of ankle– foot devices for the below-knee amputee. Thesis, MSc, University of Strathclyde, Glasgow.

University of California, Berkeley (1957) Installation of the solid ankle cushion heel (SACH) foot for adult male amputees.

Veterans Administration Prosthetic Center (1966) VAPC Research. Report Otto Bock 'Greissinger' foot and ankle assemblies (model 1A6) with compressible and non-compressible heel wedges. *Bulletin of Prosthetics Research* 10–6, 237–240.

8

The Seattle Prosthetic Foot

E.M. BURGESS

The Seattle prosthetic foot is the result of a long-term programme of research and development involving the collaboration of staff from the Prosthetic Research Study funded by the Veterans Administration (VA), the University of Washington, and local industry. The programme was stimulated by a study of the recreational activities of active lower limb amputees which was conducted in Seattle some years ago by staff of the Prosthetics Research Study (Kegel *et al.* 1980). This study revealed that the 'major specific problem' encountered by these patients in pursuing their sporting activities was in running successfully. It was apparent that this problem was directly related to the design of currently employed prosthetic feet.

In order to tackle this problem a collaborative study was initiated by staff at the Kinesiology Department of the University of Washington to collect scientific data relating to running and jumping while wearing a prosthesis. The results of this study have subsequently been published (Enoka *et al.* 1982). The study identified marked differences between the performances of normal and prosthetic feet. For example, normal foot function during running requires a significant degree of supination and pronation, which is not possible with most prosthetic feet. Of more immediate practical value was the observation that in 'running prostheses' the prosthetic foot requires to be set in an attitude of some plantarflexion rather than the 5–10° of dorsiflexion indicated for level walking. From a design standpoint one of the more important observations related to the fact that during running the magnitude of the ground reaction force may be two or three times greater than that experienced during walking. Since prosthetic feet are customarily designed for walking this results in an abnormal gait pattern.

Following the analysis of the data obtained from this study it was concluded that if an improved running performance were to be achieved it would require the design and development of an energy-storing ankle–foot unit. At this stage in the programme further assistance was enlisted from engineering consultants recruited from the local aerospace industry. The first prototype foot employed a system of layered leaf springs, of a reinforced fibreglass construction, to store the energy generated during initial loading of the foot and to release this during push-off, thus simulating the normal activity of the gastrocnemius and soleus muscles

(Burgess *et al.* 1983). Initial clinical trials with the prototype resulted in an immediate and enthusiastic response; however, a further lengthy period of development has been necessary to translate the prototype into a unit which would be both durable and relatively inexpensive. The current and now standardized foot consists of a monolithic keel made from a synthetic composite material (Delrin) which is embedded in a foam foot shape (Fig. 8.1).

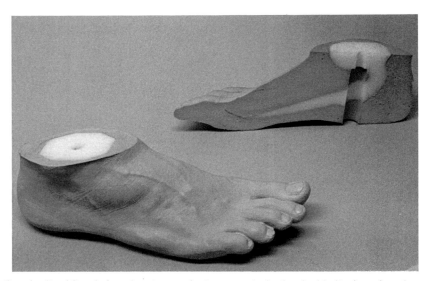

Fig. 8.1 Standardized Seattle foot showing synthetic composite keel embedded in foam foot shape.

In 1985 the developers (Burgess 1985) reported briefly the successful outcome of a local field study of 50 active patients and of progress with a more extensive national field evaluation which is being conducted by the Rehabilitation Research and Development Section of the VA Central Office in Washington D.C. The feet for this study are being fabricated by a local Seattle company which will also be responsible ultimately for commercial distribution*. The Seattle group report that they intend to continue their research programme with further applications of the concept of 'energy prosthetics'.

References

Burgess E. M. (1985) Letter to the Editor, *Prosthetics and Orthotics International* **9**, 55–56.
Burgess E. M., Hittenberger D. A., Forsgren S. M. & Lindh D (1983) The Seattle prosthetic foot — a design for active sports: preliminary studies. *Orthotics and Prosthetics* **37(1)**, 25–31.
Enoka R. M., Miller D. I. & Burgess E. M. (1982) Below-knee amputee running gait. *American Journal of Physical Medicine* **61(2)**, 66–84.
Kegel B., Webster J. C. & Burgess E. M. (1980) Recreational activities of lower extremity amputees: a survey. *Archives of Physical Medicine and Rehabilitation* **61(6)**, 258–264.

*Model and Instrument Development, 861 South Poplar Place, Seattle, Washington 98144, U.S.A.

9

Principles of Prosthetic Prescription in the Early Months after Lower Limb Amputation

J.C. ANGEL

Introduction

The change in stump shape that invariably follows an amputation means that a definitive prosthesis cannot be fitted for several months if it is to remain functional for a reasonable period of time. In the intervening period there are advantages in fitting a temporary prosthesis:

1 Stump maturation is hastened.
2 The patient's morale is boosted by his early return to walking and the restoration of body image.
3 In the geriatric patient the improved mobility may be the deciding factor in allowing discharge from hospital.
4 Muscles are strengthened.
5 Joints are prevented from contracting.
6 Joints already contracted are stretched.
7 Prosthetic adjustments, often awkward and costly in the definitive limb, can be undertaken with ease.

The disadvantages are the demands on the prosthetist's time compared to the short life of the temporary prosthesis, the compromise of cosmesis, and the discomfort caused to the recent wound.

Timing

The timing of the fitting of a temporary prosthesis is important, since if it is started too early it may rapidly become functionless, and if too late its useful life will be reduced. Fig. 9.1 shows the way in which the stump changes its shape after an amputation. The initial increase in stump circumference is due to traumatic oedema and haematoma formation. The height of this ascent is very much related to the surgeon's technique, particularly his handling of the tissues and his ability to secure complete haemostasis. The descending part of the curve is brought about by the atrophy of various tissues, together with the clearance, in the initial stages, of haematoma and oedema. Muscle atrophies through disuse, and this occurs most

63

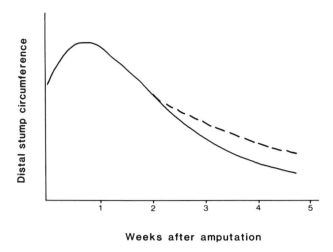

Fig. 9.1 Stump circumference plotted against time following amputation.

in well-muscled individuals. Fat atrophies through the application of pressure, and this is most noticeable in individuals with a thick layer of subcutaneous fat. The ideal amputee, from the point of view of the fitting of an early socket, is a thin man with poor muscle bulk. One can think of cases where, in the third post-operative week, the patient was supplied with a temporary prosthesis which could still be worn comfortably six months later. The least ideal is a fat woman (women usually have more subcutaneous fat) on a reducing diet and diuretic medication. In such cases the reduction in stump volume can be as high as 50% in six months. The traumatic oedema and haematoma are cleared within 15–20 days, the process being hastened by elevation and graduated pressure. It is often appropriate for the stump to be cast with a close-fitting socket at this stage. If the vascular supply is compromised, or if there is any infection, the casting will be delayed.

Social and economic factors may also have a considerable influence on the timing of the prescription of a temporary prosthesis. It needs to be brought forward for patients whose discharge from hospital is dependent upon a prosthesis. It may be delayed in the case of those who are crutch-walkers, who are already out of hospital, especially if they have difficulty in getting to and from the limb-fitting centre. Indeed, there may be some cases, for example where excessive travelling is involved or where the general health is poor, in which attempts to fit a temporary prosthesis are best abandoned altogether. Generally speaking, the more distal an amputation, the more important a temporary prosthesis is in determining the final outcome of prosthetic fitting.

Construction

The socket of a temporary artificial limb should be capable of fairly simple modification to cope with the changes in stump shape, and socket liners help towards this end. Also, it is desirable that the system used allows changes in alignment, especially if the patient is being encouraged to 'walk out' a joint contracture. Adjustability in length is also a useful feature, since patients often have a difficulty with footwear on the contralateral side. For example, an elderly patient may be able to wear only a slipper, or a trauma case may have a plaster cast and walking heel on the opposite foot for the first few weeks. The device needs to be relatively inexpensive in accordance with its short functional life, although this need not apply to components that may subsequently be incorporated into a definitive prosthesis or used again on another patient. The cost can be reduced by paying less attention to cosmesis than in a definitive prosthesis and using less durable materials. There should be good back-up from an amputee clinic team in order that the best use can be made of the temporary limb.

Post-surgical fitting and rigid dressing

The introduction of the immediate post-surgical fitting of prostheses by Weiss in Poland (1969) and Burgess (1971) and his associates in Seattle was important because it introduced plaster to amputation surgery and prosthetists to amputating surgeons. The plaster dressing, or rigid dressing, that is applied to amputation stumps is particularly helpful in controlling oedema and joint contractures, certainly from the below-knee level distally. The necessary meeting of surgeons and prosthetists in the operating theatre led to a greatly increased awareness amongst surgeons of the advantages of preserving the knee joint and a willingness to do so, even if it meant an increase in their reamputation rate.

The author is unable to agree with Dr Burgess that the fitting of an artificial foot onto the rigid dressing at the time of surgery has any advantages as regards the maturation of the stump. Much has been claimed of the psychological advantages stemming from the method, but experience suggests that the vast majority of patients are not in need of such expensive psychological support.

The mid-tarsal amputation

This controversial level can be made to yield a satisfactory amputation stump, provided it is well covered with plantar skin, has full muscle control, and has a good range of movements at the ankle and subtalar joints (Jacobs *et al.* 1977). The amputation is almost invariably performed in contaminated conditions for either trauma or the complications of diabetes, and in these circumstances it is unwise to attempt tendon suture or implantation, hence the post-operative care is of vital importance. The ankle has to be held in dorsiflexion and the subtalar joint in eversion by a rigid dressing, at least until the dorsiflexors and evertors have formed attachments to the bones of the foot. Once there is a satisfactory range of active movement at the ankle and subtalar joints, the patient can be fitted with a front opening, removable device, fitted with a rocker.

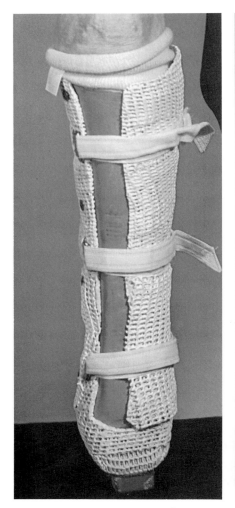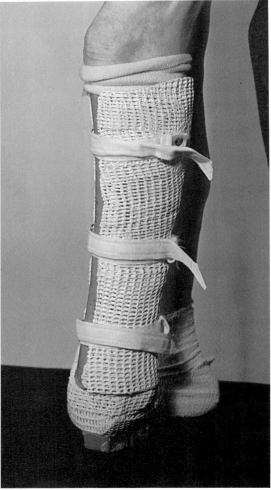

Fig. 9.2 Hexcelite rigid dressing for Syme amputation. This can be donned and doffed through a front opening. It is fitted with a rocker and packing material for optimum length.

Syme amputation

The height of the ankle joint above the ground is remarkably variable. Consequently, so is the length of the heel-pad fashioned by the standard Syme technique (Harris 1966). A short heel-pad sits firmly under the tibia after suturing, but a long one is vulnerable to displacement in either the coronal or sagittal plane. A rigid dressing is required to hold it centrally beneath the cut surface of the tibia, and this firm hold becomes even more important once the patient starts to walk, usually during the third week. This is one of the situations in which the thermoplastic bandage material, Hexcelite*, is of outstanding value. It is springy enough to allow the rigid dressing to be donned and doffed through a front opening (Fig. 9.2). The device is secured by Velcro† fastening. The majority of patients who have worn these for the first few post-operative weeks insist that they continue to be supplied with the device long after they have had their definitive limb because they find it useful as a quickly donned slipper at night and, having no foot, it is particularly comfortable to walk in. It is possible to add a foot in cases where there is limb shortening.

Below-knee amputation

At Stanmore the intention is to fit the first patellar tendon-bearing prosthesis sometime during the third week. If the patient is attending from a distance and finds travelling a problem the socket is commonly fabricated by wrapping Hexcelite directly round the stump, protecting it with two woollen stump socks, the outer one of which becomes the lining. By this means it is possible to fabricate a limb in about four hours. If it is relatively easy for the patient to attend a few days later to collect his limb then a positive cast is poured and a socket is made out of polypropylene with a P.E. Lite‡ liner. Cuff suspension rather than a patellar tendon–supracondylar prosthesis (PTS) brim offers greater security. At the moment side steels and a special uniaxial ankle unit are used together with a prefabricated cosmetic covering which has proved extremely satisfactory (Fig. 9.3a). Where it seems that healing is going to be delayed, or an unusually bulbous stump has been fashioned, then a tuber-bearing pylon is prescribed.

Through-knee amputation

An early socket with this level of amputation is unlikely to be self-suspending because of the progressive shrinking of the distal end of the stump. It must therefore be fitted with a soft waist suspension. End-bearing is important in order to toughen the healing tissues for their future load-carrying role. However, it may well be desirable to add a tuber seat to the top of the socket, especially if there is tender scar tissue in the load-bearing part of the stump. The end-bearing pad should be capable of adjustment to control the percentage of weight taken distally. The materials most commonly chosen by the author are a block-leather socket, side steels and simple ring–catch joints.

*Manufacturer : Orthopaedic Systems, Unit G22, Old Gate, St. Michaels Industrial Estate, Widnes, Cheshire WA8 8TL.
†Manufacturer: Hancock & Roberts Ltd, Stadon Road, Anstey, Leicester.
‡Manufacturer: S. H. Camp Ltd, Northgate House, Staple Gardens, Winchester, Hampshire.

(a) 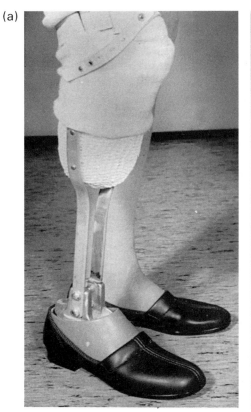 (b)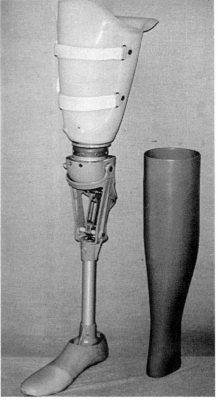

Fig. 9.3 (a) PTB pylon with Hexcelite socket. (b) 'PRIMAP' limb with prefabricated polypropylene, adjustable socket fitted on Blatchford modular assembly components.

Above-knee amputation

The use of modular components, later to be incorporated in the definitive prosthesis, has been a considerable recent advance. The socket is still an unsolved problem. The adjustable device (Fig. 9.3b) made of polypropylene is satisfactory if the change in stump shape is very small and if the dimensions are fairly standard. Unfortunately, many stumps fall outside the range of prefabricated sockets and a custom-built socket is required. As the distal end of the stump shrinks the device is supposed to accommodate this by adjustments to the Velcro fastening. Unfortunately, the shrinkage tends to occur distally, where the adjustability is least. Suspension is provided by means of a rigid pelvic band and shoulder strap. Older patients prefer to have a semi-automatic knee lock, but as they progress a stabilized knee and other mechanisms can be substituted.

There is still a place for the old-fashioned above-knee pylon fitted with a rocker end. It is particularly welcomed by the geriatric amputee who has stairs to climb, lives alone, and places more importance on function than cosmesis (Fig. 9.4a).

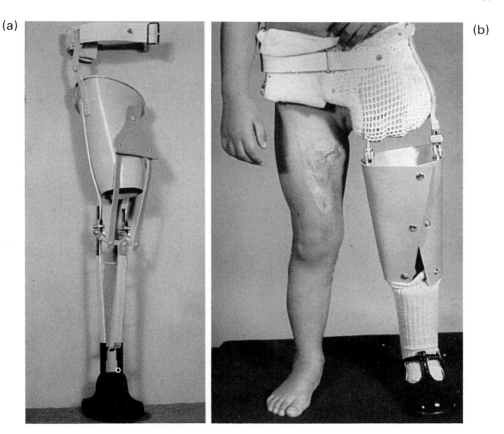

Fig. 9.4 (a) Rocker pylon for geriatric above-knee amputee. (b) Hexcelite temporary hip disarticulation prosthesis.

Hip disarticulation

The 'stump' at this level matures rapidly and there should be no need for a temporary prosthesis. However, the definitive limb requires considerable expertise of both the prosthetist and the prosthetic technician, and if this expertise is in short supply there may be a delay. This is certainly the case in the United Kingdom. Here the incorporation of modular components and the use of Hexcelite in making the temporary prosthesis have greatly improved the delivery times of the first prosthesis. The socket can be moulded directly onto an elastic support tailored to fit the body contours, although it is better wrapped onto a positive cast. Unless the patient is young and athletic the hip joint is mounted beneath the tuber and held in place with steels riveted into the Hexcelite. The knee joint has a semi-automatic lock (Fig. 9.4b).

Conclusion

It is probably fair to say that the design of temporary prostheses has not kept pace with the recent dramatic advance of their definitive counterparts. What particular features should be incorporated? The following are suggested:

1 A method of fabrication that allows the limb to be applied within three or four hours of the patient's first attendance.

2 A socket that is adjustable at least at its distal end if not the brim.

3 The alignment should be capable of subsequent modification to cope with resolving joint contractures and improvement in gait.

4 The length should be alterable and so should the set of the foot to deal with the change from slippers to shoes.

The achievement of these goals would considerably improve the quality of life in the first few months after amputation. The use of such a limb could be expected to provide the optimum means of preparing the patient for his first definitive prosthesis.

References

Burgess E. M., Romano R. L., Zettle J. H. & Schrock R. D. (1971) Amputations of the leg for peripheral vascular insufficiency. *Journal of Bone and Joint Surgery* **53A**, 874–890.

Harris R. I. (1966) The history and development of Syme's amputation. In Selected articles from *Artificial Limbs*. January 1954–Spring 1966, 233–272.

Jacobs R. L., Karmody A. M., Wirth C., & Vedder D. (1977) The team approach in salvage of the diabetic foot. *Surgery Annual* **9**, 231–264.

Weiss M. (1969) Physiological amputation, immediate prosthetic and early ambulation. *Prosthetics International* **3(8)**, 38–44.

10

Physiotherapy and the Lower Limb Amputee

M.E. CONDIE

Successful rehabilitation of the lower limb amputee depends on good co-operation between all members of the clinic team. The team will normally include:

Amputating surgeon.
Nursing staff.
Physiotherapist.
Prosthetist.
Occupational therapist.
Social worker.

A physiotherapist skilled in the treatment of amputees plays a key role within this team for several reasons. Firstly, a carefully structured exercise and mobility programme will allow the patient to achieve maximum independence after amputation. Secondly, the experienced physiotherapist's ability to assess accurately the patient's physical capabilities will contribute greatly to the decisions taken by the team in respect of prosthetic prescription and expected level of independence following rehabilitation. Thirdly, the physiotherapist will probably spend more time with the patient than any other single member of the rehabilitation team. This can allow a close relationship to develop between patient and therapist, and the patient will express fears, apprehensions, and ambitions which might not be apparent in the more formal atmosphere of a ward round or clinic. An insight can thus be gained into the patient's attitude towards his amputation, and this knowledge will in turn contribute to the team's judgement of the outcome of rehabilitation.

These points emphasize the need for experienced physiotherapists who are familiar with the particular problems associated with the treatment of amputees, and whose skills will bring about the most effective resolution of these problems. Ideally, the patient is best treated in a specialist amputee unit with a senior physiotherapist having the responsibility for the physical rehabilitation of the patient from the pre-operative state (where possible) through to the point where no further improvements will be made. A recent study at the Dulwich Hospital by Ham *et al.* (1985) demonstrates beyond doubt that this approach to amputee care, co-ordinated by a senior physiotherapist, improves the results of rehabilitation.

Pre-operative care

Early referral of the patient to the physiotherapist is extremely important if amputation is being considered. The patient is frequently extremely distressed when told of possible surgery, and will often greatly appreciate meeting an existing amputee who has had the same amputation as that proposed, and who can demonstrate the use of his prosthesis.

Patients in the older age groups suffering from vascular disease will almost always suffer from other conditions which make rehabilitation more difficult, for example arthritis, stroke, intermittent claudication of the other leg, generalized debility, failing sight, or mental impairment. Advanced vascular disease can produce pain and toxicity, which may well increase the symptoms from the conditions described above, and, whilst the patient pre-operatively may seem very ill indeed and a poor rehabilitation prospect, the post-operative picture can improve radically in a short time, and the physiotherapist should exercise caution in predicting the patient's potential level of independence.

Flexion contractures are sometimes present in one or both legs, especially in patients who have ischaemic foot pain. The leg is often held with the hip and knee flexed to allow the foot to be rubbed, or the foot is allowed to hang over the side of the bed with the knee flexed. Where possible, measures should be taken to reduce these contractures and to strengthen appropriate muscle groups. However, if the patient is unco-operative because of his physical condition, this can prove to be an impossible task.

The patient should be told what exercises and movements to perform post-operatively. He should be informed of the post-operative programme and approximate time-scale of the rehabilitation process, assuming a straightforward recovery from amputation surgery. He should also be taught to roll over in bed and to lie prone. This position removes pressure from vulnerable areas such as the heel, sacral area, and backs of elbows, and is often found to be comfortable by the patient. Lying prone will also assist in the prevention of post-operative flexion contractures at the knee (following a below-knee amputation) and hip (following a through- or above-knee amputation). The existence of some medical disorders, such as certain cardiac or respiratory conditions, is a contraindication to lying prone. It is essential to communicate continually with the patient and to keep him well informed in order to gain his full co-operation.

Post-operative care

The exercise and rehabilitation programme for each patient has to be individually planned, but a guide is given in Table 10.1. Some of these procedures require further clarification.

Table 10.1 Suggested post-operative programme.

1st post-operative day	(a)	Bed exercises in long sitting position.
2nd post-operative day	(a)	As before.
	(b)	Exercises in prone and side lying position
3rd post-operative day	(a), (b)	As before.
	(c)	Up to sit for short time with stump supported.
	(d)	Balance training in sitting position.
4th/5th post-operative day	(a), (b), (c), (d)	As before.
	(e)	Start balance and walking training with walking frame.
5th/6th post-operative day	(d), (e)	As before.
	(f)	Begin treatment in physiotherapy department.
7th–10th post-operative day	(g)	Introduce the early walking aid.

(a) Bed exercises for the below-knee amputee

(i) Active exercises to strengthen shoulder, upper limb, and trunk muscles.

(ii) Active exercises to maintain strength and mobility of remaining leg.

(iii) Static quadriceps exercises for affected leg, progressing to straight-leg raising as soon as the patient can maintain a straight knee.

It is unnecessary to emphasize active knee flexion at this early stage. A flexion contracture at this joint in not uncommon prior to amputation, and post-operatively the knee has a tendency to adopt a flexed position. It is therefore most important to emphasize knee extension, and this should be encouraged until the patient has good quadriceps power. Once this has been achieved, knee flexion exercises may be commenced.

Bed exercises for the above-knee amputee are described in a later chapter.

(b) Exercises in prone lying position

Some older patients may not tolerate this position, and it is inadvisable to insist on prone lying if the patient is unhappy.

(c) Balance and walking training with a walking frame

At this stage, the frame is the walking aid of choice for most patients because of its stability. Younger, more active patients may prefer crutches, which will permit a speedier gait.

(f) Treatment in the physiotherapy department

If the patient's condition allows it, he should be taken from the ward to the physiotherapy department. This change of environment can boost the patient's morale, and facilitates the introduction of weight and pulley exercises for the upper limbs and residual leg. These are useful physiotherapy techniques which can be easily regulated and progressed. Stump exercises and exercises to improve general strength and mobility should be continued.

(g) *The early walking aid*

The most commonly used device in the U.K. is the pneumatic post-amputation mobility aid as described by Redhead (1983), which is suitable for below-knee, through-knee, and above-knee amputees, although it will not safely accommodate a very short above-knee stump (Fig. 10.1a). The tulip limb (Liedberg *et al.* 1983) is available for below-knee amputees only (Fig. 10.1b).

(a)   (b)

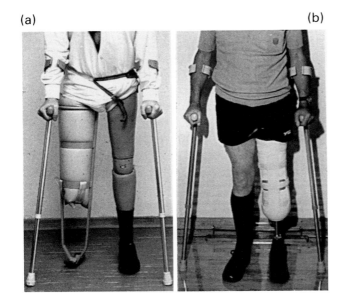

Fig. 10.1 (a) The pneumatic post-amputation mobility aid on a below-knee amputee. (b) A patient wearing the 'tulip limb'.

During training with an early walking aid, it is most important that the physiotherapist carries out regular examinations of the stump. Any area of discolouration or indication that healing is not progressing as anticipated should immediately be reported to the clinician in charge. Pain in the stump caused by the application of the device is an immediate contraindication to its use.

The early walking aid is initially used twice daily for a ten-minute period. This is rapidly increased to one hour at least twice each day. The patient should walk between parallel bars and progress to using elbow crutches. The treatment should always be conducted under supervision in the physiotherapy department. In the case of the younger amputee with no impairment of circulation, the device should be used from the seventh post-operative day. It is the author's experience that most elderly amputees who have impaired circulation may safely use an early walking aid from the tenth post-operative day, however some surgeons prefer to defer this activity until wound healing is complete. The correct use of an early walking aid produces three distinct benefits:

1 *Early training in standing balance and gait* with consequent desirable physical and pyschological effects.

2 *Control of oedema of the stump* brought about by pressure from this total-contact device and the variations in pressure achieved during walking which stimulate venous and lymphatic drainage.

3 *Assessment of the patient* as a potential user of a definitive prosthesis.

If after a period of intensive training with an early walking aid the patient cannot or will not achieve standing balance or transfer of weight from the good leg to the side of amputation, and cannot demonstrate the ability to take some steps between parallel bars, then the suitability of the patient for consideration of prosthetic restoration must be questioned. The opinion of an experienced physiotherapist in this respect is invaluable, and it may be that the patient's rehabilitation should be more realistically anticipated as being as independent as possible from a wheelchair.

Meanwhile a carefully monitored but fairly intensive programme of physiotherapy should continue. Whilst it is impossible for a physiotherapist to devote several hours each day to the treatment of one amputee, it is nonetheless possible and, indeed, desirable to draw up a daily programme of activities for the patient to follow. Occupational therapy should be introduced as early as possible into this regimen, and the amputee will thus benefit from a 'working' day which has periods of formal exercise, walking training where appropriate, and instruction in the activities of daily living.

The value of group therapy for amputees is immense. It is perfectly acceptable to include amputees of varied age, at differing stages of rehabilitation, and with assorted causes of amputation in the same group. Amputees react favourably to communication with others in the group, elderly patients are stimulated by the presence of younger people, and the young often display great kindness and encouragement towards the older amputee. Efforts should be made to involve the family of the amputee in the rehabilitation process, and, as previously stated, patients and relatives should be kept informed of progress and eventual goals. Here again the role of the physiotherapist as central to the rehabilitation process is emphasized.

Approximately three weeks after surgery, the patient will normally be ready to attend the limb fitting clinic for initial assessment by the surgeon, prosthetist, and other members of the prosthetic team.

Gait training

If the patient has made regular use of an early walking aid, he will adapt very quickly to prosthetic use. It is very important that the therapist examines the stump frequently during the early days of prosthetic wear. Steps must be taken to avoid any damage to the stump, and the patient must immediately inform the staff of any pain or discomfort.

Training should begin between parallel bars with progression to two walking sticks, then a single stick in the opposite hand, and eventually no stick where possible. Good standing balance and the ability to transfer body weight from foot to foot must be achieved prior to walking.

The patient should be instructed and well practised in the following:
1 Donning and doffing of the prosthesis.
2 Walking on slopes, uneven ground and soft surfaces, such as grass.
3 Climbing stairs.
4 Rising from the ground (e.g. after a fall).
5 Self-examination of the stump.

Where possible, the patient should remain in hospital or rehabilitation unit until he has become confident and reasonably independent in the use of his prosthesis. A prolonged period of intermittent, often irregular, and usually unsatisfactory out-patient treatment can therefore be avoided.

Final stage of rehabilitation

It is essential that the occupational therapist and the social worker are involved at an early stage to isolate and plan the long-term needs of the patient. Alterations to the house may be required, and many aids may be necessary, especially when the patient is elderly. Long-term care of the patient in some cases has to be considered.

Advice on work, transport, and many other social considerations should be available. In the case of the younger amputee, advice and encouragement on sport and recreational activities should be given. It should be made quite clear that the loss of a limb does not necessarily mean the end of all sporting and leisure pursuits. Every effort should be made to find at least one activity which the young amputee will enjoy and in which he can realistically participate. A list of organizations in the United Kingdom which can provide information on sporting facilities for the disabled, and for the amputee in particular, is given at the end of this chapter.

In conclusion, rehabilitation of the lower limb amputee provides a challenge for the physiotherapist which is both stimulating and immensely rewarding. The skills required of the therapist are much greater than those of simply planning a programme of exercise. It is particularly satisfying to be involved in a patient's rehabilitation from the pre-operative stage until the ultimate level of independence has been reached, and the opportunities to work with the patient's relatives and family, professional colleagues, and of course the amputee himself, provide a uniquely varied and enjoyable role for a caring physiotherapist.

Addresses for information on sport and leisure pursuits within the United Kingdom

British Disabled Waterski Association
18 Greville Park
Ashtead
Surrey KT21 2SN

British Ski Club for the Disabled
Corton House
Corton
Warminster
Wiltshire BA12 0SZ

The British Sports Association for the Disabled
Barnard Crescent
Aylesbury
Buckinghamshire HP21 8PP

British Amputee Sports Association
Barnard Crescent
Aylesbury
Buckinghamshire HP21 8PP

Northern Ireland Information Service for the Disabled
2 Annadale Avenue
Belfast BT7 3JH

Northern Ireland Paraplegic Association
26 Bridge Road
Helen's Bay
County Down

Scottish Council on Disability
Princes House
5 Shandwick Place
Edinburgh

Scottish Sports Association for the Disabled
14 Gordon Court
Dalcaverhouse
Dundee DD4 9DL

References

Ham R. O., Thornberry D. J., Regan J. F., Butler C. M., Lafferty K., Davis B., Roberts V. C. & Cotton L. T. (1985) Rehabilitation of the vascular amputee — one method evaluated. *Physiotherapy Practice* **1(1)**, 6–13.

Leidberg E., Hommerberg H. & Persson B. M. (1983) Tolerance of early walking with total contact among below-knee amputees — a randomised test. *Prosthetics and Orthotics International* 7, 91–95.

Redhead R. G. (1983) The early rehabilitation of lower limb amputees using a pneumatic walking aid. *Prosthetics and Orthotics International* **7**, 88–90.

SYME AMPUTATION

.

11

A Review and a Modified Surgical–Prosthetic Approach

S. SAWAMURA

James Syme, Professor of Clinical Surgery in the University of Edinburgh, first performed an amputation at the ankle joint in 1842 on a 16-year-old boy who suffered from caries of the tarsal bone. Syme found the result of this surgery very encouraging, and, as he saw it, the advantages were that the risk to life was reduced, a more comfortable stump would be provided, and the limb would be more seemly and useful for support and progressive motion. Today the first of his advantages with regard to mortality is not so important following developments in both anaesthesia and antibiotics. However, the other advantages mentioned make the Syme procedure the most useful of all levels of amputation in the lower extremity.

The technique of the classic Syme amputation is well described by Harris (1961) and by Alldredge and Thompson (1946). The most important points in the technique of the procedure in order to provide full end-bearing function of the stump are as follows. First, to ensure a broad weight-bearing surface, transection of the tibia and fibula must be made as low as possible, i.e. at the articular surface of the tibia. Second, the plane of the saw-cut must be parallel to the ground as with the patient standing. Next, by keeping the knife against bone throughout the procedure the posterior tibial artery is preserved and the blood supply to the heel-pad maintained. Moreover, the subperiosteal separation of the heel-flap from the calcaneus ensures that the anatomy of the heel-pad is preserved intact and permits proper attachment to the lower end of the tibia and fibula. Proper fixation of the heel-pad is essential to ensure firm healing and proper permanent location of the pad in relation to the bone ends. This may be achieved either by adhesive tapes, as recommended by Harris (1956), or by a rigid plaster of Paris cast. Finally, if the surgeon adheres to these principles the result is a bulbous stump which in turn provides self-suspension of the prosthesis.

The Syme amputation has been used extensively by both Scottish and Canadian surgeons. Their confidence was reinforced by the reports of Alldredge and Thompson (1946), Mazet (1968), and most particularly Harris (1961) in his magnificent and comprehensive review of Syme's amputation surgery. Over the years, since its inception in the mid-nineteenth century, a number of attempts were made to modify the procedure, mainly to avoid the bulbous end of the stump and its inevitable poor cosmetic appearance. Baudens (1842), Guyon (1868), and Elmslie (1924) amongst others contributed to this approach. In more recent time Warren *et al.* (1955) also suggested more proximal transection of the tibia. All of these efforts, with the exception of Warren's experience of six carefully selected peripheral vascular cases, failed in that the stumps did not survive. Indeed, Langdale-Kelman and Perkins (1942) condemned the Syme amputation outright on the basis of their experience. However, it is likely that their patients had been subjected to Elmslie's modification of Syme's amputation with its greatly diminished load-bearing surface area. The more recent modifications introduced by Sarmiento *et al.* (1966) and Mazet (1968) still maintain the transection of the tibia at ankle level but reduce the mediolateral diameter of the stump by trimming away the malleolar flares of the distal tibia and fibula. Further modification, developed originally by Hulnick *et al.* (1949), introduced the notion of a two-stage procedure, the objective being to clear first the infected and diseased tissues, as in war injuries or in diabetes, as described by Wagner (1977). Some six weeks later, wound healing having been achieved, the malleoli are trimmed by vertical osteotomy to reduce the mediolateral diameter of the stump through two small incisions. The opportunity is taken to remove the malleolar protrusions at the same time.

At the Hyogo Rehabilitation Centre (HRC) both surgical technique and prosthetic fitting have been modified to gain better acceptance by the patients.

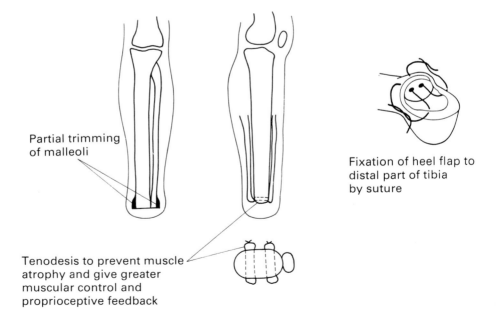

Partial trimming of malleoli

Fixation of heel flap to distal part of tibia by suture

Tenodesis to prevent muscle atrophy and give greater muscular control and proprioceptive feedback

Fig. 11.1 Modified surgical technique.

Surgical technique

The surgical procedure is performed according to the classic Syme technique, emphasizing the weight-bearing quality of the heel-pad. The modifications involve the following:

(a) Removal of a thin sliver of malleoli of both tibia and fibula to reduce the bulkiness of the bulbous end while still maintaining dimensions which ensure self-suspension. This procedure slightly reduces the capability of end-bearing of the stump. However, as pointed out by Murdoch (1976), if the prosthesis incorporates some of the principles of the patellar tendon-bearing prosthesis (PTB) the stump end is not required to sustain full end-bearing.

(b) The severed tendons are secured under physiological tension through two drill-holes located at the distal end of the tibia. This tenodesis procedure has several advantages. First, it prevents muscle atrophy. Next, it provides for better circulation, as confirmed by experimental studies conducted in Hyogo in 1971. It also provides for better proprioception, and self-suspension is augmented by the isometric contraction of the leg muscles. The heel-flap is fixed firmly to the anterolateral part of the distal end of the tibia through a drill-hole, thus preventing medial displacement of the heel-flap (Fig. 11.1).

Post-operative management

(a) A rigid plaster cast is used routinely except for infected cases. A thick sterile stockinette 'sock' is rolled over the stump under slight tension to encompass the lower leg. Two or three rolls of elastic plaster of Paris bandage are then wrapped and moulded to ensure a total-contact fitting. The moulding ensures self-suspension of the plaster cast, which is thin and light. It has proved to be comfortable for the patient and appears to enhance adherence of the heel-flap to the severed surface of the tibia and be effective in controlling oedema and preventing haematoma formation.

(b) With the exception of amputations for vascular disease, an immediate post-operative fitting regime is established. However, it is important to prevent excessive weight-bearing on the end of the stump. When this regime is followed the plaster cast is strengthened by ordinary plaster of Paris bandages and the proximal portion of the cast is moulded in a manner similar to that of the PTB prosthesis. The prosthetic foot designed at HRC is attached to the plaster cast.

(c) In those cases which are overtly infected, controlled-environment treatment (Redhead & Snowdon 1978) is the first choice.

A double-walled windowless Syme prosthesis

The original Canadian Syme prosthesis (McLaurin 1970) envisaged access for the bulbous end of the stump by means of windows either medially or posteriorly.

These prostheses, of course, pose some problems in fabrication and tend to be ugly and somewhat heavy. In an attempt to overcome these problems Mazet (1968) described a double-walled windowless prosthesis, the so-called 'balloon prosthesis'. At HRC a prosthesis has been developed constructed on the same principles (Fig. 11.2). The characteristics of this prosthesis first introduced at the Third Pan Pacific Rehabilitation Conference in Hong Kong in 1965 are:

(a) The characteristics of the PTB prosthesis are embodied in the socket design, but the posterior wall of the socket is lowered to permit the customary Japanese style of sitting. The positive plaster model has to be modified in order that there is increased force transference over the tibial condylar flare.

(b) The flexible soft inner lining is composed of sponge rubber and covered with leather.

(c) The SACH foot as used in Japan has a split between the big and second toes so that the Japanese sandal can be worn.

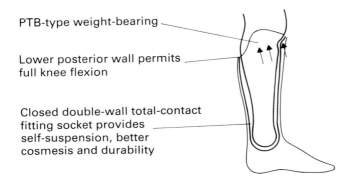

PTB-type weight-bearing

Lower posterior wall permits full knee flexion

Closed double-wall total-contact fitting socket provides self-suspension, better cosmesis and durability

Fig. 11.2 Closed double-wall socket developed at HRC.

Case material

Since 1962, 44 operations have been performed using the modified Syme amputation; of these the tenodesis procedure was performed in 15 cases (HRC group). An additional 21 cases of Syme amputation performed at another hospital are also included, making a total of 65 cases (Table 11.1). The follow-up period was from one to 22 years, with an average of ten years.

(a) Out of the total of 65 cases, five died, and revision to below-knee level was required in six cases. In four of these cases requiring revision the pathology was peripheral vascular disease, in one case trochopathia pedes myelodysplastica, and the other was hereditary sensory neuropathy.

(b) It has been recognized that peripheral vascular disease is normally seen as a contraindication to Syme's amputation. Even so, in the HRC group of 44 patients Syme amputation was carried out on four carefully selected vascular cases. All healed well at first, but subsequent breakdown occurred between two and five years later.

(c) Except for six cases, the end-bearing capability of the Syme amputation in the

Table 11.1 Causes of Syme's amputation.

	HRC	HCC	Total
Trauma and infection			
Traffic	7	7	14
Industrial	12	5	17
Miscellaneous	5		5
Malignant tumour	4	1	5
Peripheral vascular disease			
Thromboangiitis obliterans	2	3	5
Arteriosclerosis obliterans	2	3	5
Diabetes mellitus		2	2
Congenital deformity			
Defect of tibia	4		4
Defect of fibula	2		2
Miscellaneous	2		2
Trochopathia pedis			
myelodysplastica	2		2
Other	2		2
	44	21	65

HRC: Hyogo Rehabilitation Center.
HCC: Hyogo Consultation Center for Physically Disabled.

HRC group of patients was well demonstrated. In two cases there was medial migration of the heel-pad due to surgical error, and in the other four cases knee instability was present due to congenital defects of the tibia. In the second group of 21 cases, eight cases had no end-bearing capability, mostly due to impairment of the weight-bearing structure of the heel-pad, displacement of the pad, or vascular insufficiency.

(d) The double-walled windowless plastic prosthesis was well accepted by the patients. In no instance was it necessary to abandon the use of this prosthesis. In one-third of the cases, however, there were major problems in relation to excessive perspiration; this was presumably due to excessive heat building up inside the socket and the high humidity experienced in the Japanese summer. A new valve has been developed for the lower end of the socket to provide better moisture distribution.

Summary

To achieve better results from Syme amputation, modified approaches to both surgical techniques and prosthetic fitting were adopted. The technical modifications adopted ensure that the desirable end-bearing characteristics of the Syme stump are preserved. The major principles of the classic Syme amputation were maintained. The double-walled windowless prosthesis developed has been accepted well by the patients with clear advantages in cosmesis, durability, and ease of donning. Problems of excessive perspiration remain to be solved and may involve attachment of a new valve and selection of more suitable materials for the inner socket.

References

Alldredge R. H. & Thompson T. C. (1946) The technique of the Syme amputation. *The Journal of Bone and Joint Surgery* **28**, 415–426.

Baudens J. B. L. (1842) Nouvelle methode des amputations. *Premiere Memoire, Amputation Tibio-tarsienne*. Germer Baillière, Libraire, Editeur, Paris.

Elmslie R. C. (1924) Section on amputations. In *Carson's Modern Operative Surgery,* 1st Edition, Vol. 1, p. 132. London: Cassel & Co.

Guyon F. (1868) Gazette des hopitaux, p. 514, quoted from Farabeuf, *Precis de manuel operatoire* (ligatures, amputations), 1881, p. 543. G. Masson, Editeur, Paris.

Harris R. I. (1956) Syme's amputation. The technical details essential for success. *The Journal of Bone and Joint Surgery* **38B**, 614–632.

Harris R. I. (1961) The history and development of Syme's amputation. *Artificial Limbs* **6**, 4–43.

Hulnick A., Highsmith C. & Boutin F. J. (1949) Amputations for failure in reconstructive surgery. *The Journal of Bone and Joint Surgery* **31A**, 639–649.

Langdale-Kelman R. D. & Perkins G. (1942) *Amputations and Artificial Limbs*. London: Oxford University Press.

Le Blanc M. A. (1971) Elastic-liner type of Syme prosthesis: basic procedure and variations.

McLaurin C. A. (1970) The Syme type prosthesis. In *Prosthetic and Orthotic Practice* (ed. Murdoch G.), pp. 125–137. London: Edward Arnold.

Marx H. W. (1969) An innovation in Syme's prosthetics. *Orthotics and Prosthetics* **23**, 3, 131–138.

Mazet R. (1968) Syme's amputation, a follow-up study of fifty-one adults and thirty-two children. *The Journal of Bone and Joint Surgery* **50A**, 1549–1563.

Murdoch G. (1976) Syme's amputation. *Journal of the Royal College of Surgeons of Edinburgh* **21(1)**, 15–30.

Redhead R. G. & Snowdon C. (1978) A new approach to the management of wounds of the extremities. Controlled environment treatment and its derivatives. *Prosthetics and Orthotics International* **2**, 148–156.

Sarmiento A., Gilmer R. E. Jr & Finnieston A. (1966) A new surgical–prosthetic approach to the Syme's amputation; a preliminary report. *Artifical Limbs* **10(1)**, 52–55.

Sawamura S. (1967) Syme's amputation and prosthesis. *Sogo Reha* **1.11**, 1065–1079.

Wagner F. W. (1977) Amputation of the foot and ankle: current status. *Clinical Orthopaedics* **122**, 62–69.

Warren R., Thayer T. R., Achenbach H. & Kendall L. G. (1955) The Syme amputation in periperhal vascular disease. *Surgery* **37**, 156–164.

12

The Syme Prosthesis

C.H. PRITHAM

Introduction

The Syme amputation is the most distal level commonly recommended by various authorities and is spoken of by most as being the preferred level of amputation. This preference is explained by the combination of the minimal disparity in length and good distal weight-bearing capability that result. The obverse side of the coin is that its principal disadvantages also stem from these same two features (Table 12.1). The prosthetist's task is to capitalize upon the virtues of the Syme amputation, to compensate for whatever defects may present themselves, and to provide the patient with the most functional substitute for his loss. To do so requires a familiarity with the forces created during gait, structural considerations, the available feet, and alignment principles involved.

Biomechancial requirements

Radcliffe (1961) analysed the functional criteria necessary and concluded that the prosthesis must provide for three basic sort of forces.

1 Weight-bearing, whether distal, proximal or a combination of the two. Ideally all of the weight-bearing forces would be borne distally, but not all patients can cope with the distal load and in this instance some portion of the load must be borne as in a patellar tendon-bearing (PTB) prosthesis.

Table 12.1 Advantages and disadvantages of the Syme prosthesis.

Advantages	Disadvantages
Able to walk without a prosthesis	Limited room distally hinders foot selection and complicates alignment procedure.
Self-suspending	Poor cosmesis, not recommended for women
Minimal disturbance of growth potential in children	Poor structural integrity
Superior prosthetic control	Surgical results often less than optimal

(a)

(b)

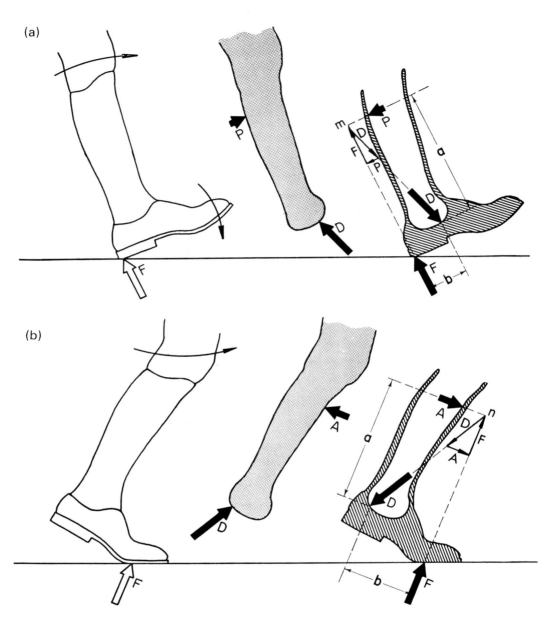

Fig. 12.1 Forces acting on the prosthesis in the sagittal plane at heel-strike (a) and toe-off (b) according to Radcliffe. (From *Artificial Limbs*, Vol. 6, No. 1, April, 1961, p. 81.)

2 One set of forces (Fig. 12.1) is created in the sagittal plane by heel-strike and another by push-off. During gait, as the centre of gravity passes forward, one set of forces gradually diminishes and the other increases. McLaurin (1970) in a similar analysis refers to the necessity for a snug fit in the sagittal plane to prevent a 'momentary loss of control at mid-stance'. Radcliffe was particularly concerned about proper contouring of the socket distally to provide for the shift of the forces in that region from anterior to posterior.

3 To stabilize the prosthesis against the torque forces in the transverse plane it is necessary to create a triangular cross-section proximally about the tibia and fibula. (Interestingly enough, McLaurin considered this a particularly vexing problem while Radcliffe was notably sanguine.)

What is of particular interest in the case of the Syme prosthesis is the high degree of compatibility among these various requirements. A PTB configuration is dictated proximally not just for weight-bearing, but also to sustain the loads created in the sagittal plane so as to avoid loading on the sensitive tibial crest and to provide rotary stabilization. The object of achieving an intimate fit is compromised by the necessity for permitting passage of the distal end. This same factor leads to socket designs that in turn compromise either structural integrity or cosmesis.

Development of the Syme prosthesis

The predominant form of construction in North America prior to World War II (Wilson 1961) featured a steel armature, moulded leather socket, and anterior lace opening. This form of construction permitted ready donning and a considerable range of adjustment in weight distribution. More than one prosthetist can ruefully testify to a patient's preference for such a prosthesis. Wilson pointed out that a comfortable fit is not always possible, and the location of the uprights medially and laterally made the prosthesis bulky and subjected them to highly repetitious cycles of compression and tension and thus failure. Both Wilson and McLaurin pointed out that uprights located anteriorly and posteriorly would be more advantageously placed to resist the imposed stresses.

Dissatisfaction with the leather and steel Syme prosthesis led to the development of the Canadian Syme prosthesis in the early post-war period. The use of a posterior opening permits ready access and control of the pressures around the tibia anteriorly. Apparently it also markedly limits the amount of proximal weight-bearing possible, because Wilson cites this as well as structural factors as motivation for the Veterans Administration (VA) version of the Syme prosthesis. The VA Syme prosthesis dates from the same period and features a medial window that does not extend proximally to the brim. This factor allows for unrestricted proximal weight-bearing. Unfortunately it does not totally resolve the question of structural integrity, although it does alter the pattern of stresses in the prosthesis.

Radcliffe (1961) analysed the situation in terms of the maximum loads imposed (those of push-off). He concluded that the free edges of the posterior opening were under tension and that similarly the edges of a medial opening were under compression. He pointed out further that, while it is possible to resist the tensile loads with materials of sufficient tensile strength, to resist the compressive loads and localized buckling it is necessary to increase the cross-sectional area of the lamination. Of course, increased proximal weight-bearing exacerbates the situation.

McLaurin, by way of contrast, concluded that the posterior edge of a medial opening was in tension instead of compression. The variation between the two analyses can presumably be explained by the fact that, while McLaurin analysed the situation solely in terms of the sagittal plane, Radcliffe also considered the frontal plane. He describes the centre of pressure as being eccentrically located not only anteriorly, but also medially, and thus imposing a lateral bow on the structure.

Socket variations

The alternative to a socket with an opening in it is a closed-wall socket. Not only is it structurally intact but the increase in diameter to allow for passage of the distal end locates the load-bearing fibres further away from the neutral axis. Apparently the first description of such a prosthesis was by Sarmiento *et al.* (1966). It consisted of a double-wall socket in which the distal inner wall was laminated and made of flexible elastomer to allow for passage of the bulbous distal end. Significantly the authors also described a modified surgical procedure to reduce the distal circumference of the limb, as the inner wall is limited in its ability to expand. This fact limits the suitability of the fabrication technique for all Syme-level amputees. Marx (1969), in an article outlining fabrication of such a prosthesis, describes the

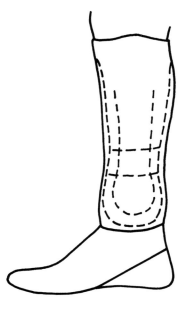

Fig. 12.2 Syme prosthesis described by Pearl and Johnson (1983). The inner wall (dotted line) is laminated with semiflexible resin and has two flaps cut in it medially and laterally to permit donning and doffing. Tension for suspension is provided by a circumferential elastic band (two parallel dotted lines). Holes are also drilled in the popliteal area to provide ventilation.

expansion as being about 1¼ – 1¾ in. Nonetheless, this variant on the Syme prosthesis has remained popular, and a variety of fabrication techniques (Eckhardt & Enneberg 1970) have been described for it, including one by Meyer *et al.* (1970), in which only the medial 'window' area is laminated with flexible elastomer.

Another variant on double-wall construction is that described by Pearl and Johnson (1983). In this approach (Fig. 12.2) the inner wall is laminated of rigid laminate, and flaps are cut medially and laterally, running from proximal to distal with the bases proximal. The flaps pivot about their bases to permit donning and doffing, and retention is provided by a circumferential elastic strap distally. Two air channels are also provided posteriorly for ventilation.

Another approach to the fabrication of a closed-wall prosthesis employs a liner built up peripherally to a cylindrical outer shape. In some instances the liner is full length (Romano *et al.* 1972) and in others it is truncated (McFarlen 1966, McLaurin 1970, Warner *et al.* 1972, Nelson 1975), bridging the concave portions of the limb only and resembling a gaiter. A number of Syme prostheses employing this design were fabricated of Surlyn by McClellan *et al.* (1984). Patients were greatly impressed with the comfort afforded by the semi-flexible walls, but durability was severely limited. This problem could doubtlessly be eliminated by the utilization of the frame construction techniques described by Kristinsson (1983). This of course brings us full circle to the leather and steel armature form of construction.

Prosthetic feet

Development of the present-day non-articulated foot, the SACH foot, was spurred on largely by the necessity of providing a satisfactory foot for the Syme prosthesis (American Academy of Orthopaedic Surgeons 1960). A number of historical precedents exist for this development (Wilson 1961), and today the SACH foot in one form or another is the foot of choice. The external keel foot suggests itself in those instances when there is ample room distally for the keel and full heel wedge. Alternatively, a special moulded SACH foot with a low-profile keel reinforced with metal and a large well in its proximal surface to accommodate the socket can be used. A variation that combines certain features of both situations is used in Memphis, Tennessee, and presumably elsewhere. The socket is sunk into a block of wood, and the foam of the moulded Syme-style SACH foot is cut flush with the top surface of the keel The two are assembled in proper configuration and the excess wood removed. The wood and socket are finished with a final lamination.

Recently a challenger to the SACH foot has appeared on the American scene. This is the stationary attachment flexible endoskeletal (SAFE) foot (Fig. 12.3) which may best be described as a SACH foot with a keel that is flexible in early stance phase and rigid in late. As with the moulded Syme SACH foot it has a well proximally to accommodate the socket. While SAFE feet offer a level of performance appreciated by amputees, they are heavy, and durability has been a problem.

The Tucker–Syme prosthesis (Cochrane & Tucker 1979) is somewhat similar. It comprises a hollow urethane foot into which a socket is mounted. The socket is laminated with an acrylic resin mixture of the ratio 60% flexible to 40% rigid. The distal portion of the socket has a length of reinforcing belting mounted to it, and is secured in the foot with flexible urethane elastomer. Two narrow openings are cut medially and laterally in the socket to permit donning and doffing. No closing windows are used. Lyttle (1984) describes the results of a small series fitted as being satisfactory, with buckling of the anterior wall or breakage of the foot occurring only after several years.

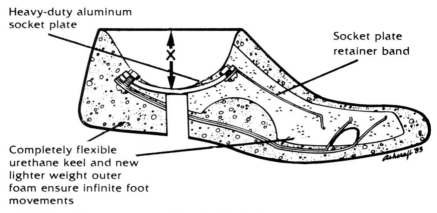

Fig. 12.3 SAFE foot. (Drawing courtesy of Campbell Childs Inc.)

The same lack of space distally that recommends the SACH foot also influences the alignment procedure. While techniques for providing some measure of flexibility during the alignment process have been described (Hampton 1960, Radcliffe 1961), it is more likely that the older technique of cut and wedge is used. Typically the amputee will be stood in the socket while proper configuration is established and recorded. Socket and foot are then assembled for dynamic alignment. In some instances temporary assembly will occur, with the socket on the standing patient as an aid in alignment. Principles of alignment have been described (Radcliffe 1961, Wilson 1961, McLaurin 1970), and it would seem that no great difficulty is found in establishing them despite the somewhat primitive means necessary. Perhaps, in this case, the length of the amputation is a positive advantage, on one hand reducing the number of variables involved, and on the other enhancing the amputee's ability to compensate.

These then are the principal factors involved in fitting the Syme prosthesis. They present the prosthetist with a unique set of challenges to be met and assets to be capitalized upon. The challenges have been met by the application of the technology that became available after World War II. Technology and materials now becoming commonplace will undoubtedly lead to further new approaches and solutions.

References

American Academy of Orthopaedic Surgeons (1960) *Orthopaedic Appliance Atlas,* Vol. 2, p. 150. Ann Arbor, Michigan: J. W. Edwards.

Cochrane I. W. & Tucker F. R. (1979). *The Tucker Syme Prosthesis Fabrication Manual,* 2nd Edition. Rehabilitation Engineering Department, Rehabilitation Centre, Health Sciences Centre, 800 Sherbrook St., Winnipeg, Manitoba, Canada R3A-1M4.

Eckhardt A. L. & Enneberg H. (1970) The use of a silastic liner in the Syme's prosthesis. *Inter Clinic Information Bulletin* **1X(6)**, 1–4

Hampton F. (1960) Recent developments in the fitting and fabrication of the Syme's prosthesis. *Orthopedics and Prosthetic Appliance Journal* **14(1)**, 45–57.

Kristinsson O. (1983) Flexible above-knee socket made from low density polyethylene, suspended by a weight transmitting frame. *Orthotics and Prosthetics* **37(2)**, 25–27.

Lyttle D. (1984) Tucker-Syme prosthetic fitting in young people. *Inter Clinic Information Bulletin* **19(3)**, 62.

McClellan B. P., Kapp S. & Stills M. (1984) The application of ionomer resins in definitive below-knee prostheses: a limited study. *Clinical Prosthetics and Orthotics* **8(3)**, 18–21.

McFarlen J. M. (1966) The Syme prosthesis. *Orthopedics and Prosthetic Appliance Journal* **20(1)**, 29–31.

McLaurin C. A. (1970) The Syme type prosthesis. In *Prosthetic and Orthotic Practice* (ed. Murdoch G.), pp. 125–137. London: Edward Arnold.

Marx H. W. (1969) An innovation in Syme's prosthetics. *Orthotics and Prosthetics* **23(3)**, 131–138.

Meyer L. C., Bailey H. L. & Friddle D. (1970) An improved prosthesis for fitting the ankle/disarticulation amputee. *Inter Clinic Information Bulletin,* **1X(6)**, 11–15.

Nelson R. A. (1975) Fabrication of a closed Syme's prosthesis. *Inter Clinic Information Bulletin,* **XIV(5)**, 11–13.

Pearl M. & Johnson R. J. (1983) An air-ventilated Syme's leg prosthesis. *Inter Clinic Information Bulletin* **18(5)**, 5–6.

Radcliffe C. W. (1961) The biomechanics of the Syme's prosthesis. *Artificial Limbs* **6(1)**, 76–85.

Romano R. L., Zettle J. H. & Burgess E. M. (1972) The Syme's amputation: a new prosthetic approach. *Inter Clinic Information Bulletin* **XI(4)**, 1–9, 17.

Sarmiento A., Gilmer R. E. & Finnieston A. (1966) A new surgical-prosthetic approach to the Syme's amputation, a preliminary report. *Artificial Limbs* **10(1)**, 52–55.

Warner R., Daniel R. & Lesswing A. L. (1972) Another new prosthetic approach for the Syme's amputation. *Inter Clinic Information Bulletin* **XII(1)**, 7–10.

Wilson A. B. (1961) Prostheses for Syme's amputation. *Artificial Limbs* **6(1)**, 52–75.

PARTIAL FOOT AMPUTATION

13

Aetiology, Principles, Operative Techniques

R.F. BAUMGARTNER

Introduction

In general, partial foot amputations have a rather poor reputation with regard to wound healing, stump performance, and prosthetic fitting. Wound healing may be delayed (or disturbed) by necrosis, gangrene, or infection, thereby necessitating reamputation at a higher level, and foot stumps may be painful and exhibit contractures that lead to varus and equinus deformities, particularly at rear-foot levels. Because of this, many surgeons still prefer a primary amputation at a below- or even an above-knee level in order to get rid of the problem, being convinced that modern prosthetics are so sophisticated as to give better satisfaction to the patient than a non-functional foot stump. Clearly they are not aware that such a decision offers the patient nothing more than a rather primitive replacement of the lower leg, ankle, and foot.

In contrast, a good foot stump always permits full end-bearing and therefore is much more physiological. A patient with a foot stump is able to walk short distances without the need of a prosthesis, e.g. from his bed to the toilet at night. Moreover, patients with toe or metatarsal amputations are often better off without any prosthesis at all, and the need for physical therapy is reduced to a minimum or none. Such foot amputees are able to walk for hours and even perform strenuous sports such as skiing and mountaineering (Wagner 1981). Moreover, the physiological proprioceptive properties of the sole are preserved. But even if sensory functions are disturbed, as in diabetes, spina bifida, or Hansen disease, a foot stump is still important in facilitating rehabilitation. In vascular patients, preservation of part of the foot is particularly important, since sooner or later the opposite leg might require an amputation too, perhaps at a higher level (Baumgartner *et al.* 1976).

The objection against poor cosmesis, particularly of rear-foot stumps, is no longer valid with proper level selection, surgery, and prosthetic technique. The physiological aspect of the loss of one or even both feet must also be considered.

Aetiology

In major limb amputations, peripheral vascular diseases are by far the main cause of amputation. In foot amputations, trauma is still of about equal importance. Comprehensive statistics on foot amputations are still not available as they are normally included with other leg or below-knee procedures.

Trauma

The foot, and particularly its distal parts, has a higher risk of trauma leading to amputation than the more proximal parts of the lower limb. The possibilities for reconstructive vascular and replantation surgery of the foot are much more limited than in the hand or leg. Primary amputations are most often caused by motorcycle, automobile, and railroad accidents, but also by lawn mowers and agricultural machines. Foot amputations are also common in war injuries.

Quite frequently a *secondary* amputation has to be performed days or months after the injury. Often one or several attempts to preserve the damaged limb have failed. Burns caused by boiling water, molten cast iron, or electricity might lead to secondary amputations as much as prolonged *exposure to cold* as encountered by mountain climbers or soldiers, for instance during the Falklands campaign. Another reason for exposure to cold which may lead to foot amputation is the abuse of alcohol or drugs.

Partial foot amputation, however, may result from a lesion of the femoral or popliteal artery when accurate diagnosis and repair have failed. Inadequate diagnosis and treatment of infected minor forefoot injuries, particularly in the area of the sole, bites by insects and snails, iatrogenic arterial obliterations after arteriography, or injection of a sclerotic agent into the artery, are rather unusual but are known to be dramatic causes of foot amputations.

Finally, microsurgical techniques permit toe transplantation to replace one or several fingers of the hand (Zhong-Wei *et al.* 1981). As the functional and cosmetic results are not as fascinating as the operative technique, this procedure has become less popular than it used to be some years ago.

Peripheral vascular diseases

Peripheral vascular diseases usually lead to gangrene and necrosis of the toes and the forefoot and to pressure sores at places with high risk, such as the calcaneum, the malleoli at the ankle, and the base of the fifth metatarsal. In diabetes and other diseases it is not only a matter of small vessel vascular disease but also sensory disturbances, and therefore, in the case of both ulcer and gangrene, infection often supervenes.

Congenital deformities

Polydactylia, bony overgrowth, and congenital lymphoedema might require a reduction of the foot to normal size by means of selective amputation. Congenital deficiencies, however, should not be regarded as amputations. Even in severe cases, the functional qualities of these stumps are superior by far to other amputations at comparable levels.

Malignancies

Malignant foot tumours are rare, but they usually lead to partial or total foot amputation.

Operative technique

As in any amputation level, one must try to preserve a maximum of tissue and still obtain a functional stump free of pain. In the foot, this task is particularly difficult due to the rather poor quality of the arterial vascular system. Gentle tissue handling is particularly important. As long as necrotic tissues are not removed, there is always an increased risk of infection of the deep tissues, abscess formation, and phlegmona. It is therefore preferable to remove necrotic tissues early. Skin incisions are, if possible, performed on the dorsum of the foot and in a longitudinal direction.

Bradytrophic tissues such as tendons, ligaments, and fascias should be excised as completely as possible. If bone is to be sectioned, it is better done through cancellous bone, as cortical bone stumps may lead to infection or may become sharp as a pencil due to tissue resorption. The bone stumps are carefully rounded, particularly on the plantar side and slightly at the dorsal edge. The length of the bone must also be carefully adapted to the adjacent bones. The bone ends should be covered entirely with the plantar soft tissues. No soft tissue tension can be tolerated. If there is insufficient soft tissue coverage, it is necessary to shorten the bone or look for secondary wound healing. Split-skin grafts should be used with great care. For major soft tissue defects, total neurovascular skin-flaps by means of microsurgical techniques are recommended. In toe and forefoot amputations, open wound treatment and avoidance of deep sutures is the method of choice. Vessels should be carefully coagulated or, if necessary, ligated with resorbable suture material. Nerve ends must be identified and shortened by a clean cut.

Amputation levels

The following levels of amputation will be considered (Fig. 13.1):
1 Distal phalanx.
2 Disarticulation PIP (hallux only).
3 Disarticulation toes.
4 Distal metatarsals.
5 Proximal metatarsals.
6 Lisfranc (1815).
7 Chopart (Fourcroy 1792).

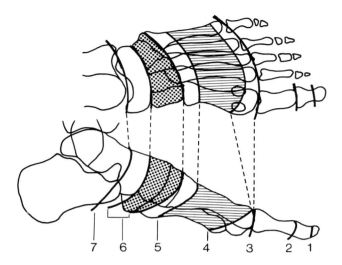

Fig. 13.1 Levels of amputation at the fore- and mid-foot.

7 6 5 4 3 2 1

At mid- and forefoot levels, the opportunity to perform an asymmetrical amputation preserving one or several metatarsal rays must be taken into consideration.

Toes

Except for the hallux, where amputations are feasible, complete disarticulation is preferred to partial toe amputation. Toe stumps often develop contractures in dorsiflexion, are non-functional, and lead to further problems. In the first ray, the disarticulation of the hallux should be completed by shaping the metatarsal head and removing the sesamoid bones.

Transmetatarsal amputations

The metatarsal bones should only be amputated through cancellous bone at the heads or at their bases, but never through the cortical diaphysis. Partial amputations give excellent stumps as long as the first metatarsal or at least two minor rays are preserved. If, for instance, in a plantar ulcer, only the metatarsal bone has to be removed, it is often possible to preserve its toe. A longitudinal incision on the dorsum of the foot exposes the bone and permits selective amputation at the base by means of an oscillating saw. The plantar ulcer is cleansed and used for drainage of the space created. In vascular disease, the chances of wound healing are better if no suture is used at all.

Lisfranc articulation

A pure disarticulation at the Lisfranc joint does not result in a good stump because of the recessed second cuneiform. However, careful alignment of every ray still gives excellent results. Care must be taken to preserve the plantar arteries which are very close to the second and third cuneiform.

Chopart articulation

As in the Lisfranc articulation, the disarticulation at this site is completed by removing the plantar and distal part of the calcaneus in order to obtain a well-rounded stump. The risk of secondary contracture leading to equinus and varus deformities is prevented by means of temporary external fixation between the calcaneus and the tibia. Neither a plaster cast nor physical therapy is effective in preventing this deformity. External fixation is particularly helpful in the case of extended soft tissue lesions and if wound healing is disturbed. In vascular patients, one should hesitate to amputate at the Chopart level and perform a Syme or even a below-knee amputation instead.

In general, Chopart amputation is preferred to Syme amputation (Harris 1966), as the physiological weight-bearing surface of the rear foot, and particularly the ankle joint, is preserved. There is no shortening of the leg. If the plantar and distal surfaces of the stump are carefully rounded, a slight equinus deformity does not diminish the quality of a Chopart stump. However, if more severe equinus deformities are faced, and particularly in the varus position, the following surgical procedures as an alternative to amputation at the Syme level should be considered.

Lateral transfer of the anterior tibial tendon

This procedure, well known in the treatment of congenital club foot, is limited to minor contractures and requires free mobility of the subtalar joint.

Lengthening of the Achilles tendon

This procedure might correct an equinus deformity by 10–20°.

Subtalar fusion with wedge osteotomy

In the case of contracture of the subtalar joint, arthrodesis combined with a wedge osteotomy to correct both varus and equinus deformities is recommended. This procedure also permits displacing the calcaneus in a ventral direction by 1 cm in order to improve the alignment between the tibia and the weight-bearing surface of the calcaneus.

Calcaneotibial arthrodesis

In case of very severe rear-foot contractures and/or extensive lack of soft tissues, the talus is removed and a fusion performed between the calcaneus and the tibia, as suggested by many authors, such as Pirogoff (1854) and Boyd (1949). Care must be taken to position the calcaneus properly in a physiological position with slight external rotation and displacement by 1 cm in a ventral direction. To facilitate prosthetic fitting it is most important to remove completely both malleoli. The tibial nerve again has to be shortened by 3 cm above the surface of the arthrodesis. In order to minimize tissue damage, external fixation by means of the Charnley compression frame for 4–6 weeks is preferred (Fig. 13.2).

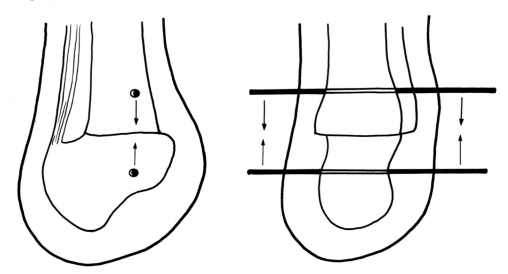

Fig. 13.2 Calcaneotibial arthrodesis with resection of both malleoli to facilitate prosthetic fitting. External fixation by means of the Charnley compression frame.

Talotibial arthrodesis

If there is rigidity of the subtalar joint, an equinus and varus deformity can also be corrected and stabilized by means of a wedge osteotomy and fusion of the ankle joint, again with complete resection of the malleoli in order to facilitate prosthetic fitting (Fig. 13.3).

Calcanectomy

Partial or total resection of the calcaneus and even of the talus might be useful salvage procedures for the foot. Even if the insertion of the Achilles tendon has to be sacrificed, the remaining foot is more functional than any prosthetic device. An ankle–foot orthosis is necessary in order to stabilize the rear foot. In cases of severe instability of the forefoot, a fusion between the anterior part of the tibia and the scaphoid and cuboid bones might be considered. Again, external fixation is a great help in post-operative treatment. The important shortening of the lower leg by 4–5 cm is a minor disadvantage compared to a total foot or even a below-knee amputation.

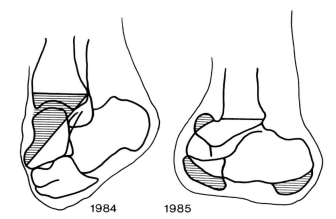

Fig. 13.3 Talotibial arthrodesis with wedge osteotomy to correct varus and equinus deformities. As the entire stump was covered by skin grafts, bony prominences were removed in a second operation.

1984   1985

Post-operative treatment

Results in foot amputation largely depend on the quality of post-operative management. Wound drainage and, in the case of the forefoot and the toes, open wound treatment are most important. Pressure sores by improper positioning or bandaging must be avoided. By placing the foot several times daily in a vertical position, and by early walking training, the danger of haematoma and stump infection is reduced. Semi-rigid orthoses made from plastic foam facilitate early ambulation, relieve excessive pressure from the stump, and protect the foot against further trauma. As in every amputation, the stump takes its final shape only after several months. Prosthetic devices and footwear therefore have to be adapted continuously during this period.

Conclusions

In using the principles of hand and reconstructive surgery, it is possible to obtain excellent foot stumps which, in combination with modern prosthetics, give much better results in function and cosmesis than any higher level amputation, including Syme amputation.

References

Baumgartner R., Brunner U. & Vaucher J. (1976) Beinamputationen nach Zwischenfallen bei Varizenbehandlung, *Phlebologie und Proktologie* **5(2)**, 136–141.

Boyd H. B. (1949) Disarticulation of the hip. In *Campbell's Operative Orthopaedics* (eds Speed J. S. & Smith H.), pp. 824–8. St. Louis: The C.V. Mosby Co.

Fourcroy A. F. (1792) La medicine éclairée par les science physiques. Vol. 4, 85–88. Chez Buisson. Contains first description of Chopart's method of partial amputation of the foot.

Harris R. I. (1966) History and development of Syme's amputation. In *Selected Articles from Artificial Limbs, January, 1954–Spring, 1966,* pp. 233–72. New York: Robert E. Kreiger Publishing Co. Inc.

Lisfranc J. (1815) Nouvelle méthode opératoire pour l'amputation partielle du pied dans son articulation tarso-metatarsienne; méthode précédes des nombreuse modifications qu'a subies celle de Chopart. Paris: Gabon.

Pirogoff N. I. (1854) Osteoplastic elongation of the bones of the leg in amputation of the foot. *Voyerno-med. Journal* **63,2 sect**. 83–100. (Pirogoff's method of complete osteoplastic amputation of the foot. German translation. Liepzig, 1854.)

Wagner F. W. (1981) The dysvascular foot; a system for diagnosis and treatment. *Foot and Ankle* **2**, 64–122.

Zhong-Wei C., Meyer V. E. & Beasley R. W. (1981) The versatile second toe microvascular transfer. *The Orthopaedic Clinics of North America, (Management of Upper Limb Amputations)* **12**, 827–34.

14

Biomechanics and Prosthetic/Orthotic Solutions

D.N. CONDIE & M.L. STILLS

Introduction

The predominance of vascular disease as the cause of lower limb amputation in the developed countries of the world has resulted in a very limited incidence of partial foot amputation with a corresponding lack of interest and development in the techniques of prosthetic management for this type of patient. It is important, however, to recognize that in the developing countries, where the causes of amputation are totally different, partial foot amputations are widely practised. It is appropriate, therefore, to examine the biomechanical factors relating to this group of amputation procedures and to consider whether the currently available technology has been applied successfully to the development of the optimal treatment for these patients.

Biomechanics

The structure and function of the foot has been described in detail by many authors; however, it is necessary to isolate the essential features which contribute to effective locomotion.

The *arch structure of the foot* with its associated maintenance mechanisms is vital, firstly during mid-stance when the ground reaction forces are shared between the naturally adapted tissues on the heel and metatarsal heads as the body pivots over the ankle joint, and, secondly, from heel-off when the foot acts as a lever maintaining the elevation of the body during the push-off phase.

The most important role of the *foot joints* is undoubtedly the supination and pronation movements of the subtalar joint, which are associated with absorption of the longitudinal rotations of the leg which occur when walking and the compensatory twisting of the forefoot which maintains even contact across the foot throughout the stance phase.

When considering the design of a prosthetic replacement it is necessary to assess, for each level of amputation, the extent to which each of these vital functions will be disrupted. The challenge facing the prosthetist is to design prostheses which can compensate for the loss of the foot and its functions, and which can be interfaced effectively with the stump without restricting the functions of the ankle joint.

Amputation of toes

Amputation of the toes will have little or no influence on foot function, apart from the loss of the final push-off associated with extension of the great toe. Prosthetic replacement is essentially cosmetic and is simply achieved by supplying a shoe filler.

Transmetatarsal amputation

Transmetatarsal amputation involves the removal of the anterior pillars of the arch structure, effectively destroying the weight-bearing mechanism of the foot. Loss of joint function is minimal. The prosthetic replacement must therefore be designed to reconstitute the arch structure and function, requiring the use of a forefoot filler, a longitudinal arch support, and a plantar stiffener. The maintenance of such a prosthesis in relation to the stump is simply achieved by the use of footwear with a sufficient vamp.

Lisfranc amputation (tarsometatarsal)

The damage to the weight-bearing structure of the foot is more extensive following this amputation; however, the requirements for its prosthetic replacement are essentially the same as following transmetatarsal amputation. In contrast, it is no longer reasonable to depend upon the patient's shoe to maintain the relationship of the prosthesis to the stump, and alternative techniques must be employed.

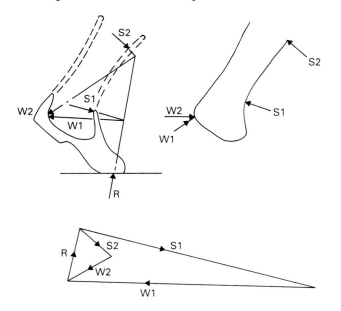

Fig. 14.1 Biomechanical analysis of the interface forces on the socket of a Lisfranc prosthesis.

A hypothetical analysis of the interface forces on the socket of a Lisfranc prosthesis serves to highlight the dilemma facing the prosthetic designer (Fig. 14.1). During push-off the dorsiflexion moment generated by the ground reaction force will tend to cause the prosthesis to rotate in an anticlockwise direction, which will result in a marked gait deviation. Two methods of overcoming this situation are analysed, the first of which depends on the generation of an effective counterforce on the very limited dorsal aspect of the stump using a short socket, and the second of which requires that the socket is extended proximally to create the required counterforce on the anterior aspect of the leg. Clearly, the latter approach is technically much more easily achieved and will result in lower contact pressures, however the cost of this solution must be recognized as the total elimination of motion at the proximal joints.

Chopart amputation

These factors become even more severe when considering the interface conditions following Chopart amputation. In this case it is virtually inconceivable that an adequate counterforce could be generated without recourse to an extended socket. An alternative biomechanical solution, however, has been proposed, which achieves its stabilizing effect by virtue of the counterforce generated on either side of the malleolus by a close-fitting socket (Fig. 14.2). An analysis of the forces which would be generated in this situation, however, demonstrates that this solution is not practical in view of the very small surfaces on the stump available to transmit the high resulting forces.

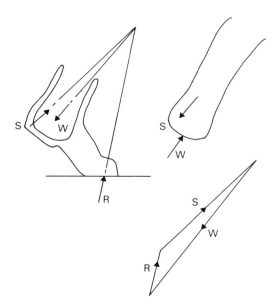

Fig. 14.2 Biomechanical analysis of the interface forces on the socket of a Chopart prosthesis.

One further possibility must be recognized when analysing this problem. The tendency for rotation to occur between the prosthesis and the stump will only arise as the patient transfers his weight onto the forefoot prior to heel-off. It is quite feasible for an amputee to modify his weight-bearing pattern to avoid this weight transfer; however, this manoeuvre will require significant compensatory adjustment in the pattern of knee and hip motion if the appearance of a relatively normal gait pattern is to be achieved.

Function of the foot joints

From the previous discussion it will be clear that the critical factor in relation to the retention of normal ankle joint function will be the method adopted to obtain a satisfactory fit between the prosthesis and the stump. If the prosthesis can be confined to the foot, normal or at least adequate ankle and subtalar function can be retained, even in the more proximal partial foot amputations. Unfortunately, no mechanisms exist which will compensate for supination and pronation of the forefoot. The most serious consequence of this functional limitation will, however, be avoided if the forefoot is constructed from a relatively flexible material and is wedged laterally to ensure that contact is maintained across the forefoot during the final phase of foot contact.

Prosthetic/orthotic designs

It is generally agreed that an amputation occurring distal to the mid-metatarsal level can be managed with a shoe filler or a plantar surface device with a soft foam shoe filler attached. Amputations proximal to the mid-metatarsal level, however, generally require a device, whether it be called prosthetic or orthotic, secured to the foot, and which *may* or *may not* extend above the ankle joint.

Above the ankle

It is the belief of many that proper management of mid-transverse metatarsal amputation (or above) must include an extension above the ankle. Many of these designs take the form of an ankle–foot orthosis, which may be constructed from a thermoplastic material (polypropylene) or thermoset plastic (polyester or acrylic), or be incorporated into a conventional metal and leather type of system. Those devices fabricated from thermoplastic and thermoset materials are generally formed over a positive model of the amputated extremity. The portion of the device in contact with the foot is designed to achieve total contact and is generally lined with a soft interface material to increase comfort. The normal profile of the foot may be restored during the initial fabrication process or achieved later by a build-up of foam. This foot build-up may act to extend the foot lever arm, but in some instances may only act as a shoe filler. In the latter case the shoe is modified to include a full-length spring steel shank and rocker sole. It is considered that this combination of prosthesis and shoe will provide a smooth transition from foot-flat to heel-off and permit an effective push-off.

Tarsometatarsal amputations may require a solid ankle device (Fig. 14.3). These designs employ similar methods of construction with the addition of an anterior section, extending from a level equal to the height of the posterior section distally to the dorsum of the foot. This addition acts to lock the foot and lower leg into the posterior section and eliminate ankle motion. The proximal region of the anterior section may take the form of a patellar tendon-bearing socket, extend to mid-calf, or originate just above the ankle. Variations of all three exist, and the amount of ankle control will be determined by the design selected. In designs where ankle motion is to be limited, further modifications to the shoe are required to achieve a normal gait. A cushion heel applied to the shoe will permit a smooth transition from heel-strike to foot-flat. Prosthetists who routinely employ these systems report good results with successful ambulation.

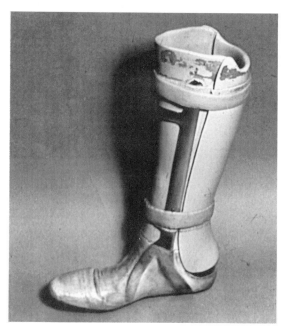

Fig. 14.3 Solid ankle prosthesis for a tarsometatarsal amputation.

Below the ankle (slipper type) (Fig. 14.4)

A number of designs exist that do not extend above the ankle. They appear to be divided into the following categories:
1 Rigid.
2 Semi-rigid.
3 Semi-flexible.
4 Flexible.

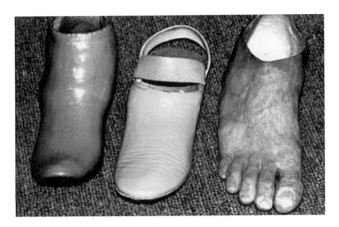

Fig. 14.4 Examples of slipper-type prostheses.

All of the above systems are fabricated on a positive model of the stump. The positive model is modified to increase loading on good tissue and to relieve or decrease pressure on sensitive areas prior to the formation of the definitive socket.

The *rigid* and *semi-rigid* systems are based on a laminated or thermoformed socket formed over the positive model. Limited flexibility can be built into the system by using flexible resins for this portion of the device. A foam lining is generally employed to act as an interface between the rigid walls of the sockets and the skin of the stump. The profile of the foot is restored with a build-up added to the socket. Complications may be encountered in using the rigid/semi-rigid designs when motion occurs inside the socket, resulting in skin breakdown on the distal plantar surface of the stump. These complications have led to the development of semi-flexible and flexible designs.

Semi-flexible designs utilize a combination of materials; however, the basis is generally a urethane elastomer. One such semi-flexible system utilizes a laminated, rigid, University of California–Berkeley shoe insert as its base. The insert is bonded to a modified monoelastic cushion-heel foot and the entire system is laminated together with a urethane elastomer*. The resulting system does not interfere with normal ankle motion and has gained good acceptance.

Another semi-flexible design uses solely urethane elastomer for fabrication of the socket and foot. This design is referred to as the slipper-type elastomer prosthesis (STEP). The STEP design is somewhat complex in its design and fabrication. Permananent tooling is developed for each individual patient and is retained by the patient for possible fabrication of a replacement device at a later date. This tooling consists of a permanent polyester resin positive model of the stump and a negative mould of the finished artificial foot. The device is fabricated using a semi-flexible urethane elastomer.† If a pressure point is noted on use it is

*Lynadure — Medical Center Prosthetics, Inc., Houston, Texas.
†Calthane 1900 — Cascade Orthopedic Supply, Chester, California.

suggested that material be removed from the exterior of the prosthesis to increase socket flexibility. Good results have been reported from this prosthesis.

Flexible foot prosthesis (Fig. 14.5)

A flexible, cosmetic prosthetic foot which utilizes reinforced silicone materials has recently been developed. A negative weight-bearing alginate impression is made of the stump and contralateral foot. An exactly detailed dental-stone positive model of the stump is made from this impression. A wax check socket is fabricated on the model and checked for comfort on the patient. Modifications are made to relieve sensitive areas and to load the appropriate areas. A mirror-image model of the sound foot is sculptured from wax and checked for sizing against the patient. A negative model of the sculptured foot is then made using the lost wax method. The resulting negative model of the foot may then be used in conjunction with the rectified model of the stump to produce the prosthesis. The material employed is a pure reinforced silicone that is precolour-matched to the patient's skin tones. At fitting, the detailed colour matching is achieved using the sound side as a model.

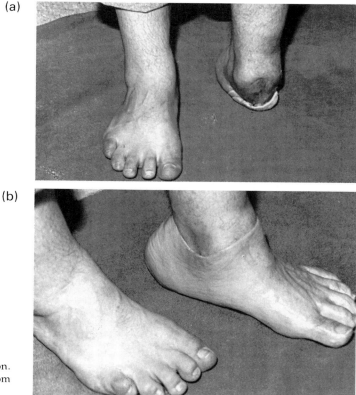

(a)

(b)

Fig. 14.5 (a) Patient with tarsometatarsal amputation. (b) Patient wearing a custom flexible foot prosthesis.

To date only approximately 50 patients have been fitted with the flexible silicone cosmetic prosthetic foot; however patient acceptance has been nearly unanimous. The developer* initially intended the prosthesis solely as a cosmetic restoration, however the resulting increase in function soon became apparent. Requests for cosmetic restoration by males are almost equal in number to those requested by females. The psychological effects of cosmetic restoration have not yet been evaluated, however it is probable that this has some influence on the functional acceptability of the prosthesis by the patient. Many of the patients fitted with the flexible silicone cosmetic prosthetic foot had previously been fitted with partial foot prostheses of the types previously described. Biomechanical comparisons of the functions of these various designs would be valuable.

Summary

A balanced foot is a necessity for the successful fitting of any prosthetic system. Trauma-related amputations apparently do well with the slipper-type prosthesis, and the developer of the silicone system reports successful fittings of diabetic patients. The need for the prosthesis to extend above the ankle appears to be limited to those patients with very short amputations, and even then successful fittings have been demonstrated with the slipper-type, using ankle straps for suspension.

In conclusion, it is believed by many that partial foot amputation can offer significant functional improvement over Syme amputation and that the use of these surgical techniques requires to be re-evaluated in the light of the new technologies and materials available today for providing these patients with functional prostheses.

Acknowledgements

The following individuals have contributed material and their considerable talent and understanding of this subject. The authors sincerely thank them for their assistance: John H. Bowker MD; Horst Buckner CDT; Ernest M. Burgess MD; Darrell R. Clark CO; Frank L. Golbranson MD; Frank Gottschalk MD; Vert Mooney MD; Alvin L. Muillenburg CPO; Charles H. Pritham CPO.

References

Childs C. & Staats T. (1983) The slipper type partial foot prosthesis. In *Advanced Below-Knee Prosthetic Seminar: Fabrication Manual.* California: UCLA Prosthetic and Orthotic Education Program.

Fillauer K. (1976) A prosthesis for foot amputation near the tarsal-metatarsal junction. *Orthotics and Prosthetics* 30:3, 9–11.

Hayhurst D. J. (1978) Prosthetic management of partial foot amputee. *Inter-Clinic Information Bulletin*

*Mr H. Buckner, Life-Like Laboratory, Dallas, Texas.

17(1), 11–15.

Lunsford T. (1980) Partial foot amputations—prosthetic and orthotic management. In *Atlas of Limb Prosthetics: Surgical and Prosthetic Principles* (American Academy of Orthopaedic Surgeons), pp. 320–5. St. Louis: C. V. Mosby.

Wilson M. T. (1979) Clinical application of RTV elastomers. *Orthotics and Prosthetics* **33(4)**, 23–29.

ABOVE-KNEE AMPUTATION

15

Surgery

G. NEFF

Introduction

If one looks at modern textbooks of surgery, the first impression is that despite all the progress of medicine during the last decade amputation surgery has become of negligible importance and can be restricted to a few pages among many hundreds. The second impression concerns the common opinion that there is nothing new in amputation surgery to be reported. The third impression is that above-knee amputation is recommended as 'the safest level' — especially for dysvascular patients — which could not be further from the truth (Fig. 15.1). At the same time it is seen to be the most simple procedure to be done easily by the least experienced doctor on duty in a surgical ward. No doubt it can be performed quickly and without hesitation by these junior colleagues, but they have no understanding whatsoever of what will happen afterwards with the patient; certainly not when he is about to be fitted with a prosthesis. This regrettable attitude corresponds precisely to the conviction of the overwhelming majority of otherwise experienced surgical colleagues, namely that amputation is some kind of 'bankruptcy'.

Even today the philosophy of how to cut off a leg as fast as possible and how to make a 'frog-mouth' incision through all the soft tissues by single anterior and posterior bold cuts influences the amputation procedure; this technique was obligatory in the past, when poor asepsis and inefficient and dangerous anaesthesia forced the surgeon to operate with speed in order to save his patient's life. All the benefits of modern medicine are available; why can today's patients not benefit from them when amputation becomes necessary? Furthermore, the application of modern prosthetics, such as total-contact sockets, depends to a large extent on proper amputation techniques to create well-shaped powerful osteomyoplastic above-knee stumps. It is essential to recognize this interdependency if amputation surgery is practised, and especially so at the above-knee level.

The relationship between causal condition and operative technique

The techniques for above-knee amputation may vary widely depending on the

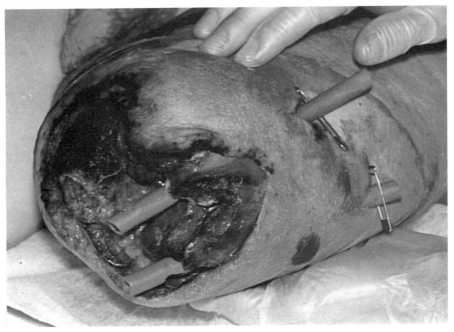

Fig. 15.1 Severe infection and necrosis after a so-called 'safe' above-knee amputation in a dysvascular patient.

aetiology. In the dysvascular patient the surgeon must try very hard to avoid above-knee amputation in favour of the through-knee disarticulation or below-knee amputation to preserve all the advantages of end-bearing or those of retention of the knee joint with the increased possibility for locomotion and a return to the community (Table 15.1) (Baumgartner 1973, 1979, Burgess & Matsen 1981, Dederich 1970, Murdoch 1975, 1984, Neff 1981a, b, Stirnemann & Althaus 1983, Stirnemann *et al.* 1987). In contrast, trauma or tumour amputees may profit from all of the sophisticated techniques, such as the osteomyoplastic procedures enabling optimum prosthetic fitting and rehabilitation (American Academy of Orthopaedic Surgeons 1980, Burgess *et al.* 1969, Murdoch 1968, Neff 1985, Sommelet *et al.* 1964 Weiss 1968, Wilson 1963).

Osteomyelitis may necessitate a two-stage procedure employing open flaps (Fig. 15.2) followed by secondary suture later on under aseptic conditions. In certain circumstances a semi-open technique may be applicable with excellent results (Dederich 1970, 1983, Neff 1981a). In congenital above-knee stumps osseous overgrowth may be a significant problem necessitating one reamputation after another. A more fruitful procedure is stump capping (Fig. 15.3), as developed by Marquardt (Marquardt 1976, 1980, 1980/81). This procedure prevents further osseous overgrowth, and in addition may gain in length depending on the growth capacity of the remaining proximal femoral epiphyseal plate.

Table 15.1 Comparison of above-knee, through-knee, and below-knee amputation due to peripheral arterial insufficiency with respect to progress after amputation and rehabilitation after wound healing (n=413). Modified from Stirnemann *et al.* (1987).

Progress	AK (n=124) (%)	TK (n=93) (%)	BK (n=196) (%)
Primary wound healing	55	44	40
Secondary wound healing	14	22	35
Reamputation	1	25	16
Mortality (30 days)	30	9	9
Rehabilitation after wound healing	AK (n=85)	TK (n=62)	BK (n=147)
Walking with prosthesis	22	66	84
Wheelchair	48	18	14
Bedridden	30	16	2

AK, above-knee; TK, through-knee; BK, below-knee.

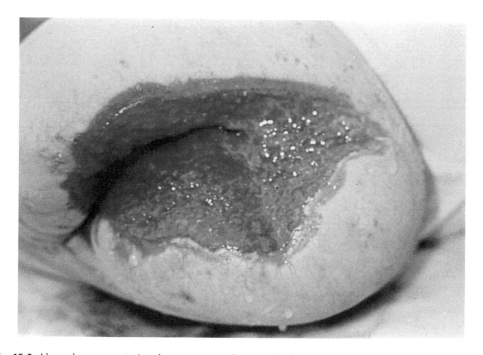

Fig. 15.2 Above-knee amputation due to osteomyelitis; result after three weeks of open treatment.

(a)   (b)

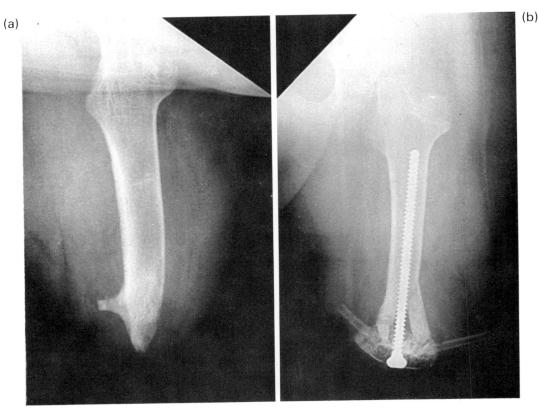

Fig. 15.3 Pre-operative (a) and post-operative (b) situation after stump capping with a cartilage/bone graft to prevent osseous overgrowth.

Acute traumatic amputation seldom offers the opportunity of free choice of flap design. Sometimes lack of skin may be seen as a reason for further shortening of the stump. There is seldom any excuse for this with the available techniques of modern plastic surgery. In particular, mention can be made of the use of mesh graft transplants, whether from the amputated part of the same leg or from another part of the body, or even free vascular musculocutaneous grafts which may provide the opportunity for excellent healing and preservation of most of the initial stump length (American Academy of Orthopaedic Surgeons 1980, Dederich 1970, Murdoch 1975, 1984).

Surgical technique

How should the above-knee amputation be performed? There are many approaches and it is most probable that every surgeon has his own preferences. For this reason it seems appropriate to point out some ideas which may prove helpful in performing this procedure. As general and vascular surgeons continue to perform amputations on their dysvascular patients in many parts of the world, the most common reason for above-knee amputation presenting to the orthopaedic surgeon is malignancy with osteogenic sarcoma in the first instance. Due to the young age of such patients everything is in the surgeon's favour to apply all the variety of procedures to create perfect above-knee stumps. In accordance with the recommendations of Enneking *et al.* (1980; Enneking 1983) radical amputation plus chemotherapy ensures the best chance of survival (Neff 1985).

Position and preparation of the patient

The usual position is supine with a cushion of at least 10–15 cm thickness under the buttocks so as to prevent the formation of a flexion contracture. As an alternative, Kuhn (personal communication) has proposed a side position, which allows for free movements in the hip joint as well as a neutral position during osteomyoplastic sutures. If possible, a tourniquet is applied, but eschew the use of a rubber bandage to evacuate the blood from the entire leg as this may well harm the tumour and predispose to the distribution of tumour cells; thus the leg is elevated and then the tourniquet is inflated. When amputating at a level proximal to mid-thigh a tourniquet may interfere with sterility and may have to be abandoned.

Incision

The operation begins with a circular incision of the skin and the subcutaneous tissues; at the same level the soft tissue is cut step by step with precise haemostasis, preferably by ligature of bleeding vessels; the large vascular elements and the major nerves are clamped until later. The leg is severed by a transverse osteotomy. Only in cases with a short remnant of the femur due to the involvement of tumour in the diaphysis of the femur is an attempt made to preserve more soft tissue by dissecting carefully, step by step, long anterior and posterior musculocutaneous flaps well away from the tumour area of the bone and the adjacent soft tissues. The bone is divided at the definitive level with respect to the type and degree of malignancy of the tumour as referred to above.

Osteoplasty

Incisions are made medially and laterally through the skin and subcutaneous tissue to create one dorsal and one ventral flap; then the muscle groups are divided from each other and the bone exposed. The periosteum is divided and pushed proximally with a raspatory. Definitive shortening of the bone takes place at a length of half the diameter of the thigh at the amputation level to allow for a myoplasty and wound closure without too much tension. The bone is divided by a saw and the sharp anterior edge removed with a bone nibbler; further smoothing of the bone is performed with a bone rasp or file. This is necessary as painful bursae may form if a sharp edge is left. Next the periosteum is pulled down (Fig. 15.4), the ends are turned outside in, and the the tube of periosteum is closed with a few stitches. Thus there will be no remaining periosteum to create bony spurs outside the bone. Moreover, as Dederich (1970, 1983) has demonstrated, the intramedullary vascular system is kept separate from the parosteal vascular system. Otherwise the differential pressure in a situation of direct anastomosis between the systems is thought to be a cause of severe pain.

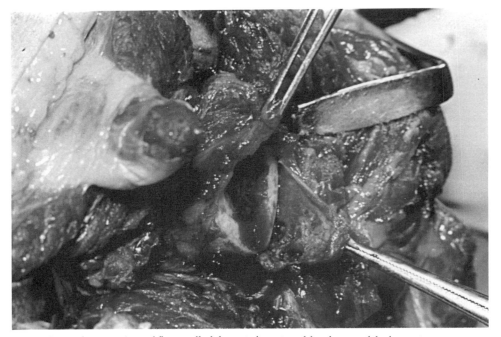

Fig. 15.4 Osteoplasty: periosteal flaps pulled down to be sutured for closure of the bone stump.

Vascular bundle

Arteries and veins are separated carefully, the big veins being ligated twice, just as with the artery, which in addition should be severed by a through-and-through stitch ligature. If the larger arteries and veins are not ligated separately, there is an increased risk of an arteriovenous fistula forming with all its disadvantages. The vascular ligature should be at least 1–2 cm shorter than the level of the bony end. Small blood vessels may be cauterized, although a ligature is preferred. In dysvascular patients cauterization is contraindicated because of the production of necrotic tissue.

Nerves

Nerves also require definitive treatment. Small nerves like the saphenous nerve or cutaneous branches are selected, clamped, pulled down gently, and then squeezed gently with forceps and resected with a sharp scalpel. The sciatic nerve is prepared likewise, the surrounding tissue being retracted proximally for at least 3–4 cm. The nerve should also be ligatured because the accompanying small vascular bundle (Fig. 15.5) may be the cause of significant bleeding, especially in dysvascular patients. Proximal to the ligature the nerve is squeezed three times with decreasing force, as recommended by Lenggenhager (1959), who noted that the neuroma which will inevitably develop will be distributed over a larger or smaller area according to the differential pressure of the forceps with more or less severe destruction of the axons. Finally the nerve is cut distal to the ligature and the stump of the nerve allowed to retract deeply into the muscles approximately 3–4 cm proximal to the bony stump end and safe from involvement in distal scar tissue.

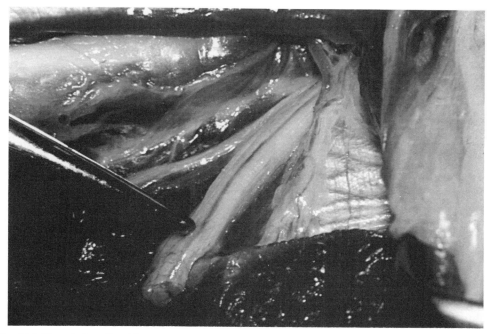

Fig. 15.5 Vascular bundle of the nerve, a source for haematoma unless ligated.

Myodesis and myoplasty

The definitive treatment of muscles may be described as myodesis and myoplasty. Myodesis is the attachment of the muscles to the femoral stump and requires initially the drilling of four holes about ½–1 cm proximal to the cut end of the femur. These four holes are threaded with four strong non-resorbable sutures. It is very important to attach only the inner layers of the muscles to the bone and to avoid strangulation of the entire muscle belly by all-enclosing sutures (Fig. 15.6).

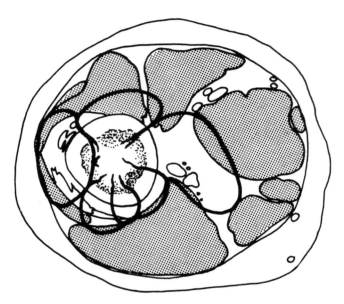

Fig. 15.6 Myodesis: attachment of inner layers of muscles to the bone. From Neff (1981a); modified from Wilson (1963).

The first closed suction drain should be located in this area. Myodesis is followed by myoplasty, the end-to-end suture of antagonistic muscle groups, first abductors and adductors, then the hamstrings and quadriceps (Fig. 15.7). In extremely short femur stumps it is not possible to achieve this, because of the traction of the pelvitrochanteric muscles and the iliopsoas muscles, which will unavoidably result in a flexion–abduction contracture due to the loss of most of the hamstring and adductor muscles. Emphasis must be placed on the importance of achieving a well-balanced tension in the different muscle groups when suturing, preferably with the hip joint in the neutral position.

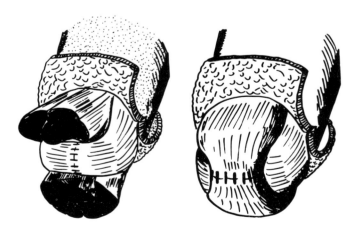

Fig. 15.7 Myoplasty: suture of antagonistic muscle groups. From Neff (1981a); modified from Sommelet *et al.* (1964).

If a tourniquet is used, it should be removed as soon as the treatment of nerves and vessels is completed followed by precise haemostasis, preferably by ligatures and only exceptionally by cauterization.

Even today there are advocates of a so-called slim and conical stump shape by thinning out the muscles. This is not necessary. Indeed, there is no reason to do so, because the amputee will require all his remaining muscle forces for proper fitting of the prosthesis and for optimal control (Fig. 15.8).

(a)

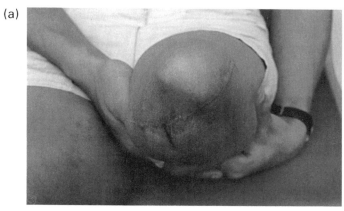

(b)

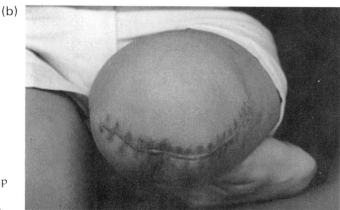

Fig. 15.8 Above-knee stump before (a) and after (b) osteomyoplastic correction.

Superimposed sutures of the fascia support the myoplasty. In the case of amputation in dysvascular patients fascial suture may replace major myoplastic procedures and still maintain a reasonable stump shape.

Suture

A second closed suction drain is placed superficially along the wound before the skin flaps are cut to size and sutured. One should not hesitate to have the skin suture running directly across the end of the stump; the location as well as the direction of the scar is insignificant so far as prosthetic fitting is concerned. It is important for wound healing in critical cases that there should be an optimal ratio of the base to the length of the skin flaps.

Special procedures

In dysvascular patients who have had previous vascular surgery it is worth considering removal of any artificial substitute for the superficial femoral artery as the first step to above-knee amputation. Dacron vascular prostheses in the groin sometimes cause trouble to the patient by pressure of the socket rim on this sensitive area.

In arteriosclerosis all tissues have to be treated gently, skin flaps should be bent only over a layer of gauze to prevent the arteriosclerotic vessels from cracking. Holding sutures and retractors must be used carefully. The skin should not be squeezed in forceps, but lifted gently for counterpressure while suturing. A non-touch technique will do the least harm in borderline situations.

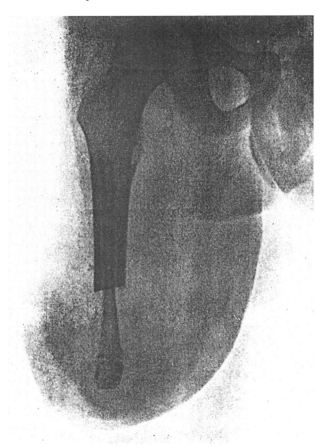

Fig. 15.9 Elongation of a short femoral stump by implantation of part of the fibula. From Kristen *et al.* (1975).

A very short proximal femur amputation, but with a reasonable amount of soft tissue remaining, might be an indication for elongation of the remaining femur, using either part of the tibia connected to the femur by plates and screws, or part of the fibula implanted into the marrow cavity (Fig. 15.9). Alternatively, a ceramic endoprosthesis may be used to gain additional length, with satisfying results, as reported by Kristen *et al.* (1975) and Salzer and Knahr (1978). Even the total replacement of the femur by an entire endoprosthesis to stabilize the soft tissue of an above-knee amputation stump has been performed. Kuhn (1978) reported a surprisingly good result of a prosthetic fitting with an above-knee prosthesis fitted to a lady whose femur had disarticulated in the hip joint; there remained a reasonable long above-knee 'fillet stump', which was pulled down into the prosthetic socket by a tube of gauze, offering sufficient hold to control the prosthesis.

In children, Marquardt and Correll (1984) have demonstrated that in Marquardt's technique of stump capping with the growth plate intact there is not only solid fusion between the stump and the graft but that the growth plate appears to remain open (Fig. 15.10). This provides the expectation of a possible contribution to length which is, of course, a very important factor in those children.

Lengthening of a short femoral stump by means of an external fixator apparatus, with or without interposition of bone grafts, may yet improve the situation of the above-knee amputee with respect to future prosthetic fitting.

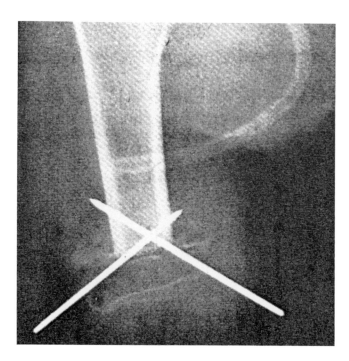

Fig. 15.10 Stump capping with distal tibial epiphysis including the growth plate. From Marquardt & Correll (1984).

Conclusion

Even if more distally located amputation levels are usually preferred, there is no doubt that above-knee amputation is still the correct level in a significant number of individuals, and, if certain principles are respected, according to the individual situation, aetiology, age, and life expectation, the result can be optimal.

References

American Academy of Orthopaedic Surgeons (AAOS) (1980) *Atlas of Limb Prosthetics: Surgical and Prosthetic Principles*. St. Louis: C. V. Mosby.

Baumgartner R. F. (1973). *Beinamputationen und Prothesenversorgunbei arteriellen Durchblutungsstorungen*. Stuttgart: Enke, Verlag.

Baumgartner R. F. (1979). Knee disarticulation versus above-knee amputation. *Prosthetics and Orthotics International* 3, 15-19.

Burgess E. M. & Matsen F. A. (1981) Current concepts review determining amputation levels in peripheral vascular disease. *Journal of Bone and Joint Surgery* 63A, 1493–1497.

Burgess E. M., Romano R. L. & Zettle J. H. (1969) Amputation management utilizing immediate postsurgical prosthetic fitting. *Prosthetics International* 3, 28–37.

Dederich R. (1970) *Amputationen der unteren extremitat. Operationstechnik und prothetische Safortversorgung*. Stuttgart: Thieme.

Dederich R. (1983) Indikationen zur Amputation sowie die stumpfversorgung bein Knocheninfekt der unteren extremitat. *Orthopade* 12 (4), 235–255.

Enneking W. F. (1983) *Musculoskeletal Tumor Surgery*. New York: Churchill Livingstone.

Enneking W. F., Spanier S. S. & Goodmann M. A. (1980) A system for the surgical staging of musculoskeletal sarcoma. *Clinical Orthopaedics* 153, 106–120.

Kristen H., Knahr K. & Salzer M. (1975) Atypische amputations-formen bei knochentumoren der unteren extremitat. *Archiv fur Orthopaedische und Unfall-Chirurgie* 83 (1), 91–107.

Lenggenhager K. (1959) Zur verhinderung der postoperativen phantomschmerzen nach amputationen. *Helvetica Chirurgica Acta* 26, 559–561.

Marquardt E. (1976) Plastische operationen bein drohender knochendurchspieBung am kindlichen oberarmstumpf. *Zeetschift fur Orthopaedie und ihre Grenzgehete* 114, 711–714.

Marquardt E. (1980) The multiple limb deficient child. In *Atlas of Limb Prosthetics: Surgical and Prosthetic Principles* (American Academy of Orthopaedic Surgeons), pp. 627–630. St. Louis: C.V. Mosby.

Marquardt E. (1980/81) The operative treatment of congenital limb malformation. *Prosthetics and Orthotics International* 4, 135–144 (part I); 5, 2–6 (part II); 5, 61–67 (part III).

Marquardt E. & Correll J. (1984) Amputations and prostheses for the lower limb. *International Orthopaedics* 8, 139–146.

Murdoch G. (1968) Myoplastic techniques. *Bulletin of Prosthetics Research* 10 (9), 4–13.

Murdoch G. (1975) Research and development within surgical amputee management. *Acta Orthopaedica Scandinavica* 46, 526–547.

Murdoch G. (1984) Amputation revisited. *Prosthetics and Orthotics International* 8, 8–15.

Neff G. (1981a) Amputationen und prothesen. In *Chirurgie der Gegenwart, Bd.V. Bewegungsorgane* (eds Zenker B., Deucher F. & Schink W.). Munich: Urban & Schwarzenberg.

Neff G. (1981b) Die amputation im kniegelenk — chirurgische und prothetische gesichtspunkte. *Orthopadie Technik* 32, 24–29.

Neff G. (1985) Therapie maligner knochentumoren. Amputation und orthopadie-technische Versorgung. *Therapiewoche* 35, 5195–5201.

Salzer M. & Knahr K. (1978) Die operative therapie der malignen knochentumoren. *Zeitschrift fur Orthopadie und ihre Grenzgebiet* 116(4), 517–525.

Sommelet J., Paquin J. M. & Fajal G. (1964) *Problemes d'Amputation. Atlas d'Appareillage Prothetique et Orthopedique*. Nancy: Faculte de Medecine.

Stirnemann P. & Althaus U. (1985) Die transgeniculare amputation: Ein alternative zur oberschenkel amputation? *Chirurg*, 54 (3), 170–174.

Stirnemann P., Mlinaric Z., Oesch A., Kirchhof B. & Althaus U. (1987) Major lower extremity amputation in patients with peripheral arterial insufficiency with special reference to the transgenicular amputation. *Journal of Cardiovascular Surgery* **28**, 152–158.

Weiss M. (1968) Physiologic amputation, immediate prosthesis and early ambulation. *Prosthetics International* **3**, 38–44.

Wilson A. B. (1963) Limb prosthetics today. *Artificial Limbs* **7(2)**, 1–42.

16

Biomechanics of Above-Knee Prostheses

N.A. JACOBS

The biomechanics of the above-knee prosthesis has been well documented by Radcliffe (1955, 1970, 1977) amongst others. This chapter is an attempt to summarize their findings.

Socket design

Success in fitting an above-knee amputee is based on providing a suitably shaped socket that offers a good environment for the stump. It should also transmit comfortably the forces which are produced between the stump and the socket in weight-bearing and which are required for stability and control. It is now generally accepted that a total-contact socket provides the best 'container' for the above-knee stump. As well as controlling oedema, it provides better force and pressure distribution possibilities, and improves the proprioception of the user. The material of the socket also has a bearing on the stump environment, and different materials are used, all of which offer some advantage or other to the user. The leather socket is probably the most sympathetic to the patient; the wooden socket is comfortable in both warm and cold climates, does not corrode, and is easily adjustable; the metal socket is light and easily adjustable; the rigid plastic socket is quick and cheap to manufacture and can conform to a rectified shape; and the flexible plastic socket developed by Kristinsson (1983) is comfortable to the user and light in weight.

Regardless of the material, however, the socket must be designed to transmit forces and pressures comfortably. To achieve this, the socket must be designed to support the mass of the body. As the above-knee stump is not capable of end-bearing, other parts must be used for this purpose. The most important of these are the ischial tuberosity, the gluteal fold, and the rest of the flare of the socket brim. If the socket is designed for total contact, a little further weight-bearing will be found at other sites. Foort (1979) identified 13 different portions of the stump that can contribute to weight support, including the end of the stump.

The next biomechanical factor of the socket to be considered relates to medio-lateral stability and the use of the hip abductors in stabilizing the pelvis during walking. In the normal subject the pelvis tends to fall on the unsupported side walking, however the hip abductors of the supporting limb are active in controlling this tendency (Fig. 16.1). This is possible because the foot is planted firmly on the ground and the structures of the leg allow it to be used for this purpose. In the case of the above-knee amputee wearing an ischial-bearing socket (Fig. 16.2) the pelvis pivots about the support point (S). For the abductors to stabilize the pelvis, the socket must prevent the femur moving laterally more than a very small distance, and be so designed that the force distribution will not be uncomfortable or painful. If the socket cannot provide this lateral stabilization force, there will be excessive movement of the end of the femur until it contacts the socket. The lateral force will be applied over a relatively small area, resulting in unduly high pressure and pain at the distal end of the stump. To reduce this pain the amputee would react by widening his walking base and swaying his trunk over the prosthesis with each step; this would help bring the weight line over the support line and reduce the need for abductors to stabilize the pelvis. For the socket to be able to provide lateral stabilization a counter force, M, must be applied on the medial side of the socket situated proximally. Care should be taken not to carry any vertical force on the medial brim of the socket as it would be likely to cause pain.

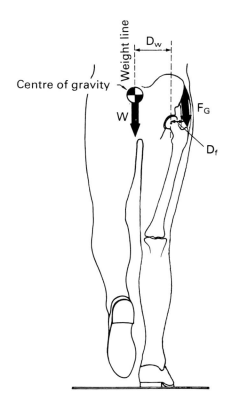

Fig. 16.1 Stabilization of the pelvis in the normal subject.

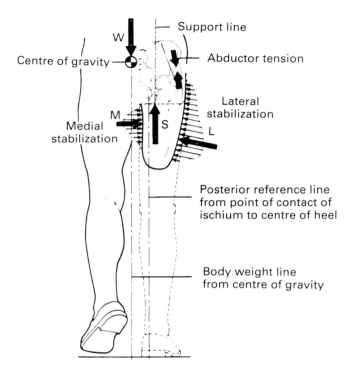

W

Support line

Centre of gravity

Abductor tension

Lateral
stabilization

M

Medial
stabilization

S

L

Posterior reference line
from point of contact of
ischium to centre of heel

Body weight line
from centre of gravity

Fig. 16.2 Use of the hip
abductor musculature for lateral
stabilization of the pelvis in the
above-knee amputee.

It has been suggested that the design of the flexible socket which uses a medial
structural support does not stabilize the femur, as a flexible material cannot provide
the force required. This is not the case. When the stump is in the socket, the socket
becomes almost rigid, allowing only the small deformations that are required to
improve comfort. The overall biomechanics do not change. Kawamura and
Kawamura (1985) reported on their experiences in measuring movements of the
end of the femur in both rigid and flexible sockets. They concluded that there was
no appreciable difference in movement of the femur in the flexible socket as
compared to the rigid socket.

In the anteroposterior plane the socket should be designed so that the amputee
is able to control the stability of the knee joint and also influence movements of
the knee joint during swing phase. An elderly infirm amputee would not be capable
of controlling knee function, and thus a locked or safety knee would probably be
prescribed. However, a young active amputee would be expected to use his hip
musculature to control the prosthetic knee joint.

Fig. 16.3 shows the anteroposterior force distribution during the stance phase
of walking that can be expected when a young above-knee amputee wears an
ischial-bearing total-contact socket with a simple uniaxial knee joint. The knee is
set in such a position that it can be stabilized during the major part of the stance
phase but is able to flex at push-off to initiate the swing phase. At heel-strike the

hip extensors are active in stabilizing the knee joint. Such activity will bring the ground reaction force ahead of the knee joint axis so that the knee will not flex. For this to be achieved without excessive movement of the femur within the socket there must be counter-forces from the socket at A_1 and P_1. During mid-stance the hip extensors are not very active, however the ground reaction is still passing in front of the knee joint, stabilizing it, and also producing forces at A_2 and P_2 on the stump in a pattern similar to that at heel-strike. At push-off the amputee should begin to flex his hip joint in order to initiate flexion of the knee for the following swing phase. This changes the pattern of stump/socket force distribution and the anterior force A_3 moves distally and the posterior force P_3 moves proximally.

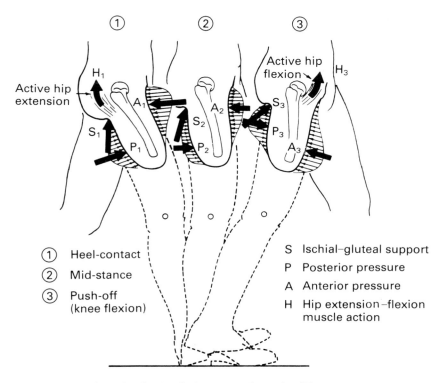

Fig. 16.3 Anteroposterior force distribution during stance phase of walking.

When determining the final shape of the socket, consideration must be given to the stump shape and the forces that can be anticipated between the stump and the socket during weight-bearing and locomotion. Additionally, the prosthetist should be aware of the anatomy of the stump in order to produce a well-shaped socket. This is particularly true at brim level, where the majority of the vertical forces are carried. A cross-section of the socket at brim level (Fig. 16.4) shows its shape to accommodate the complexity of the stump's anatomy. Reliefs for the hamstring tendons and the gluteus maximus, rectus femoris and adductor longus muscles need to be accommodated by the shape of the brim. Additionally, the soft area over Scarpa's triangle needs to be compressed to help ensure that the ischial tuberosity is maintained on the ischial seat.

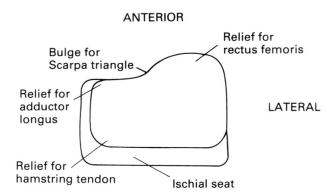

Fig. 16.4 Cross-section of socket at brim level.

Of course, different-shaped stumps require different-shaped brims, and these general principles need to be adapted to the individual patient. Fig. 16.5 gives an indication of the way that different stumps can be accommodated. The lateral wall of the socket should be kept as high as possible to distribute the lateral force over as large an area as possible. The medial wall should be low enough to avoid painful contact with the pubic ramus. The posterior brim should be kept parallel to the ground, and the anterior wall should be kept as high as possible to help maintain the ischial tuberosity on the ischial seat, but not so high as to be uncomfortable for sitting. In general, a well-fitting socket will distribute forces over as large an area as possible, thus reducing pressures on the stump. This is the rationale behind the design of the quadrilateral socket, but any above-knee socket must incorporate these biomechanical principles in order to fit comfortably and for the amputee to have a good gait pattern.

Alignment

The alignment of the above-knee prosthesis is carried out on the bench, statically with the patient standing in the prosthesis and dynamically with the patient walking. By alignment is meant the relative position and orientation of the socket, knee, and foot. Alignment has an important influence on the forces generated between the stump and the socket, as well as on the performance of the amputee when walking. It is of prime importance when considering knee stability, and thus the knee axis should always be located in a position such that the load carried by the prosthesis during walking passes ahead of the knee axis, preventing it from flexing.

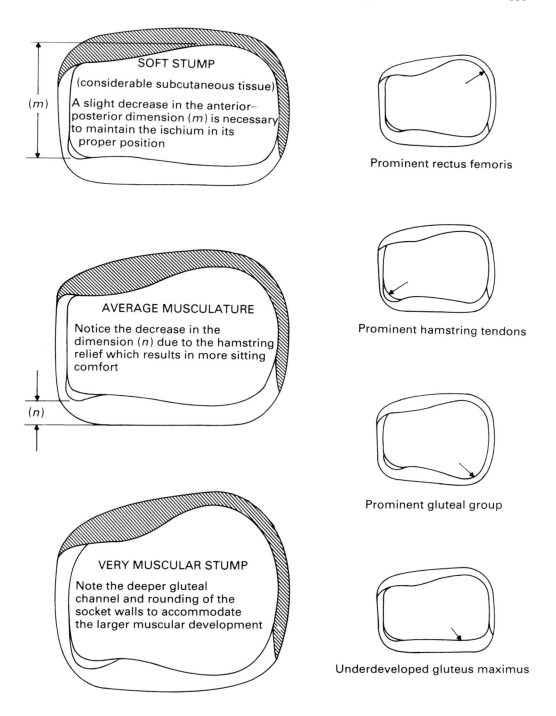

Fig. 16.5 Variation of quadrilateral socket shape for different types of stump.

Different bench alignment systems exist to enable the prosthesis to be set up to achieve this alignment stability. The German system (Fig. 16.6a) uses a plumb-line which passes from a point in the centre of the socket brim through or adjacent to the bisector of the length of foot with the knee joint well behind this line; the United States advocates a plumb-line from the trochanter passing through the ankle joint, with the knee joint on or behind this line, and is commonly known as the TKA line (Fig. 16.6b). A modified system is the MKA line, where the medial location of the knee joint is placed on the line between the bisector of the medial wall and the ankle joint (Fig. 16.6c). Because the knee joint is placed in about 5° of external rotation, the lateral location of the knee joint is behind this line. All these alignments produce a similar result in stabilizing the knee. A good final alignment may only be achieved after the patient has worn the limb and walked on it, allowing the prosthetist to carry out a static and dynamic alignment. Some general principles of alignment are well agreed upon nonetheless.

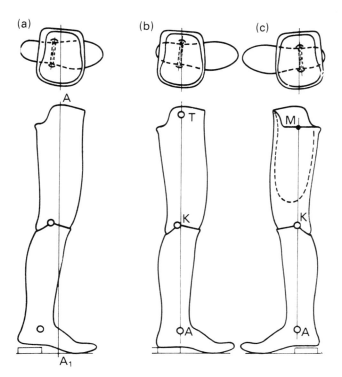

Fig. 16.6 Bench alignment systems. (a) German system, (b) TKA reference, (c) MKA reference.

For an average length of stump the socket is slightly adducted (Fig. 16.7). This will help place the hip abductors in an advantageous position to stabilize the pelvis. The foot may have to be placed laterally, especially in the case of elderly amputees. The socket is also set in an initial flexion of about 5° which allows the hip extensors to be placed in an advantageous position to help control the stability of the knee

SHORT FUNCTIONAL LENGTH

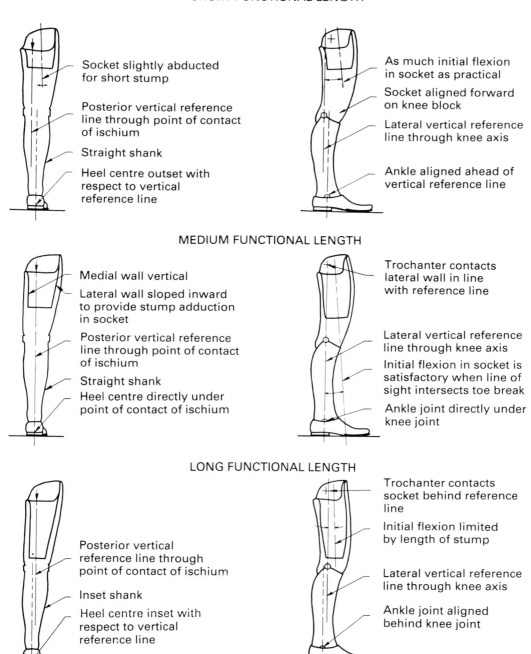

Socket slightly abducted
for short stump

Posterior vertical reference
line through point of contact
of ischium

Straight shank

Heel centre outset with
respect to vertical
reference line

As much initial flexion
in socket as practical

Socket aligned forward
on knee block

Lateral vertical reference
line through knee axis

Ankle aligned ahead of
vertical reference line

MEDIUM FUNCTIONAL LENGTH

Medial wall vertical

Lateral wall sloped inward
to provide stump adduction
in socket

Posterior vertical reference
line through point of contact
of ischium

Straight shank

Heel centre directly under
point of contact of ischium

Trochanter contacts
lateral wall in line
with reference line

Lateral vertical reference
line through knee axis

Initial flexion in socket is
satisfactory when line of
sight intersects toe break

Ankle joint directly under
knee joint

LONG FUNCTIONAL LENGTH

Posterior vertical
reference line through
point of contact of ischium

Inset shank

Heel centre inset with
respect to vertical
reference line

Trochanter contacts
socket behind reference
line

Initial flexion limited
by length of stump

Lateral vertical reference
line through knee axis

Ankle joint aligned
behind knee joint

Fig. 16.7 Alignment variations to accommodate stumps of different functional length.

at heel-strike and throughout the stance phase. The knee joint is set on the trochanter–ankle line. In addition, initial flexion of the socket helps to maintain the ischial tuberosity on the ischial seat; transfers part of the support on the ischial tuberosity to the hamstring tendon; places the gluteus maximus in a better position to sit on the posterior brim; and minimizes the development of lumbar lordosis, especially where there is some flexion contracture.

For a short stump the socket is slightly less abducted. The adductors of the hip joint are likely to be weakened by the amputation, and although the hip abductors are unaffected they cannot be fully employed in stabilizing the pelvis because of uncomfortably high pressures created between the end of the femur and the lateral socket wall. As explained earlier, to reduce this pressure the foot is placed laterally and the patient would be expected to walk with his trunk swaying over the prosthetic leg. The hip extensors may also be affected by the amputation with a possibility of flexion contracture. To make the extensors as effective as possible in stabilizing the knee, as much initial flexion of the socket as can be allowed is built into the prosthesis; initial flexion may be as high as 20°. The knee joint position is also placed behind the trochanter–ankle line in order to be more easily stabilized by the hip extensors during the stance phase.

For a long stump the socket is adducted and the foot can be placed medially so that the patient can walk with a narrow heel base. Although this has the effect of increasing the lateral force on the femur, this is counteracted by its larger lever arm which tends to reduce the magnitude of the force and hence the pressure on the tissues. Because the stump is long and powerful the amputee can stabilize the knee joint quite easily without it being necessary to build too much flexion into the socket. In any case, flexion possibilities are limited for cosmetic purposes. Additionally, it may be possible to place the knee joint slightly ahead of the hip–ankle line because of the ease of controlling knee stability, and also to help with smooth knee flexion at the push-off phase.

The principles of alignment provide guidelines in fitting in the widely varying situations found with different amputees. An elderly amputee with a medium stump would have to be considered differently from a young amputee with similar length of stump. The younger amputee would be considered to have a functionally longer stump than the elderly patient. Additionally, the use of different knee or ankle components will have a bearing on the alignment of the limb.

Quadrilateral sockets have customarily been aligned using an alignment jig, which has the disadvantage of not having the same mass characteristics or components of the finalized limb. Modular prostheses allow the limb to be aligned without transferring out the alignment components, and employ the knee components that are to be used in the finished prosthesis. This is desirable in achieving a good final alignment.

This chapter has attempted to outline the basic biomechanics of above-knee prosthetics. Regardless of the philosophy of cast-taking and alignment, if these requirements are met, the resulting prosthesis will be satisfactory and the amputee should be able to walk comfortably and well.

Acknowledgements

The author is grateful to the Editors of *Prosthetics and Orthotics International* for permission to reproduce Figs 16.2, 3, 5 and 6 and to the Editorial Board of *Artificial Limbs* for the use of Fig. 16.7.

References

Foort J. (1979) Socket design for the above-knee amputee. *Prosthetics and Orthotics International* **3**, 73–81.

Kawamura I. & Kawamura J. (1985) A biomechanical evaluation of the ISNY socket. Presentation to Orthopadie and Reha-Technik '85 International, Essen, Federal Republic of Germany, June, 1985.

Kristinsson O. (1983) Flexible above-knee socket made from low density polyethylene suspended by a weight transmitting frame. *Orthotics and Prosthetics* **37(2)**, 25–37.

Radcliffe C. W. (1955) Functional considerations in the fitting of above-knee prostheses. *Artificial Limbs* **2(1)**, 35–60.

Radcliffe C. W. (1970) Biomechanics of above-knee prostheses. In *Prosthetic and Orthotic Practice,* (ed. Murdoch G.), pp. 191–198. London: Edward Arnold.

Radcliffe C. W. (1977) Above-knee prosthetics. *Prosthetics and Orthotics International* **1**, 146–160.

17

Socket Design for the Above-knee Amputation

H. PFAU

Introduction

Any discussion about good functional design for a prosthetic above-knee (AK) socket is as old as the history of making artificial limbs. Textbooks from 1894 (Hoffa) and 1915 (Ritschl) show that the shape of the socket in former times seemed not to be very important. The prosthesis was made of leather with a soft cushion and suspended on the body by shoulder straps (Fig. 17.1). At the time when the wooden AK socket was made so that it became airtight with a distal vacuum, there grew up the realization of the importance of a good functional socket design, and different socket shapes were employed (Pfau *et al.* 1937). Accordingly the functional requirements, the anatomical considerations, and the problems of force transference in determining the correct AK socket design should be examined. On principle the author believes that the point of the body weight-bearing is located at the ischial tuberosity. Next, both the anatomical circumstances and the physical demands are considered from three different viewpoints. These are lateral, anterior and horizontal.

The importance of socket shape

The shape of the socket has functions of importance as illustrated from each aspect. First, the anatomy requires more detailed analysis. The ischial tuberosity is the lowest point of the pelvis. Its purpose is to support the body weight of the amputee during the stance phase. The greater trochanter on its lateral side is prominent. There is little or no cushion of muscle or tendon. Most of the muscles of the upper leg have been divided at the amputation. If the point of insertion has been lost by the amputation the muscles lose their function and the muscles atrophy. This is certainly the case in the majority of amputations performed by the conventional method with simple division of the muscles. In the author's experience only in a few cases has a myoplastic procedure been performed in which the antagonists are sutured together. In this way an artificial insertion is established and thereby the muscles maintain their activity, resulting in improved blood supply (Dederich 1967).

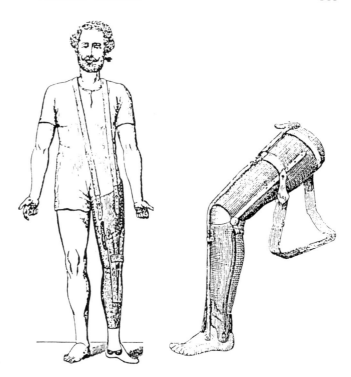

Fig. 17.1 Early prostheses.

Clearly these several techniques of amputation in different patients ensure that each stump exhibits individual characteristics. Even when stumps seem at first sight to have the same shape, any one stump is unlike any other. Therefore the use of prefabricated socket formers for taking the measurements should be handled with care, especially when they are hard and not elastic. The author prefers to make the plaster cast without the aid of any former, but on the few occasions when seating rings are used those made of elastic material are employed.

Returning to the different aspects of the socket:

1 In the frontal view of the seating, recognizing that the position of the ischial tuberosity is the lowest point of the pelvis, the need is for a good, well-defined ischial seat which should be horizontal (Fig. 17.2).

2 Medially a mould to encompass the perineum is necessary, otherwise the patient will experience pressure pain on this sensitive area.

3 Laterally the brim should be as high as possible to prevent any tilt of the pelvis in a lateral direction. It is essential to provide enough relief for the prominent part of the greater trochanter which makes a rolling movement during the swing phase.

In viewing the interior of the socket in its middle area there must be a clear convex lateral support plane; this is necessary to ensure that abduction movement of the stump during the stance phase is controlled. The abduction of the stump against the lateral support maintains the pelvis in a horizontal position. In the swing phase of the healthy leg, if there is not enough lateral support and the stump

is not controlled by contact against this area, a Trendelenberg phenomenon will
be seen. The lower third of the socket should accurately reflect both the shape and
volume of the distal stump. If the socket end portion is too large there will be
proximal constriction and the stump end will become oedematous and badly
discoloured. In the lateral view, the upper brim as mentioned presents the ischial
seat as the point of weight-bearing; just distal to the ischial seat the socket invests
the stump closely.

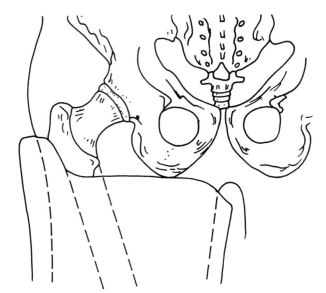

Fig. 17.2 Horizontal ischial
seat.

   To ensure that the seating posteriorly is maintained, the anterior brim of the
socket must be high enough to provide a counterforce and prevent the stump
sliding forwards off the ischial seat. If the anterior socket brim is too low then the
ischial tuberosity will certainly lose contact with the brim. On the other hand, if
the anterior socket brim is too high, the patient will have difficulties when sitting
with the prosthesis. The middle part of the socket must be close-fitting but also
provide space for enlargement of muscles in contraction, thus providing intimate
contact between stump and prosthesis during the swing phase. It is not so much
the vacuum at the stump end which keeps the prosthesis on the stump but rather
the contraction of the stump muscles against the walls of the socket which ensures
suspension of the prosthesis. In the horizontal view, especially with respect to the
seating, the muscles in the stump vary according to the surgery employed, and
may be bulky and active or atrophied.
   The strongest muscle posteriorly is the gluteus maximus. The gluteus maximus
with its full capability of contraction can bring about a lot of painful problems,
especially in the area of the adductor longus, if the seating and upper part of the
socket does not provide for enlargement of the gluteus maximus (Fig. 17.3).

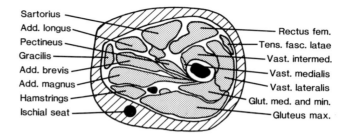

Fig. 17.3 Cross-section of the socket at the ischial seat.

The anatomical relationship of the muscles, which is constant, encourages the development of theories of socket design, but the variation from patient to patient and the effect of surgery merit care in the application of any theory.

The individual characteristics of each case are, of course, dependent on a number of factors, such as the age and sex of the patient, the type of amputation, the length of the stump, the condition of the patient, and those muscles in the stump which are still active. Once the anatomical circumstances are analysed and the physical demands on the stump are understood, then a socket shape may be envisaged based on the theoretical system but modified by individual characteristics.

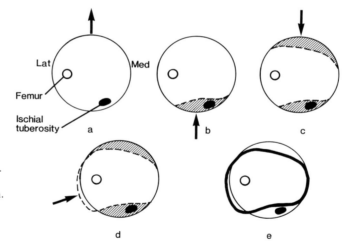

Fig. 17.4 Functional socket shape. (a) Undeformed stump. (b) Bulge under ischium. (c) Pressure from anterior brim. (d) Allowance for gluteus maximus. (e) Resultant socket shape.

In the horizontal view the outline of the stump, as long as it is not deformed, is a circle. However, the need for a horizontal ischial seat and the counterforce of the anterior brim, and not least the requirement to accommodate the bulk of the gluteus maximus, has already been acknowledged. Accordingly the circle of the undeformed stump must now be modified. In Fig. 17.4a the plain outline of the undeformed left stump is seen with, in the lateral area, the femur and in the posteromedial area the ischial tuberosity. In Fig. 17.4b the bulge for the ischial seat is provided and in Fig. 17.4c the high anterior brim provides an opposing force to maintain the ischium on the seat. Finally in Fig. 17.4d allowance is made for the gluteus maximus while maintaining the volume requirements. The three main changes of the original circle produce a resultant shape (Fig. 17.4e) which is called a 'cross-oval' socket. This is the basis of the system but, to repeat, the individual circumstances of the stump must be recognized and the socket modified to meet them.

The work of Müller and Hettinger (1954), which analysed pressure situations with different configurations, confirmed that the support beyond the ischial tuberosity, the high anterior brim, and relief of the gluteus maximus leads to a good functional socket design. If the system described is used, and if the individual circumstances of the stump are recognized, a socket design will be produced which allows the amputee to walk with his prosthesis without pain.

References

Dederich R. (1967) Technique of myoplastic amputations. *Annals of the Royal College of Surgeons* **40**, 222–227.

Hoffa A. (1894) *Lehrbuch der Orthopadischen Chirurgie,* 2nd edition. Stuttgart: Ferdinand Enke.

Muller E. A. & Hettinger T. (1954) Die Messung der Druckverteilung im Schaft von Prothesen. Zeitschrift Orthopadie-Technik Nr. 9, Essen.

Pfau H., Engelke & Thomsen (1937) *Lehrbuch fur Bandagisten und Orthopadiemechaniker.* Berlin: Otto Elsner.

Ritschl A. (1915) *Amputationen und Ersatzglieder an den unteren Gliedmassen.* Stuttgart: Ferdinand Enke.

18

The Flexible Above-Knee Socket

O. KRISTINSSON

Introduction

This chapter describes a new concept in socket technology for above-knee amputees — the flexible above-knee socket with an external weight-transmitting frame.

The flexible socket system consists of two separate parts: (a) a pliable, transparent or translucent socket for tissue containment; and (b) a rigid, external supporting frame for weight transmission (Fig. 18.1). The socket is vacuum-formed from thermoplastic sheet material, over a plaster of Paris model. The frame is laminated over the socket. It consists of a cup covering the socket end, a medial strut, and a brim which extends around three-quarters of the socket circumference. The use of carbon fibre and glass fibre, in a sandwich-type laminate, makes this structure stiff and strong, and thus capable of transmitting the body weight to the prosthetic system. Properly designed, the frame does not bend under the loads involved and is reasonably resistant to torsion. The new socket is now available to patients at many centres all over the world.

The flexible socket was developed in co-operation with Een-Holmgren in Sweden. New York University Medical School (NYU), in co-operation with Ossur hf. in Reykjavik and Een-Holmgren, Stockholm, has prepared a worldwide introduction of the concept, and thus the socket has become known as the ISNY (Iceland–Sweden–New York) socket.

Experiments with flexible sockets were initiated in 1971, when attempts were made to fit a bilateral amputee who had previously used laced leather sockets with total-contact suction sockets. Although the new sockets were quite comfortable while standing and walking, they were, compared to his old ones, extremely uncomfortable on sitting. He was used to a somewhat loose fit in the sitting position and above all the soft feeling and tactile feedback provided by the leather sockets. Because of this the patient rejected the new sockets, and asked for replacements similar to his old ones. It was quite obvious that if the sockets were to be made to his requirements (leather was considered unacceptable) they had to be flexible over as large an area as possible. They also had to be relatively resistant to stretching so that their volume would not be significantly changed during loading, and they had to be sufficiently well supported so that the body weight could be effectively transmitted to the prosthetic system. The materials tested were soft laminating resins like silicone, polyester, epoxy, acrylic, polyurethane, and Lynadure. Eventually this led to the fabrication of a pair of prostheses with silicone sockets, partially covered by supporting, rigid frames, and the patient was satisfied. Those sockets would probably be classified now as window sockets. They were successfully used during a period of no less than seven years.

Although it is true that the soft, pliable socket is not a new idea, the problem of combining a soft socket with a stiff supporting structure has restricted the use of the common test sockets as definitive sockets. The need for sufficient support has often required the test socket to be covered entirely with a rigid shell.

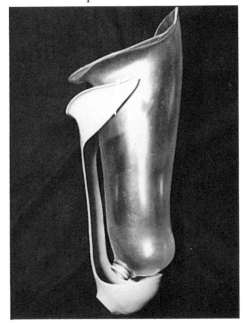

Fig. 18.1 The flexible socket and the rigid frame. A new or modified replacement socket can be fitted to the same frame if the model has not been altered in regions where the frame and socket meet.

Materials and methods

Vacuum-forming a socket from a thermoplastic sheet material over a plaster of Paris model is a relatively simple and easy procedure. The experienced technician soon discovers how to match sheet material thickness and frame size to model length to get even socket wall thickness. The thermoplastic materials most widely used for flexible sockets are low-density polyethylene (LDPE) and Surlyn (Thermovac).

Workstation model preparation

A vacuum-forming stand is easy to fabricate and use. The stand accepts the pipe mandrel and has a round platen 34 cm in diameter. The moulding frames most commonly used are made from 5 mm aluminium sheet and have an inside diameter of 36 cm. However, by keeping a set of, say, four frames, sizes 20, 25, 30 and 35 cm inside diameter, and interchangeable platens, and by varying sheet material thickness, socket wall thickness can be predetermined, so that the small investment in making several sizes of frames may well be a wise one. The positive model is prepared according to conventional methods. The use of a valve specially designed for thermoplastic sockets is recommended.

Vacuum-forming

For heating the plastic sheet either an air-circulating oven, preheated to 150 °C, or an infrared oven can be used. The author uses an air-circulating household oven for this purpose with good results. The model is placed upside down on the vacuum stand. In order to give some space between the model and the platen, and to assist air evacuation, a soft foam pad may be used. The hot plastic sheet is draped slowly over the model. When a seal between the plastic and platen is secured, the evacuation process is started. While carefully inspecting for wrinkles, the plastic should be manually manipulated until it totally conforms to the model.

Frame-trimming

The distal cup should cover the end of the socket up to where the radius meets the lateral wall. The medial bar should be approximately 60 mm wide. The anterior and posterior extensions should follow the proximal borderlines, extend to the anterolateral and posterolateral corners, sweeping down from the corners to meet the medial bar approximately 50 mm below the medial brim edge.

The model with the socket in place is mounted on a laminating stand. The valve is fitted and the housing is surrounded with clay to prevent undercuts in the laminate. A 5 mm Pelite sheet is backed with two-sided adhesive tape and cut to strips 6 mm wide. The tape backing is peeled off and the strip is then stuck to the socket to indicate the future outlines of the rigid frame. The purpose of using the Pelite strip is twofold. Firstly, it is of great help when cutting the laminate after the resin has set; secondly, it gives the edges an inside flare which ensures that sharp edges will not cut the flexible socket during use. One layer of nylon stockinette (NS) is then pulled over the socket and tied off over the valve. A PVA bag is pulled over the nylon-covered socket, tied off, and the air evacuated.

Carbon and glass fibre lay-up

The lay-up for the medial bar consists of four layers of 50 mm carbon fibre tape (CF) (Fig. 18.2a); 12 layers of glass fibre (GF) (100 mm wide folded lengthwise in thirds and sewn down the centre); and a further four layers of CF. A similar lay-up is used for the anterior and posterior extensions. The lay-up can be altered according to socket length and patient weight. Two layers of NS are used underneath, and two layers on top of, the combination of carbon and glass fibre. The main purpose of the GF is to separate the two CF bodies, thus creating a profile using the stiffness of the CF (Fig. 18.2b). As a general rule it can be said that the greater the distance between the two CF bodies the stiffer the laminate will become.

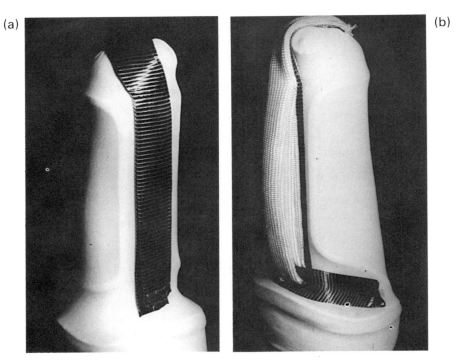

(a)   (b)

Fig. 18.2 (a) Lay-up, the four innermost carbon fibre tapes. (b) Glass fibre is used to separate the two carbon fibre bodies.

Lamination and trimming

When the lay-up is completed, a PVA bag is pulled over, tied off below the model and at the top, and the air evacuated. Both 100% rigid polyester and acrylic resins can be used. It is essential that the CGF should be thoroughly saturated, therefore the resin should be worked vigorously into the lay-up.

After the resin has set, the laminate is cut, using the bulge over the Pelite as a guideline. Care must be taken not to damage the socket during this operation. The frame and socket are pulled off the model. The frame is trimmed, following the lines previously mentioned. A distal extension in the form of either a rigid foam or a wooden block is applied, and the socket is ready for initial alignment.

The socket and frame are secured to each other with the help of double-sided adhesive tape, or by the socket being folded proximally over the frame edges, thus creating rounded edges and locking the socket on the frame. In order to do so the edges are heated and a 10 mm overhang folded down.

Finishing

The prosthesis is finished in much the same way as a conventional rigid-socket prosthesis. If an endoskeletal system is used, the foam cover can be extended to the desired proximal level. When using an exoskeletal system the thigh may be covered with Plastazote and hide, or similar cushioning and protecting materials.

Discussion

For the last four years Surlyn or Thermovac has been used as a socket material. The proximal edges were cut 2–3 mm outside the frame edges. The socket and frame were secured to each other with double-sided adhesive tape. This occasionally led to pinching of the skin and hair between the socket and the frame. Socket breakdowns occurred but were rare. In 1984 the NYU modification of folding the socket over the frame was adopted.

If the lateral anteroposterior region of the proximal socket opening is not properly supported, its form will change during the stance phase due to the action of the gluteal muscles and rectus femoris. The double-curved flares are vulnerable to stress, resulting from repeated flexing. Should the frame extensions be too short or too weak and thus allow too much lateral AP dimensional distortion, there is a risk of splitting occurring, especially in the anterolateral corner. Experience suggests that socket wall thickness has little or nothing to do with this phenomenon. Folding the edges may further exaggerate the risks, and great care should be taken to make the transition from a folded to an unfolded edge as smooth as possible.

Different approaches to fit will not be further discussed. The flexible socket can be used for various spatial socket designs and fitting techniques with, perhaps, minor modifications of the frame. The advantages are threefold. Firstly, from the patient's point of view the socket is, being pliable, susceptible to shape variations of the residual limb, thus giving greater freedom of muscle activity during ambulation and better conformity during suspension and rest (Fig. 18.3a). The socket is soft to the touch and yields to external forces, thus offering the wearer more tactile feedback than the rigid socket. Suspension is enhanced due to both the nature of the material used and the fact that the socket walls tend to collapse inward during the suspension phase. Secondly, from the viewpoint of the prosthetist, the transparent or translucent socket offers excellent possibilities for visual inspection through the walls, thus making judgement of fit an easier task (Fig. 18.3b). About 70–75% of the socket area can be altered, without interfering with surfaces where socket and frame meet, either by local reheating of areas of the existing socket or by making a new one over an altered positive. Most problems

(a)   (b)

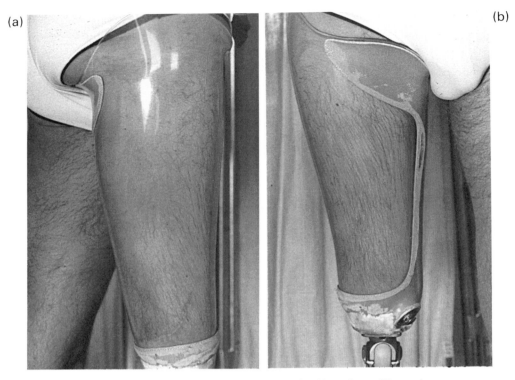

Fig. 18.3 (a) Lateral view. The large area covered only by the flexible socket wall is an advantage, especially for amputees with long residual limbs. (b) Anterior view. The transparent socket permits visual inspection of the residual limb during load-bearing.

of inexact fit or atrophy, for example, can be overcome easily and inexpensively. Thirdly, from an economic standpoint, the socket is much more easily and quickly fabricated, modified, and replaced than a conventional socket. These factors should make for a better service for the amputee. The co-operation between Ossur hf. in Reykjavik and Een-Holmgren in Stockholm has now led to the emergence of prefabricated components that will, in most cases, eliminate the need for individually made rigid frames. The components are (a) a distal cup for connection to the knee set-up by bonding and lamination; (b) a medial strut connected to the cup by screw-in components; and (c) a brim, that comes in nine sizes, right and left, connected to the medial strut by a slide-on female box. The rigid frame as designed fixes the socket distally by a screw-in valve housing fixation. The socket and the rigid frame can be detached from the knee set-up by disconnecting the two screw-in components. Now both the socket and the frame can be replaced without the alignment being lost. The frame components are manufactured to high industrial standards and have been designed to withstand loads exceeding the accepted international standards.

Acknowledgements

The author would like to thank Mr Sveinn Finnbogason CPO and the staff at Ossur hf. in Reykjavik, Mr Sture Carlsson CPO and Mr Bo Klasson at Een-Holmgren in Stockholm for their help and contribution to the development, and Dr S. Fishman and his staff at the New York University Medical School for the development of a manual and educational programme.

Bibliography

Foort J. (1979) Socket design for the above-knee amputee. *Prosthetics and Orthotics International* **3**, 73–81.

Holmgren G. (1979). The interface between the body and the above-knee prosthesis. *Prosthetics and Orthotics International* **3**, 31–36.

Irons G., Mooney V., Putnam S. & Quigley M. (1977). A lightweight above-knee prosthesis with an adjustable socket. *Orthotics and Prosthetics* **31(1)**, 3–15.

Koike K., Ishikura Y., Kakurai S. & Imamura T. (1981) The TC double socket above-knee prosthesis. *Prosthetics and Orthotics International* **5**, 129–134.

Kristinsson O. (1983) Flexible above-knee socket made from low density polyethylene suspended by a weight-transmitting frame. *Orthotics and Prosthetics* **37(2)**, 25–27.

Lehneis H. R., Chu D. S. & Adelglass H. (1984) Flexible prosthetic socket techniques. *Clinical Prosthetics and Orthotics* **8(1)**, 6–8.

Mooney V. & Snelson R. (1972) Fabrication and application of transparent polycarbonate sockets. *Orthotics and Prosthetics* **27(3)**, 1–13.

Pike A. C. & Black L. K. (1982) The Orthoglas transparent test socket — an old idea, a new technology. *Orthotics and Prosthetics* **36(4)**, 40–43.

Radcliffe C. W. (1955) Functional considerations in the fitting of above-knee prostheses. *Artificial Limbs* **2(1)**, 35–60.

Redhead R. G. (1979) Total surface bearing self suspending above-knee sockets. *Prosthetics and Orthotics International* **3**, 126–136.

Van Rolleghem J. & Berteele X. (1979) Socket fabrication. *Prosthetics and Orthotics International* **3**, 68–72.

Volkert R. (1982) Frame type socket for lower limb prosthesis. *Prosthetics and Orthotics International* **6**, 88–92.

19

Knee Components for the Above-knee Amputation

K. E T. ÖBERG & K. KAMWENDO

Introduction

This chapter is directed to orthopaedic surgeons, orthopaedic engineers, and physiotherapists dealing with lower extremity amputees. It has grown out of the authors' experience of the difficulty in obtaining comprehensive information on prosthetic knees available on the market. It is intended to facilitate the job of the rehabilitation team in assessing the patient's needs and to provide the physiotherapist with the information necessary to plan appropriate gait training.

To have better understanding of different designs of prosthetic knee joints and their function, one should be aware of the difference between prosthetic and normal walking, and the effects of the prosthesis on the patient. Function codes have been developed according to an international model presented in studies on prosthetic knee joints by Radcliffe (1970) and Hägglund and Öberg (1980). Since the codes were first published in detail, they have been simplified further in order to make them more clear-cut. A new grading scale for describing the stabilization effect of a prosthetic knee joint is presented, along with guidelines for selection of the most appropriate prosthetic knee function with regard to the stabilization effect of the joint, the level of amputation, and the activity of the amputee. These guidelines are intended to facilitate team discussions, but not to be followed blindly. The issue of the weight of knee joints has not been addressed because of their diversity and thus the difficulty in comparing semi-manufactured and complete components. Equally, durability and repair problems have not been considered because representative basic material on these issues is not available.

Normal and prosthetic walking — a comparison

In normal walking the knee is almost straight at heel contact. It then flexes to 20° in early stance in what is called stance-phase knee flexion. This flexion angle at the beginning of the stance phase is, however, dependent on walking speed, an increased walking speed implying an increased flexion angle. The stance-phase knee flexion decreases the upward displacement of the body centre of mass in the vertical plane. During mid-stance the knee extends again and then during terminal stance, or 'push-off', it starts to bend again in preparation for toe-off. The knee flexes to its maximum (about 65°) during the swing phase. Observe that when the toe leaves the ground, and the stance phase thus ends, the knee has already flexed to about 40°. Thus, the swing phase is well prepared for and the leg can swing without dragging against the ground and without energy-demanding extra movements such as vaulting or circumduction. At about 30% of the swing phase the knee starts to extend again, and upon heel contact it achieves full extension. Upon heel contact the leg is affected by an external force, namely the floor reaction force (Fig. 19.1). In normal walking this force passes behind the knee, thereby initiating the above-mentioned stance-phase knee flexion. Whenever the floor reaction force line passes in front of the knee joint rotation centre, it causes extension of the knee (Fig. 19.1).

Stability of the knee in the stance phase requires that the external flexing force is counteracted by an internal extending force. In the normal leg this is brought about by muscular activity, mainly by quadriceps. Note that the muscles 'permit' a controlled knee flexion (the quadriceps contracts while lengthening).

The walking pattern of above-knee amputees is considerably different from that of normal walking due to the absence of essential muscle groups. Due to loss of

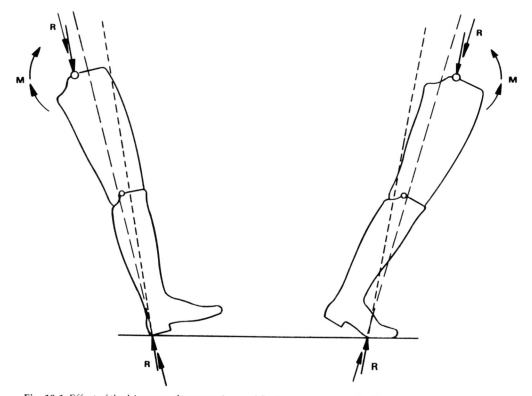

Fig. 19.1 Effect of the hip muscular extension and flexion moments on the floor reaction vector.

knee muscles the patient can no longer flex or consequently actively extend the knee under load. Today there are only experimental prosthetic knees, so-called 'bouncy knees', that are similar to the normal knee in this aspect (Fisher & Judge 1985). By different brake mechanisms it is now possible to prevent, with more or less security, collapse of the knee during the stance phase. In other words, different levels of stance phase stability can be achieved. In general, however, the above-knee amputee must be sure that the prosthetic knee is fully extended at heel contact in order to ensure stability. The knee stays straight during a large period of the stance phase. If the knee joint mechanism is very stable, it is not possible to flex the knee before the toe is off, i.e. when the stance phase ends. Absence of knee flexion at the beginning and end of the stance phase implies a higher energy demand on the amputee's walking.

Earlier, it was pointed out that after heel contact the knee joint is exposed to a flexion force, i.e. the ground reaction force. The patient can affect this by contracting the hip extensors so that the force line moves towards the knee centre, which implies that the flexion moment decreases and the knee stability increases. For knee joints without stabilization mechanisms, stance phase stability is completely dependent on the patient being able to activate the hip extensors in such a way that the ground reaction force line passes ahead of the knee centre, thus causing extension of the joint. By the end of the stance phase, the patient can, on the other hand, modify the direction of the ground reaction force so that it again passes behind the knee centre. This is done by activation of hip flexors. If the knee lacks stabilization mechanisms, it sometimes can be flexed while the prosthesis is still loaded, which facilitates the initiation of swing phase.

During the swing phase the hip joint is flexed, mainly by contraction of iliopsoas. Due to the moment of inertia of the shank and foot, these tend to 'lag behind' the accelerated knee centre, which results in knee flexion and a backward and upward swinging of the shank and foot. Even with considerable changes in the walking speed, the maximum flexion angle in the normal knee stays constant at about 65°, mainly as a result of the retarding effect of the quadriceps extending action.

For above-knee amputees, the size of the flexion angle depends on the swing phase control with which the knee mechanism is equipped. There are available mechanisms which give a relatively good imitation of the normal knee movement during the swing phase. Note that adequate control of maximum knee flexion at different speeds requires some type of velocity-dependent or 'viscous' damping of knee swing.

Functional classification — codes of joint types (Fig. 19.2)

Single axis (C)

The rotation centre of the joint is fixed in one point in all angular positions of the knee.

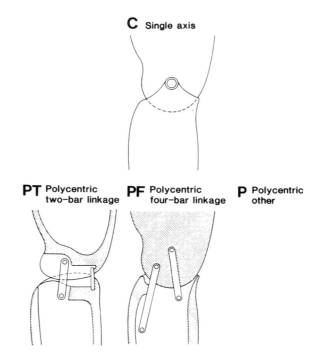

Fig. 19.2 Functional
classification — types of joints.

Polycentric joint

The rotation centre has different locations in different angular positions of the knee
i.e. there are many (poly) joint centres. Different prosthetic knee designs have
been developed to imitate the polycentric human knee joint, or alternatively to
provide polycentric action quite different from the normal knee.

Polycentric two-bar linkage (PT)

Refers to a knee where the stump and shank glide against each other. This
constitutes a link which rotates with the thigh as well as with the shank, thus
making two joints.

Polycentric four-bar linkage (PF)

Refers to a knee where the stump and shank are joined by two links. The links
bend at each of their ends with the thigh as well as with the shank, thus making
four joints. The four-bar linkage mechanisms are the most frequently used
polycentric joints.

Polycentric — other (P)

Includes polycentric joints which are not of the two- or four-bar linkage type, such as polycentric condylar, or designs with more than four joints.

Functional classification — codes of stance phase stabilizing mechanisms (Fig. 19.3)

None (N)

No stability mechanism. The knee joint is stabilized by extension of the hip or by the knee being in an overextended position.

Hydraulic (H)

The knee is locked by the oil flow in a hydraulic system being shut off.

Mechanical lock (L)

The knee joint is locked during the whole walking cycle, i.e. the patient walks

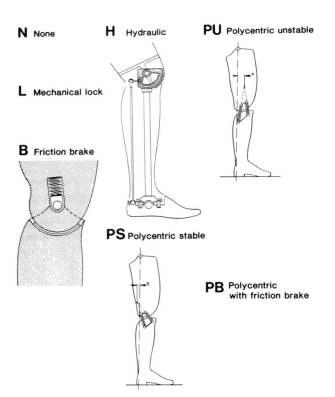

N None

H Hydraulic

PU Polycentric unstable

L Mechanical lock

B Friction brake

PS Polycentric stable

PB Polycentric with friction brake

Fig. 19.3 Functional classification — stance phase stability.

with a stiff knee. The locking procedure takes place in an extension position and is most often an automatic one. Unlocking is done manually.

Friction brake (B)

Weight-bearing load of the prosthesis causes certain components of the knee to be deformed so that a braking friction moment arises. Technically, this can be formed in different ways, e.g. with a metal clamp or a brake band around the knee axis.

Polycentric stable (PS)

The rotation centre, while the knee is extended, lies always behind a reference loading line joining the hip joint and the heel. The ground reaction force line at the instant of heel contact causes the knee to extend, and thus the knee is stable without activation of hip extensors.

Polycentric unstable (PU)

The rotation centre, while the knee is extended, lies above the level of the normal knee and in front of a reference load line joining the hip joint and the heel. The ground reaction force at the instant of heel contact is thus inclined towards the knee joint and the knee is stabilized by activation of hip extensors by the patient. Extension of the hip affects the resultant force line of the ground reaction force so that it passes in front of the effective knee centre, causing the knee to extend.

Polycentric with friction brake (PB)

Upon loading, the condyle-like surfaces in the knee are pushed against each other, which induces a braking effect. This, together with the elevated position of the rotation centre of the polycentric knee, provides good stabilization of the knee in an extension position. The hip extensors in this case do not need to be activated.

Functional classification — codes of swing phase control mechanisms (Fig. 19.4)

None (N)

No resistance (counteracting moment) in joint movement.

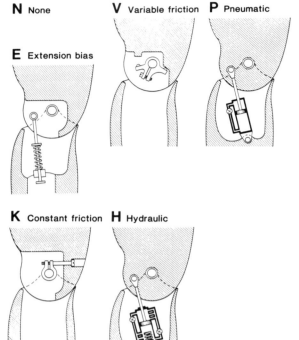

N None **V** Variable friction **P** Pneumatic

E Extension bias

K Constant friction **H** Hydraulic

Fig. 19.4 Functional classification — swing phase control.

Extension bias (E)

An elastic restraint provides a progressive resistance (counteracting moment) against knee flexion and helps in its extension. The restraint consists usually of a metallic spring or an elastic band.

Constant friction (K)

This provides a constant resistance (counteracting moment) in the joint which reflects the normal swing function of the knee in a simplified way.

Variable friction (V)

This provides increments increasing resistance (counteracting moment) according to the position of the knee. However, the mechanism does not adjust itself according to the walking speed.

Hydraulic (H)

The resistance (counteracting moment) increases with the walking speed, thus presenting a good imitation of the normal knee moment. Resistance arises from an oil flow in a system of orifices.

Pneumatic (P)

The resistance (counteracting moment) increases with the walking speed. This arises by resistance to flow in orifices and compression of air at the same time. It provides a good imitation of the normal knee movement. Examples of knee mechanisms are shown in Figs 19.5, 19.6 and 19.7.

Stabilization levels (Table 19.1)

0 Unstable

Upon normal adjustment the knee joint is stabilized by hip extension even though the knee is fully extended. The knee collapses if it is loaded in a flexed position. The knee is easily flexed while the hip flexors during load are in an extended position, which facilitates preparation for the swing phase.

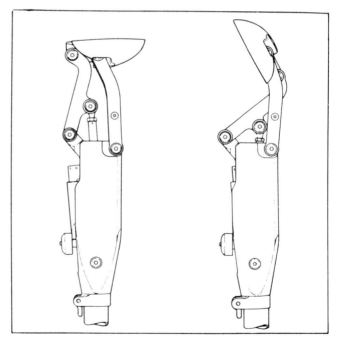

Fig. 19.5 Knee mechanism — OHC disarticulation knee.

PF – PU – H   1

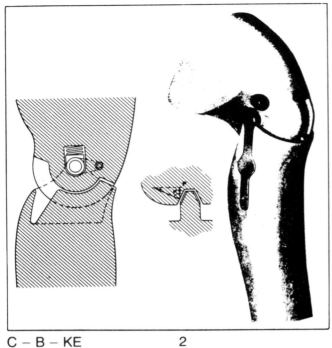

C – B – KE   2

Fig. 19.6 Knee mechanism — Otto Bock Jüpa knee 3P23.

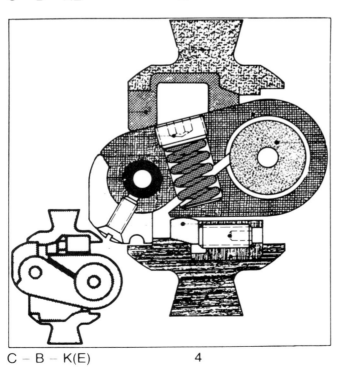

C – B – K(E)   4

Fig. 19.7 Knee mechanism — Otto Bock modular brake knee 3R15.

Table 19.1 Knee stability levels.

0 Unstable
1 Low instability
2 Stable
3 High stability extended
4 High stability
5 Mechanical lock

1 Low instability

The knee must be stabilized by hip extension, even when it is fully extended. Compared with the stabilization level '0', the need for hip extension is reduced. The knee collapses if it is loaded in a flexed position. The knee can be flexed with hip flexors while still under load, which facilitates preparation for the swing phase.

2 Stable

When the knee is fully extended, no hip extension is required to preserve stability. If the knee is loaded by the whole body weight in a flexion position, it collapses. The knee can flex with hip flexors while under load in an extended position but with certain difficulties. This makes preparation for swing phase difficult.

3 High stability at extension position

When the knee is fully extended, no hip extension is needed to preserve stability. The knee collapses if it is loaded by the whole body weight in a flexed position. The knee can *not* flex with hip flexors while under load in an extension position, which prevents any knee flexion before toe-off.

4 High stability

Refers to the maximal sensitivity adjustment of the knee for activation of brake effects. Hip extension is not needed in flexed or extended positions in order to preserve stability. The knee can thus be loaded in a moderate flexed position without collapsing. The knee cannot be flexed with hip flexors while under strain, which prevents any knee flexion before toe-off.

5 Locked knee

The knee is locked during the whole gait cycle and the patient walks with a stiff knee.

The amputation level, as well as the level of the patient's activities, must form the basis for judgement about the patient's need of a knee function. This function dependence is described in Fig. 19.8. Even though other factors, like occupation, leisure time interests, and personality type, can affect the kind of knee function, albeit to a lesser extent, and the distinctions between different activity levels are not sharply defined, function limits are drawn so that alternative functions are available for a given combination of amputation and activity levels.

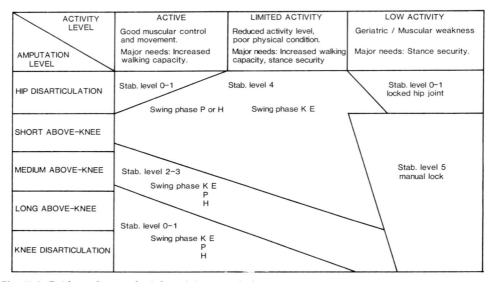

Fig. 19.8 Guidance for prosthetic knee joint prescription.

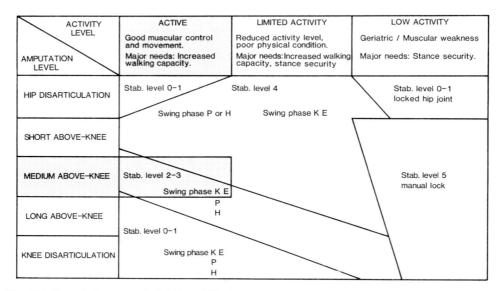

Fig. 19.9 Prescription example: Medium AK, active.

Different types of swing phase control are also presented in Fig. 19.8, for emphasis on these important functions to be considered upon selection of the knee joint. In general, it can be said that the more active the patient is, the greater is the need for a more dynamic swing phase control, such as pneumatic or hydraulic.

Example 1: interpretation of the diagram (Fig. 19.9)

An active patient with a medium above-knee stump lies in the shaded rectangle. The greatest part of the rectangle relates to stabilization levels 2 and 3. Most patients with this combination of levels can achieve their optimal walking capacity with knee mechanisms of stabilization level 2 or 3. The top right-hand corner of the rectangle is a smaller part relating to stabilization level 4. A fewer number of patients are thus in need of knee mechanisms of stabilization level 4 in order to achieve their optimal walking capacity. Finally, the left-hand corner of the rectangle relates to stabilization level 0–1, i.e. very few patients are suggested to achieve optimal walking capacity with knee mechanisms of stabilization level 0 or 1.

Example 2 (Fig. 19.10)

The patient has a medium stump, but his activity level can be considered limited. This covers the shaded rectangle appearing in the diagram. The greatest part of the rectangle relates to stabilization level 4. Most of the patients with this level combination can thus achieve their optimal walking capacity with knee mechanisms of stabilization level 4, while few patients can achieve this with stabilization levels 2 or 3.

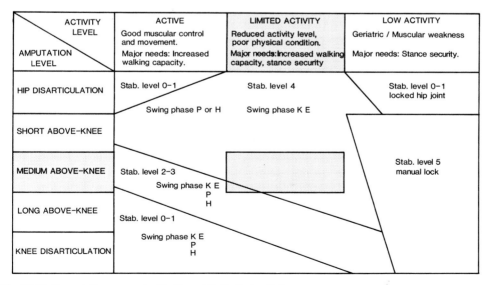

Fig. 19.10 Prescription example: Medium AK, limited activity.

Bibliography

Fisher L. D. & Judge, G. W. (1985) Bouncy knee: a stance phase flex-extend knee unit. *Prosthetics and Orthotics International* **9**, 129–136.

Hägglund L. & Öberg K. (1980) Prosthetic fitting of KD, AK and HD amputees related to type of knee mechanism: a survey in Sweden. 1980 World Congress, International Society for Prosthetics and Orthotics (abstract), 107.

Öberg K. (1981) Quantitative analysis of gait disorders. Doctor's thesis. Uppsala: University of Uppsala.

Peizer E., Wright D. W. & Mason C. (1969) Human locomotion. *Bulletin of Prosthetic Research* **10 (12)**, 48–105.

Radcliffe C. W. (1970) Prosthetic-knee mechanisms for above-knee amputees. In *Prosthetic and Orthotic Practice* (ed. Murdoch G.), pp. 225–249. London: Edward Arnold.

20

Prescription Criteria, Fitting, Check-out Procedures and Walking Training for the Above-knee Amputee

R.G. REDHEAD

Introduction

A below-knee amputee has lost only the foot and ankle. Fitted with a modern patellar tendon-bearing (PTB) limb the patient's hip and knee can act normally while walking, and all that is lacking is an active 'push-off' from plantar flexion of the ankle. The situation is very different for the above-knee amputee. In both structural and functional terms the major part of the leg is lost. An above-knee prosthesis has therefore to replace the foot, the ankle, and the knee joint. The majority of modern above-knee sockets are based upon an ischial-bearing brim design, thus diverting a proportion of the axial compression load away from the hip joint when the patient is standing or walking, so disturbing the normal proprioceptive pathway. If the above-knee amputation has had to be performed in the proximal part of the thigh, or if the surgeon has failed to achieve a satisfactory myoplasty/myodesis, there may be an unbalanced muscle action about the hip that will interfere with the normal action of the joint. It is clear therefore that an above-knee amputation results in a major loss of function of the normal living limb. The patient's ability to achieve a successful rehabilitation as an above-knee amputee will be very dependent upon good amputation surgery, a prosthesis which has been manufactured to an appropriate prescription, correct fitting and alignment, and adequate training (Redhead 1984).

Prescription criteria

The selection of an appropriate prescription for a prosthesis for a patient should result in the supply of a limb that will satisfy the needs of that patient after he has been discharged from hospital, taking into account his mental and physical abilities, the length, configuration, and power of the stump, and any occupational, recreational or special environmental activities. These needs will vary from those of the young healthy person who has lost his leg as the result of an accident and who will be returning to active work to the elderly patient who has had an amputation because of peripheral vascular disease and who may have had additional complications such as a cardiac infarct. Successful rehabilitation for a patient such as this is for him to achieve sufficient independence to enable him to return to his own home. The young active patient is therefore seeking a limb that will give him as normal a gait pattern as possible, will impede the speed of his activities to a minimum extent, will be strong enough not to let him down, and will have an acceptable cosmetic appearance. The older patient needs a limb that he can put on and take off by himself, that will give him maximum security against having a fall, that is simple for him to understand, light enough for him to use, and has an acceptable cosmesis.

The most important factor for all amputees being fitted with a prosthesis is a comfortable socket that does not cause stump complications. To arrive at a prescription for a suitable limb for a patient the prescribing physician or prosthetist needs to work to a logical scheme. The approach outlined in Table 20.1 ensures that each of the major options is considered as the prescription is drawn up.

Table 20.1 Prescription options.

TYPE OF LIMB		Modular endoskeletal Metal-stressed skin Wood
SOCKET	*Material*	Laminated plastic Hard thermoplastic Flexible thermoplastic Wood Metal

	Design	Ischial-bearing
		    quadrilateral socket
		    British 'H' socket
		 Conventional (trumpet) ischial/gluteal-bearing
		 Ischial-bearing total-contact socket
		 Total surface-bearing socket (Redhead 1979)

SUSPENSION	*Self-suspending*	Suction/muscle hold socket

	External suspension	Hard
		    multiaxial hip joint and pelvic belt
		    uniaxial hip joint and pelvic belt
		 Soft
		    silesian belt and its variants
		    various combinations of waist belt, down straps
		       and shoulder braces

KNEE JOINTS	*Articulation*	Single-axis joint Multibar link joints
KNEE CONTROLS	*Stance phase controls*	Alignment and no lock Hand-operated optional lock Semi-automatic non-optional stance/swing phase lock Fully automatic stance phase lock allowing a free knee in the swing phase

Table 20.1 *Cont'd.*

KNEE CONTROLS	*Stance phase controls*	Stance phase flexing knee controls 'Bouncy knee' (Judge & Fisher 1981, Fisher & Judge 1985)

	Swing phase controls	Dampers
		  friction
		  pneumatic
		  hydraulic
		Extension bias
		  external elastic
		  internal mechanisms

ANKLE JOINTS		None Simple uniaxial Multiaxial Adjustable for shoe heel height
FEET		Solid ankle cushion heel (SACH) Moulded plastic Wood Felt (for small children)
COSMESIS		Hard shape Soft shape Two-piece cover One-piece cover continuous over the knee
EXTRAS		Shin rotators (only on endoskeletal tubular shins) Protective covers/pads, as appropriate for the ischial seat, knee joint and ankle joint Socket end-support/bearing pad

Using this scheme a prescription for a limb for the young active adult amputee can be arrived at. If it is assumed that the patient lives near a limb-fitting facility that has the necessary resources the limb might be built up as follows:

Type of limb	Modular
Socket material	Flexible thermoplastic
Socket design	Ischial-bearing quadrilateral total-contact
Suspension	Self-suspending suction/muscle hold socket
Knee unit	Uniaxial
Swing phase control	Pneumatic damper. No extension bias mechanism
Stance phase control	Fully automatic stabilizer
Ankle	Multiaxial
Foot	Moulded plastic
Cosmesis	One-piece cosmetic cover over a soft shape

The above prescription will not result in the lightest limb but is an example of the type of specification that should be considered for a high-activity patient. If the scheme is used to arrive at a specification for a limb for an elderly patient with peripheral vascular disease and a history of having had a coronary infarct (living near limb-fitting facility) the result could be the following prescription:

Type of limb	One of the lightweight modular designs
Socket material	Hard thermoplastic
Socket design	Ischial-bearing quadrilateral or 'H' socket to be worn with a stump sock and fitted with a soft stump end-support pad
Suspension	Uniaxial hip joint and pelvic belt
Knee unit	Uniaxial
Stance phase control	Semi-automatic non-optional stance/swing phase lock
Swing phase control	None
Ankle	Uniaxial
Foot	Moulded plastic
Cosmesis	One-piece cover over a soft shape

This prescription will result in a lightweight limb that is simple and easy for the older patient to put on and take off without help. The uniaxial hip joint will provide good hip stability in the stance phase and guide the limb through the swing phase. The semi-automatic knee lock will limit the patient to a fixed knee gait, but this will ensure security against the knee 'giving way' under the patient.

Fitting procedures

These may start as soon as the wound has healed and the stump dimensions show signs of stability. This may be as early as two weeks after surgery, while in other cases the start of fitting may have to be delayed for clinical reasons. The ideal is that it should be possible to measure/cast the stump, provide the socket, assemble the limb, fit the limb to the patient, and finish the limb for delivery, all on the same day. Such a procedure may be possible if the centre has the resources, the number of patients is not too great, and they all arrive at the centre early enough in the day and are prepared to stay for a sufficient length of time for the work to be completed. The service can be provided for one or two patients arriving early in the day but it is easily overwhelmed if the number of patients increase, some of them arriving later in the day. Even using premade adjustable above-knee sockets, the 'one day delivery' of limbs has not proved practical under routine working conditions in limb centres in England. Economic reasons make it impossible to raise the level of the workshop resource and increase the number of staff to cope with peak conditions, which would leave them underutilized at other times.

A more practical programme for supplying the limb is to measure/cast the stump at the first visit and then to see the patient again at a second visit 7–10 days later to fit the limb and finish it for delivery. If the prescription is for a non-modular type of limb then, in the majority of cases, it will require the patient to make a minimum of three visits, thus leading to a delay that may amount to several weeks before the limb can be delivered. To achieve the two-visit service the first critical factor is the socket. The simplest solution is to use a premade adjustable socket selected from a range of such sockets. Though this solution is not applicable to all patients, if the dimensions of the stump fall within the size range of such a system it can produce satisfactory results for a first prosthesis. If a cast of the stump is to be used, the system of casting should result in a positive cast that needs no major rectification, and the subsequent fabrication of the socket should be possible on a wet cast. The CAD/CAM system for designing and manufacturing sockets may be an alternative method for the rapid production of sockets in the future (Klasson 1985). The second critical factor for the two-visit fitting/delivery service is the method of producing the structure of the limb. In practical terms this usually means assembling the limb from prefabricated components and using some form of external cosmetic shape and cover. A number of modular limb assemblies that satisfy this requirement are now available.

Check-out procedures

A limb should be checked at two stages. It should be done first at the end of the fitting stage. If any faults are identified they can then be corrected without too much work, as the various fastenings in the limb have not been finally secured and there is no cosmetic cover on the limb. The second check should be made when the limb is finished and is to be delivered to the patient. At this stage the correction of any major fault is not easy, and in many cases will require major dismantling of the limb and its cosmetic cover. Thus the final examination at delivery should only be to check small items such as the set of the ankle, that no minor adjustments are required to the socket, and that the knee controls are functioning correctly.

The check-out of a prosthesis should start with an examination of the stump to identify any existing evidence of previous problems. The limb is then examined off the patient to check that it has a sensible bench alignment, i.e. the ankle is set at a correct angle so that the limb stands up straight, the knee extension stop is set correctly, and the knee controls can be operated. The socket should be examined to assess its general features and to see that there are no obvious faults in its design or fabrication. The patient should then be asked to put the limb on and a check made with the patient standing to see that the limb is the correct length, that if a free knee is fitted the joint is adequately stable, and that the patient has safe standing balance. A laser vector system such as the one being devised in the Bioengineering Centre, Roehampton, will be a very useful device in the future for assessing the relationship between the vertical ground reaction force vector and the axis of rotation of the knee joint (Wilson et al. 1979). The lateral stability of the limb should be examined and the patient asked to lift the foot off the floor to test the efficiency of the suspension.

Having completed the static check the patient should be asked to walk on the limb. The stride length should be observed from the side; if the socket is set in too much flexion the prosthetic stride will be short, while if the socket is in excessive extension the stride will be overlong. The movement of the knee in the swing phase is best seen from the side, when the action of the knee damper and extension-assist mechanism can be assessed and if necessary adjusted. The ankle action should be such that the foot comes to the floor smoothly after heel contact and that the ankle dorsiflexion control acts adequately leading up to toe-off. The patient should then be seen walking from the front and from the back to assess the lateral stability of the limb, to ensure that there is no 'whip' in the swing phase and that the toe out of the prosthetic foot matches that of the normal foot.

The patient then sits down and the fit of the socket is checked to see that there are no pressure points around the socket brim. The limb is then removed and the stump examined for unexpected pressure marks.

Walking training

Walking training should start before the amputation is performed. The main contraindications include severe pain that cannot be controlled with drugs, toxaemia due to ischaemic tissue and/or infection that renders the patient too ill to co-operate, and other medical/surgical complications. The majority of patients having a planned amputation benefit enormously from undergoing a programme of physical and mental preparation for about a week prior to surgery. This should include learning the regimen of exercises they will be expected to carry out after the amputation, and treatment to reduce any joint contractures that are present. With a suitable dressing on the lesion on the leg to be amputated, and if necessary using adequate analgesic cover, the patient should be stood up to practise standing balance and, if possible, walking between walking rails.

Walking training in the generally accepted sense should start 5–10 days after surgery using a pneumatic walking aid (Little 1971, Redhead *et al.* 1978, Redhead 1983). Patients with longer above-knee stumps can use this type of walking aid satisfactorily, while those with shorter stumps may need the stability provided by a more positive socket, for instance an adjustable plastic socket mounted on a simple temporary limb structure. If the patient is making good progress and the stump is healed, manufacture of the first definitive limb may begin during the third week after surgery. If the amputation was necessary because of peripheral vascular disease it is always wise to wait until 21 days after surgery before casting/fitting the stump with a definitive socket.

After delivery of the first definitive prosthesis the patient will need a period of instruction in the rehabilitation department, where he will be taught how to put the limb on and take it off himself. He will be shown how to balance standing between rails and how to transfer weight from one side to the other. He will practise lifting the prosthesis off the floor and simulating a stride from toe-off to heel contact. When he has mastered these skills the therapist will start him walking between rails, making sure that he has a good stance and gait pattern. From there the patient will progress to walking out of the rails using appropriate aids as necessary. If the patient has learned to walk with a locked knee and subsequently progresses to a limb with a free knee he will need a further period of training to learn to use the new limb safely.

Conclusion

The stages of rehabilitation of the above-knee amputee that have been considered are only part of the total care programme for the patient. Success depends very much upon free and adequate communication between all members of the team and proper assessment of the patient and all his needs right from the start of treatment. It is vital that the surgeon performing the amputation realizes that when fashioning the stump he is producing the first component of the prosthesis, the motor that will drive the new limb; and that the prescription for the rest of the prosthesis will depend very much upon the success of his efforts. If the surgery has resulted in undesirable limitations on the choice of the prescription there may be problems obtaining a satisfactory fitting, and subsequently the patient may fail to achieve the expected degree of activity and independence. All the members of the team must understand fully the role they have to play and present to the patient a positive approach. In this way the patient will come to have confidence in the staff looking after him and so be best-placed to realize his ambition to return to as normal a life as possible.

References

Fisher L. D. & Judge G. W. (1985) Bouncy knee: a stance phase flex–extend knee unit. *Prosthetics and Orthotics International* **9**, 129–136.

Judge G. W. & Fisher L. D. (1981) A 'bouncy' knee for above-knee amputees. *Engineering in Medicine* **10(1)**, 27–32.

Klasson B. (1985) Computer aided design, computer aided manufacture and other computer aids in prosthetics and orthotics. *Prosthetics and Orthotics International* **9**, 3–11.

Little J. M. (1971) A pneumatic weight-bearing temporary prosthesis for below-knee amputees. *Lancet* **1**, 271–273.

Redhead R. G. (1979) Total surface bearing self-suspending above-knee sockets. *Prosthetics and Orthotics International* **3**, 126–136.

Redhead R. G. (1983) The early rehabilitation of lower limb amputees using a pneumatic walking aid. *Prosthetics and Orthotics International* **7**, 88–90.

Redhead R. G. (1984) The place of amputation in the management of the ischaemic lower limb in the dysvascular geriatric patient. *International Rehabilitation Medicine* **6**, 68–71.

Redhead R. G., Davis B. C., Robinson K. P. & Vitali M. (1978) Post amputation pneumatic walking aid. *British Journal of Surgery* **65**, 611–612.

Wilson A. B., Pritham C. & Cook T. (1979) A force-line visualization system. *Prosthetics and Orthotics International* **3**, 85–87.

21

Physiotherapy and the Elderly Above-knee Amputee

M.E. CONDIE

The amputee presenting the greatest rehabilitation problem for the physiotherapist is the elderly patient with an above-knee amputation. Approximately 66% of all lower limb amputees referred to limb-fitting centres in England and Wales have their amputations because of peripheral vascular disease, and around 78% of the referred patients are over the age of 60 (DHSS 1984). In Scotland, where a similar pattern exists, a recent study showed that almost one-third of all lower limb amputations and disarticulations (including amputation of toes) are at the above-knee level (Scottish Health Service Common Services Agency 1982). A personally conducted, unpublished survey of lower limb amputations carried out in a district general hospital from January 1977 to December 1979 shows slightly fewer above-knee than below-knee amputations in the first year, but slightly more above-knee in the next two years. The average number of amputations in each year was 33. Whilst the desirability of preserving the knee joint is now well documented (Burgess & Marsden 1974, Murdoch 1975), and although improved assessment techniques help to achieve this aim, it can be seen from these figures that a considerable number of above-knee amputations are still being performed.

In general, the younger, more active above-knee amputee will learn to use his definitive prosthesis without much difficulty and will be able to return to an acceptable lifestyle fairly soon after amputation. His problems are likely to be prosthetic rather than physical, and are often encountered when the function of the artificial limb fails to match that of a 'real' leg during sporting or recreational activities. The elderly, above-knee amputee, on the other hand, often has problems in adapting to even limited prosthetic use. Skilled and accurate assessment of the patient's capabilities is vital to establish a realistic rehabilitation goal. All too often in the past such patients have been referred for prosthetic fitting regardless of their physical condition, including exercise tolerance, mental attitude towards the loss of a limb, and appreciation of the hard work required in learning to use an artificial leg.

The energy cost of ambulation by amputees has been well documented, and in a literature review of the subject by Fisher and Gullickson (1978) spanning the previous 40 years, it is suggested that the average above-knee amputee expends

89% more kcal/m than the normal person. Some patients, especially those with additional medical problems, will be unable to produce the extra energy required to ambulate independently, no matter how intensively they are trained.

It is particularly important that the patient displays enthusiasm for the proposed rehabilitation programme and the will to work hard. Even the most skilled and energetic physiotherapist will be unable successfully to train an amputee to achieve independent gait using a prosthesis if the patient is unco-operative. For some elderly people, especially those with a chronic disability or disease, walking and leading a functionally independent life with normal legs is an extremely difficult task. It is unreasonable to expect such people to become independent artificial limb users, and it makes no sense to commit expensive therapy time and expertise to attempting to restore walking ability in patients who will spend most of the day in a chair.

Close collaboration between all members of the clinic team is vital if satisfactory and appropriate rehabilitation is to be achieved. The patient's immediate family and, of course, the patient himself must be involved in discussions on his future lifestyle. The decision to abandon any attempt at prosthetic fitting and subsequent walking training should only come after careful evaluation of the patient, however the suggestion will often come first from the amputee himself. If ambulation with a prosthesis is not considered possible, then a cosmetic, non weight-bearing prosthesis can be prescribed, which may make the patient's self-image more acceptable.

Pre-operative care

The aims of pre-operative physiotherapy are as follows:
(a) To maintain or improve strength and mobility.
(b) To prevent or reduce a flexion contracture at the hip.
(c) To inform the patient and his family of the proposed rehabilitation plan following amputation.
To achieve these aims, the procedures described in the chapter on physiotherapy and the lower limb amputee should be followed as closely as possible.

Hip flexion contractures are often present in this category of patient; however, as previously stated, the prone lying position may not be tolerated. Where this is the case, the patient should be placed in side lying on the unaffected side, thus allowing hip extension to be carried out, either actively by the patient or passively by the physiotherapist. This position also relieves pressure on vulnerable areas of skin which, in the case of the elderly patient, can quickly break down.

The older patient who is about to undergo above-knee amputation will often have difficulty in moving about the bed. A monkey-pole and a rope-ladder attached to the bed will help to reduce this problem. This equipment will also be very helpful in the early post-operative period.

Post-operative care

For the first two to three weeks after surgery physiotherapy should be intensive and enthusiastic. Except in a very few cases, it is difficult to judge at this early stage which amputees will not achieve independence with a prosthesis. In addition to techniques designed to strengthen muscle and maintain full joint mobility, respiratory physiotherapy should be carried out regularly to reduce the risk of post-operative chest infection. A guide to the early post-operative programme is given in Table 21.1. Most of these procedures have been clarified in the previous chapter on physiotherapy but further details are given below:

Table 21.1 Suggested post-operative programme.

1st post-operative day	(a)	Chest physiotherapy.
	(b)	Bed exercises in long sitting.
2nd post-operative day	(a), (b)	As before.
	(c)	Exercises in side lying (patient lies on non-amputated side).
3rd post-operative day	(a), (b), (c)	As before.
	(d)	Up to sit for a short time.
	(e)	Balance training in sitting position.
4th/5th post-operative day	(b), (c), (d), (e)	As before.
	(f)	Start balance and walking training with walking frame.
5/6th post-operative day	(e), (f)	As before.
	(g)	Begin treatment in physiotherapy department.
	(h)	Begin prone lying if the patient's condition will allow it.
7th–10th post-operative day	(i)	Introduce the early walking aid.

(b) Bed exercises for the above-knee amputee

1 Active exercises to strengthen shoulder, upper limb, and trunk muscles.
2 Active exercises to maintain strength and mobility of remaining leg.
3 Static or resisted exercises for the hip extensors. These should be carried out with the patient lying as flat as possible on his back with one pillow beneath his head. The patient then pushes his stump down against the bed, or alternatively against manual resistance given by the physiotherapist.
4 Active and resisted exercises for the hip abductors and adductors with emphasis on the adductors.

There is a tendency for the stump to adopt a flexed, abducted position, and it is therefore unnecessary to encourage active hip flexion at this stage. Great emphasis should be placed on hip extension, and this should be continually encouraged throughout the rehabilitation programme.

(i) The use of the early walking aid

A summary of the benefits derived from its use are:
1 Early training in standing balance and gait.
2 Control of oedema of the stump.
3 Assessment of the patient as a potential user of a definitive prosthesis.
Particular points in relation to its use by the elderly above-knee amputee are described below.

The only device which is regularly used for the above-knee amputee in the U.K. is the pneumatic post-amputation mobility aid (Redhead 1983). It is not suitable for the very short stump as the stump tends to slide out of the pneumatic bag when the patient flexes his hip to initiate the swing phase of walking. Additional suspension by means of a shoulder strap or harness should be used. This strap also assists the patient to swing the device clear of the floor during walking.

The value of the early walking aid in the assessment of the patient's capabilities is enormous, and it is at this stage of the rehabilitation programme that the decision should be made to proceed with prosthetic manufacture and training, or to aim for as much independence as possible from a wheelchair. The judgement of an experienced physiotherapist who has strived to encourage standing balance, weight transference, and walking using the early walking aid, and who has been unsuccessful in achieving these aims, will normally be that the patient is unsuitable for training with a definitive prosthesis. This clinical judgement, along with assessments from the other members of the rehabilitation team, will allow the team to set a realistic rehabilitation goal for the patient.

It is not within the scope of this chapter to describe training in wheelchair use, however it is important to say that although the patient will spend most of the day seated in the chair he should be encouraged to make independent transfers from chair to chair, bed to chair, and chair to toilet, and to make use of a walking frame for a one-legged gait if at all possible.

Gait training

As with the below-knee amputee, the patient will adapt fairly quickly to his prosthesis if he has made good use of the early walking aid. The patient is first taught to don and doff the prosthesis correctly. If the amputee is confused, or has a further physical disability such as a hemiplegia, and cannot dress himself, it is unlikely that he will cope with donning his prosthesis unaided.

Walking training begins with the patient seated between parallel bars, and he is shown how to stand and sit safely. If the knee mechanism is semi-automatic, then the knee should be locked prior to standing and unlocked before sitting down. Balance training in standing is then given; the amputee is taught to transfer weight from one leg to the other and is encouraged to sit on the ischial flare of the prosthetic socket when bearing weight on that side.

Walking should not be allowed until the amputee can achieve standing balance and weight transference with minimal assistance. Gait training begins between the parallel bars and progression should be to the use of two walking sticks. Occasionally an amputee may prefer the stability of a walking frame, but this device does restrict the length of stride which can be taken and hinders a smooth, swing-through gait. Ideally, the patient should eventually discard one walking stick, retaining the stick held in the contralateral hand to the side of amputation. This allows one hand to be free for other purposes such as carrying objects and opening doors. The amputee should be taught to climb stairs, walk over uneven ground and soft surfaces, such as carpet, and negotiate small objects in a confined space, such as would be created by furniture in his own home. It is also important that he is shown how to rise from the floor if a fall occurs. This is best done by 'bumping' along the floor to the nearest stable chair or couch, and then pulling up onto the chair.

It is unlikely that most elderly above-knee amputees will walk great distances. For them, stability, and the ability to transfer safely from chair to chair and to walk with confidence around the house, is more important than having the stamina to walk for miles in a straight line.

Final stage of rehabilitation

A suitable home environment is essential if the elderly amputee is to return there from hospital. A 'home visit' should therefore be made by the appropriate staff (usually the occupational therapist and the physiotherapist) at an early stage of the patient's rehabilitation. Problems, say in the kitchen and bathroom, can be identified, and appropriate modifications made prior to the amputee being sent home. Ease of access to the home should be ensured, and this may mean fitting handrails and stair ramps. A further home visit by the amputee and therapists prior to final discharge is strongly recommended in order that areas of difficulty are clearly established and appropriate training given and/or adaptations made to overcome these.

Finally, it is important that after the amputee's eventual discharge from hospital neither he nor his immediate carers feel cut off from the rehabilitation team. It may be that a period of out-patient physiotherapy will be necessary, or, perhaps even better for the elderly amputee, a period of domiciliary physiotherapy could be considered. Certainly the amputee should be given a name and telephone number for immediate contact should a problem arise. Personal experience has shown that the physiotherapist, having established a long-standing relationship with the amputee and his family, is best suited to the task of accepting such queries.

The care of these patients is a long-term process requiring much knowledge, skill, and patience on the part of the physiotherapist. A real team effort is essential if the amputee is to achieve his full potential, and the opportunity to play a key role in such a team should be accepted eagerly by the physiotherapist.

References

Burgess E. M. & Marsden F. W. (1974) Major lower extremity amputations following arterial reconstruction. *Archives of Surgery* **108**, 655–660.

Department of Health and Social Security. Statistics and research division (1984) Amputation statistics for England, Wales and N. Ireland. Stanmore: DHSS.

Fisher S. V. & Gullickson G. (1978) Energy cost of ambulation in health and disability: a literature review. *Archives of Physical Medicine and Rehabilitation* **59 (3)**, 124–133.

Murdoch G. (1975) Below-knee amputation and its use in vascular disease and in the elderly. In *Recent advances in Orthopaedics* No. 2 (ed. McKibbin B.), pp. 152–172. Edinburgh: Churchill Livingstone.

Redhead R. G. (1983) The early rehabilitation of lower limb amputees using a pneumatic walking aid. *Prosthetics and Orthotics International* **7**, 88–90.

Scottish Health Services Common Services Agency (1982) Scottish hospital in-patient statistics. Edinburgh: SHS.

THROUGH-KNEE AMPUTATION

22

Surgery, Including Transcondylar and Supracondylar Procedures

J. STEEN JENSEN

Introduction

In amputations of the lower limb, much emphasis has been placed on preserving the knee with the purpose of improving gait and control of the prosthesis, preserving shock absorption, and reducing energy consumption. There is no doubt that in young people function is outstanding following below-knee amputation for tumour, trauma, congenital deformities, or other causes. In the author's opinion it is doubtful whether the above considerations apply to elderly patients suffering from peripheral vascular disease.

Level selection

Unfortunately, the knee disarticulation procedure seems to be forgotten in most clinics performing amputation surgery. This is reflected by the vast majority of recent papers reporting below-knee (BK) amputation rates of 50%, or, in the most outstanding and specialized clinics such as that of E. M. Burgess, Seattle, as high as 80%, the remainder being amputated at above-knee (AK) level. The pattern presented by Ebskov (1983) from the Danish Amputation Register seems to be representative of the western world in spite of active attempts since 1980 to reintroduce the through-knee (TK) level through scientific papers and meetings. It is pleasing to note that in Denmark the percentage of TK amputations increased from about 2% in 1978 to 7% in 1983, although some 50% are still amputated above the knee, and only 41% below the knee.

The situation in Denmark is typical of that found in a country without specialized clinics. This means that the amputation surgery is most often performed by surgeons in training, i.e. those with the lowest possible level of qualification, and because of the economic restrictions in modern hospital service the majority of amputations are performed at the end of the daily operation lists and even during the night. Unfortunately, this practice also reduces the quality of supervision and education, because the amputations are in competition with more sophisticated traumatology. Much has been said about the value of exact level assessment by technical methods, but the vast majority of amputations are performed after clinical assessment by surgeons with limited experience.

This is in no way an apologia, but simply a reminder that more effort should be concentrated on teaching the value of level assessment and the importance of considering levels other than AK and BK with regard to amputation for ischaemic gangrene in elderly people.

In spite of these rather depressing circumstances it was possible in Knud Jansen's department to obtain in a series of dysvascular patients the pattern of primary level selection shown in Table 22.1. In this series the number of stump complications was rather high, 20% (Table 22.2) being reamputated after primary TK or BK amputations, leading to the final distribution of levels demonstrated in Table 22.3. The explanations for the high complication rates are improper surgery or inaccurate level assessment, but also that prophylactic antibiotics were not used in this series, or indeed generally throughout Denmark up to 1984.

Table 22.1 Primary levels of amputation in dysvascular patients.

Above-knee	111	(35%)
Through-knee	66	(21%)
Below-knee	143	(45%)

Table 22.2 Stump complications after amputation in dysvascular patients.

Above-knee	2	(2%)
Through-knee	13	(20%)
Below-knee	28	(20%)

Table 22.3 Final levels of amputation in dysvascular patients.

Above-knee	116	(44%)
Through-knee	48	(18%)
Below-knee	101	(38%)

The author's reasons for being a strong advocate for TK amputations since 1980 are based on two observations. The first is that salvage of a BK stump with infection or gangrene nearly always resulted in an AK amputation. The second is the success rate obtained in ambulating those patients with TK amputation.

The most interesting series are those which study patients who were ambulators prior to amputation. With regard to patients living in nursing homes information of this kind is rather uncertain. Consequently only patients admitted from their own homes will be reported here. The striking feature of the results is that successful rehabilitation after TK amputation exceeds or at least equals that obtained with BK amputations (Table 22.4). In consequence of these observations it is strongly advocated that a TK amputation be performed instead of a BK in all cases with doubtful level assessment and in all feeble geriatric patients with weak muscles and poor balance or with contralateral ischaemia. TK amputation is also recommended in those cases usually subjected to AK amputation if the skin is viable, even when some doubt remains.

Table 22.4 Rehabilitation of dysvascular amputees admitted from home.

	Ambulating with prosthesis	Wheelchair-bound	Discharged to nursing home
Above-knee	43 (47%)	25	23
Through-knee	28 (75%)	1	8
Below-knee	64 (70%)	13	14

The only relevant problem in TK prosthetics seems to be the cosmesis, which to some extent is solved by the four-bar knee mechanism. The advantages are, however, very considerable, as the stump is end-bearing, muscle balance is not interrupted, and a strong lever arm for the muscles is preserved. In addition the stump profile ensures rotational stability.

Operative technique

The operative technique is rather simple and can be easily learned by doctors in training. The skin incision is made circumferentially 8–10 cm below the knee joint, or 3–5 cm below the tibial tuberosity, extending through the muscular fascia. The skin-flaps are not marked out initially, but tailoring delayed until skin suture, although later stages require a vertical incision of the patellar tendon. The patellar tendon, the collateral ligaments, and the hamstring tendons are detached from their insertions at the shank. A subfascial dissection anteriorly and on both sides is followed by a broad capsulotomy below the menisci with wide exposure of the joint, as the patella is turned upwards (Fig. 22.1). The cruciates are divided at their distal attachments, the knee is flexed, and the strong posterior capsule divided. Both heads of gastrocnemius are divided 2 cm below joint level in order to preserve the superior geniculate artery.

The popliteal vessels are divided at joint level, whereas the lateral and medial popliteal nerves are pulled gently down, ligated to create a circumscribed neuroma, and finally divided. The menisci are removed, but no bone surgery or synovectomy is performed with the purpose of reducing bleeding. After insertion of an intra-articular suction drain the collateral ligaments are stitched to the cruciates.

The next step is probably the most important in the myodesis, as it concerns the patellar ligament, which is also stitched to the cruciates. The importance lies in the placement of the kneecap, which should be pulled down until the apex of

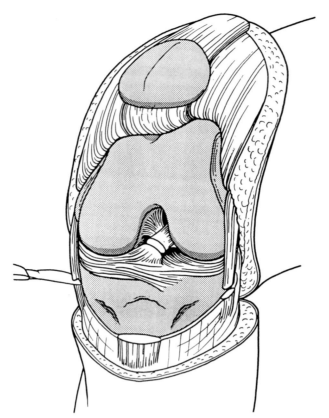

Fig. 22.1 Through-knee amputation technique; ligaments and joint capsule divided close to tibial attachment.

the patella is level with the condyles (Fig. 22.2). This creates a triangular bone profile, which secures the rotational stability and allows end-bearing. It is important not to pull the kneecap any further distally to avoid skin problems over the apex of the patella. Baumgartner (1979) leaves the patella undisturbed, but the loss of power of rectus femoris as a hip flexor must be considered.

Finally, the wound is closed with interrupted stitches using resorbable material subcutaneously and monofilaments in the skin. It is preferable to trim the skin in the manner of sideflaps, as originally described by Kjolbye (1970). This is to place the scar in the unloaded, intercondylar area, and also to avoid skin problems over the prominent medial condyle. These skin-flaps also place less demand on skin below the joint level.

A reamputation rate of 20% was encountered in the author's series, caused by skin necrosis or infection or both. A number of synovial fistulas in the wound between the condyles might be expected. These, however, proved to be a minor problem, as they can be treated conservatively with dry dressing and need not

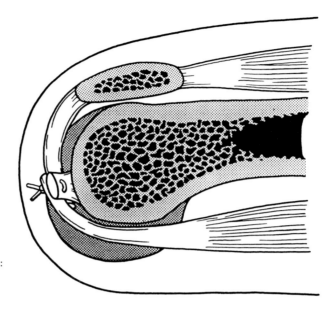

Fig. 22.2 Apex of patella at same level as femoral condyles: patellar tendon sutured to cruciate ligaments.

delay prosthetic fitting. It is the author's belief that the number of skin breakdowns can be diminished by applying prophylactic antibiotics and by avoiding skin tension over the medial condyle. The obvious surgical advantage in the procedure described is the avoidance of bone transection, as bleeding is much less and hence the risk of deep infection is reduced.

Alternative procedures

Several other procedures have been described over the years for amputations in this area. One of these is the Gritti–Stokes procedure (1857, 1870), which involves bone resection through the condylar area and of the ventral aspect of the patella, which is finally transplanted and secured to the exposed condylar bone area. This technique has gained little popularity, probably because of the bone surgery involved and the requirements of almost the same skin length as in TK amputations. Furthermore, the loads at the end of the stump are distributed over a smaller area.

Other procedures are variants of transcondylar amputations. Among these is included the Mazet technique (1968), which involves trimming the posterior part of the condyles vertically in order to avoid a bulbous stump. Once again bone surgery is performed, with the attendant risks already mentioned. Furthermore, the end-bearing area is reduced and suspension made more difficult. The technique should, however, be kept in mind for use in those cases where the skin tension is too pronounced after regular TK performance. This is sometimes experienced in cases with severe pre-operative knee contracture, where shaving, especially of the medial condyle, may be indicated for salvage of the limb at this level.

Further transcondylar or supracondylar techniques are not described as they are considered inappropriate, and in the view of the author do not constitute relevant alternatives to either the TK or a well-performed AK amputation.

Acknowledgement

The illustrations were drawn by Bo Jespersen.

References

Baumgartner R. F. (1979) Knee disarticulation versus above-knee amputation. *Prosthetics and Orthotics International* **3**, 15–19.

Ebskov B. (1983) Choice of level in lower extremity amputation: a nationwide survey. *Prosthetics and Orthotics International* **7**, 58–60.

Gritti R. (1857) Dell' amputazione del femore al terzo inferiore e della disarticolazione del ginocchio. *Annales Universitatis Milano* **161**, 5–32.

Kjolbye J. (1970) The surgery of the through-knee amputation. In *Prosthetic and Orthotic Practice* (ed. Murdoch G.), pp. 255–257. London: Edward Arnold.

Mazet R. (1968) Syme's amputation, a follow-up study of fifty-one adults and thirty-two children. *Journal of Bone and Joint Surgery* **50A(8)**, 1549–1563.

Stokes W. (1870) On supra-condyloid amputation of the thigh. *Medical Chirurgical Transactions, London* **53**, 175–186.

23

The Knee Disarticulation Prosthesis

P. BOTTA & R.F. BAUMGARTNER

Introduction

Through-knee amputations were not performed very frequently until 1970, when special attention was given to the knee disarticulation for vascular patients and special prosthetic fitting techniques were developed. Until these developments conventional prostheses were all mere modifications of above-knee prostheses; the socket was made from a leather corset with lateral steel bars. They rarely took advantage of the special biomechanical features of the through-knee compared with the above-knee stump. Furthermore, comfort, cosmesis, weight, and durability of these prostheses were unsatisfactory.

A socket for a through-knee stump must fulfil the following requirements:

1 There must be total surface contact between the stump and the socket in the upright and in the sitting position.

2 The stump end must be fully end-bearing, as the femoral condyles are designed by nature to put full weight on the tibial plateau and vice versa. By virtue of this, a knee disarticulation stump has excellent proprioception.

3 No ischial seat is provided, and therefore free range of motion of the hip joint in every direction must be possible.

4 The patient must be able to doff and don his prosthesis in the sitting position. This procedure must be easy to learn and be safe, even for geriatric patients in poor physical and mental condition.

5 The socket must not contain windows, straps, laces or belts, and must still provide a snug fit between the stump and the prosthesis.

6 There must be little or no additional length or breadth when compared to the normal anatomy of the thigh and knee.

7 The socket design must permit connection with any suitable prosthetic knee joint designed for through-knee amputation, particularly those with lock mechanisms or with hydraulic swing phase control.

8 The prosthesis should not require special clothing adaptation, nor should it cause increased wear.

9 Cleansing and maintenance of the socket and the prosthesis must be simple.

10 The prosthesis should be as light as possible without loss of safety and durability with regard to the patient's physical activities.

11 Once the socket has been fitted, minor alterations should be possible with a minimum of cost and labour.

12 The manufacturing technique of the socket and the prosthesis must be standardized and readily taught to any qualified prosthetist who is aware of the special anatomy of the stump and the use of plastic materials in prosthetics.

13 The cost of a through-knee prosthesis should not be higher than that of a conventional above-knee prosthesis.

Manufacturing technique

Plaster negative mould

The success of the prosthetic fitting depends largely on the quality of the negative plaster mould. Particular attention must be paid to the weight-bearing area at the end of the stump. In knee disarticulation, both femoral condyles, including the intracondylar notch and the patella, have to be carefully moulded. An exact replica of the weight-bearing area is also necessary in any type of transcondylar amputation. For many years, the authors have used a simple technique which does not require extra effort on the part of the patient. The patient lies in a supine position and has his hip flexed at an angle of about 70°. This technique is safer and more comfortable for the patient and better for the prosthetist than taking the mould in a standing position, as Lyquist (1983) suggests.

First, the skin is covered generously with grease and then with an elastic tube stocking (Tubigrip), prepared for the stump's requirements by suturing its end and by enlarging the proximal half which will cover the thigh, as shown in Fig. 23.1. A snug fit of the Tubigrip is very important in order to obtain an exact plaster replica of the stump. A strip of plaster is prepared to fill first the intracondylar notch and the groove behind the condyles. A second strip of plaster is then placed transversely behind the condyles so that the ends of the strip terminate on both sides at the rim of the patella. These strips are just laid on the stump without any external pressure. As soon as these plaster strips are ready for setting, some layers of plaster of Paris bandages are added, first in a longitudinal direction in order to cover the entire stump end. Only now is a thin layer of circular bandage added, strictly avoiding any constricture. The plaster negative is modelled with both hands, particularly in the area between and above the condyles. Gentle modelling is important proximally, and not on the condyles (Fig. 23.2a). In the same way, the proximal end of the patella is modelled. Even the most sophisticated stump end cushion is unable to compensate for errors made in taking the plaster negative mould.

The socket always goes as high as about one inch (2–3 cm) from the groin in order to provide good stability of the socket in the frontal and transverse planes.

The positive plaster mould obtained with this method usually does not need further correction.

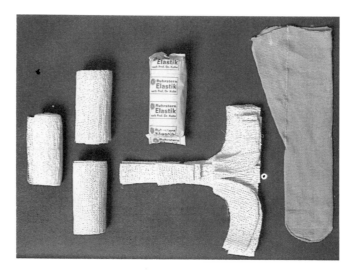

Fig. 23.1 Material needed for the negative mould: elastic plaster bandages, plaster strips, Tubigrip stocking.

(a)   (b)

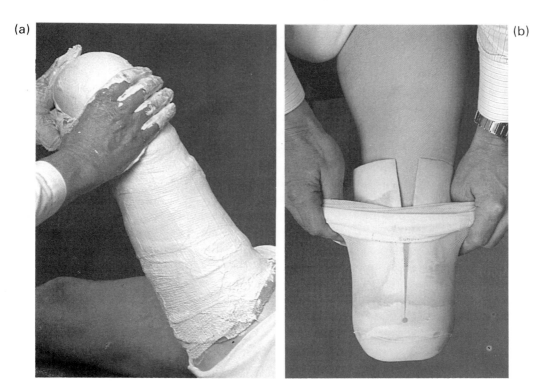

Fig. 23.2 (a) Left hand is modelling the intracondylar notch while the right hand is placed at the dorsal side of the supracondylar area. (b) Patient donning his soft socket.

Socket

The socket is made of two parts, an inner soft liner and an outer socket made of plastic resin. The soft socket serves as an intermediate layer between the bulbous shape of the stump and the conical shape of the outer liner. Furthermore, it serves as a cushion to the distal part of the stump where the bone is covered only by skin. The soft socket also permits easy adaptations to further shrinkage of the soft tissue.

The soft socket is made from closed-cell polyethylene foam. In slim patients, the authors prefer to make the soft socket somewhat longer than the outer liner. If necessary, a slit with holes of 8–10 mm punched at its ends makes doffing and donning of the soft socket easier. In obese patients, or to improve cosmesis, it is sufficient to make the soft socket just for the distal half of the stump (Fig. 23.2b).

Only the distal half of the laminated resin socket is made of hard plastic, whereas the proximal half is made of soft plastic. This gives extra comfort, as the socket adapts closely to the various shapes taken up by the stump in the standing and particularly in the sitting position.

An ischial seat is only indicated if the stump end does not tolerate full end-bearing. With adequate surgical technique, a through-knee stump should be able to tolerate full weight-bearing once the wound has healed. The opportunity to avoid an ischial seat is another great advantage of through-knee compared to above-knee amputation.

Knee joint

There is no ideal knee joint that can be universally employed. In geriatric patients the authors use knee locks with optional locking. New types made from polyethylene or carbon fibres are not heavier than 160–200 g. In younger and active patients, however, these knee joints are not durable enough. The authors therefore use the four-bar linkage knee joints with or without hydraulic swing phase controls which are commercially available, i.e. from Otto Bock or U.S. Manufacturing. Even so, most sophisticated knee joints for knee disarticulation cause a slight overlength of the thigh which must be compensated for by a shortening of the lower leg. This might lead to a loss of contact with the floor in the sitting position. This disadvantage can be neglected in younger patients. In geriatric patients, however, any overlength is avoided if possible. In these cases, the simple solution is a single-axis lateral knee joint as used in upper leg braces. As the soft tissues of the through-knee stump shrink by 1–2 cm, the extra width caused by these joints is tolerable.

In order to save weight the ultralight SACH foot is used. A heavy-duty through-knee prosthesis should not exceed 2200 g. For geriatric patients, the weight can be reduced to 1600 g.

Doffing and donning

Even the geriatric patient is able to doff and don the prosthesis while sitting without any help, even if one arm is paralysed due to hemiplegia. One or two stump socks of nylon, or nylon and wool, must first cover the stump. The soft socket is put on and covered by another nylon stump sock. The patient is then able to fit his stump into the prosthesis without any special effort. In geriatric patients, it is recommended that the anterior part of the soft socket and the prosthesis be marked in order to facilitate correct donning. Finally, the patient is given an instructional leaflet explaining how to handle, wash, and maintain his artificial limb.

Reference

Lyquist E. (1983) Casting the through-knee stump. *Prosthetics and Orthotics International* 7, 104–106.

Further reading

Baumgartner R. (1984) Die Exartikulation in Kniegelenk bei geriatrischen patienten: Indikation, operative Technik und Nachbehandlung. (Through-knee amputation in geriatric patients.) *Medizinisch-orthopädische Technik* **104**, 5–7.

Botta P. & Baumgartner R. (1983) Socket design and manufacturing technique for through-knee stumps. *Prosthetics and Orthotics International* 7, 100–193.

Botta P. & Baumgartner R. (1984) Prothesenversorgung nach Knieexartikulation. (Prosthetic fitting following knee disarticulation.) *Medizinisch-orthopädische Technik* **104**, 8–10.

International Society for Prosthetics and Orthotics (1983) Special issue: through-knee amputation surgery and prosthetics. *Prosthetics and Orthotics International* **7(2)**.

24

The Knee Unit Dilemma with Respect to the Knee Disarticulation Procedure

E. LYQUIST

Introduction

The through-knee (TK) amputation, when performed correctly, provides a long and powerful stump with a bulbous distal part, which is capable of total end-bearing. In spite of obvious advantages, such as length, power, and end-bearing, this level of amputation suffered a lack of popularity until only a few years ago.

As a consequence of stump length, until about 15 years ago none of the prosthetic knee mechanisms available could meet even reasonable cosmetic requirements, nor could they meet the functional demands of the young active amputee. In the past the most commonly used prosthesis for knee disarticulation incorporated a leather socket with side bars and joints identical to those used for conventional below-knee prostheses. The shank was normally made of wood or aluminium (Fig. 24.1). The knee width of such design is significantly increased in relation to the normal knee and becomes cosmetically unacceptable. Furthermore, this type of knee joint does not incorporate a swing phase control, as required for the young and active amputee.

Knee mechanisms designed for the above-knee prosthesis have been used in some instances; the use of such knee mechanisms eliminates the problem of increased knee width, and a swing phase control may also be incorporated. However the length of the prosthetic thigh is increased by some 10–15 cm compared to the normal thigh. Consequently the length of the shank must be reduced correspondingly. This situation influences not only cosmesis but also sitting comfort and gait performance.

The requirements of the TK knee mechanism

A prosthetic knee mechanism for the knee disarticulation must be so designed as to increase the length of the prosthetic thigh no more than 25–35 mm. This increase will not significantly influence cosmesis when the amputee is seated with the knee flexed 90° or more, as no-one sits in a completely symmetrical posture for any significant period of time. Any increase in knee width must be kept to a minimum.

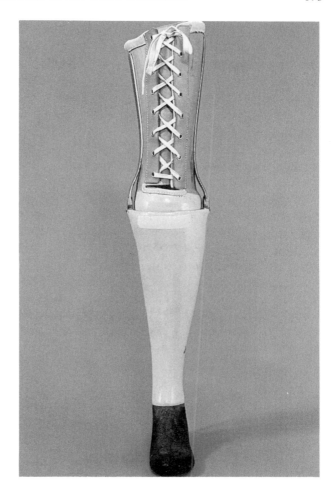

Fig. 24.1 Through-knee prosthesis with leather socket and uniaxial side steels.

As the femoral condyles are left untouched by the amputation a small increase cannot be avoided, but it should be limited to the thickness of the socket material only.

The requirements thus cited indicate that the knee mechanism must be positioned distal to the socket and designed to let the shank move in and under the thigh when the amputee sits. The long and powerful stump dictates that a high degree of voluntary control may be expected, and, furthermore, that a swing phase control will be required by a large number of amputees in order to achieve maximum gait performance. The geriatric amputee, who nowadays represents a large group, may not always be able to control the prosthetic knee, unless it is designed with a high degree of stability; indeed, in some cases a knee lock must be incorporated. In spite of the excellent suspension, which is a product of the anatomy and can be achieved in most cases, the weight of the knee mechanism may present a problem to the geriatric amputee.

Knee mechanisms specially designed for the TK prosthesis

In recent years a number of polycentric knee mechanisms have been specially designed for the knee disarticulation prosthesis. The functional characteristics, advantages, and disadvantages of polycentric knee mechanisms have been described by Radcliffe (1957, 1970), and will not be discussed in any detail in this chapter. One of the advantages of these mechanisms, and in particular of the four-bar linkage, is that the location of the centre of rotation makes it possible to place the device in the shank distal to the socket. Furthermore it can be so designed as to make the shank move in and under the thigh when the knee is flexed.

The first polycentric knee designed for the TK prosthesis was developed at the Orthopaedic Hospital Copenhagen (OHC) and presented in prototype form at the Conference on Priorities in Prosthetic and Orthotic Practice in Dundee in 1969. The OHC knee, manufactured by the United States Manufacturing Company (USMC), is produced in two versions. One version (Fig. 24.2, left) incorporates the USMC Dyna-Plex hydraulic swing control, the second version (Fig. 24.2, right) a pneumatic swing control placed in the tube connecting the knee unit to the foot. Both versions provide good stability but differ in swing phase characteristics and durability. The better swing phase control and durability is offered by the hydraulic-controlled

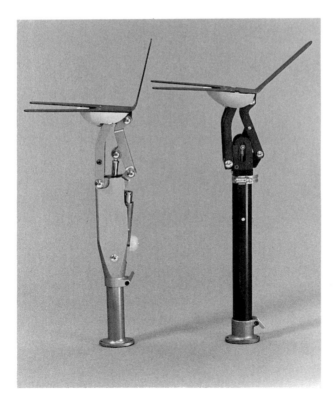

Fig. 24.2 Left, USMC OHC knee incorporating hydraulic swing control. Right, OHC knee with pneumatic swing control.

version. The disadvantages of the OHC hydraulic version is that the Dyna-Plex unit occupies a length of shank such that it cannot be used by the small adult patient. In addition, the space required for the unit makes it difficult to achieve proper cosmesis if the circumference of the calf is less than 30 cm. The OHC hydraulic knee unit is heavy but is nevertheless preferred by many patients. The OHC pneumatic version has smaller dimensions and less weight but is less robust and should not be used for the heavy amputee. With both versions it is possible to keep the increase in thigh length down to 25–30 mm. The cosmesis is acceptable.

A few other mechanisms for knee disarticulation prosthesis are now commercially available, for example the Otto Bock modular polycentric knee (Fig. 24.3), which can be delivered with a knee lock, and the IPOS–Balgrist knee (Fig. 24.4). Recently the Hanger Company has produced a small lightweight four-bar linkage, which may be used even for children. There is no doubt that the improvements in the design of knee mechanisms which have taken place over the last 15 years will increase the popularity of the through-knee amputation and make this level more common.

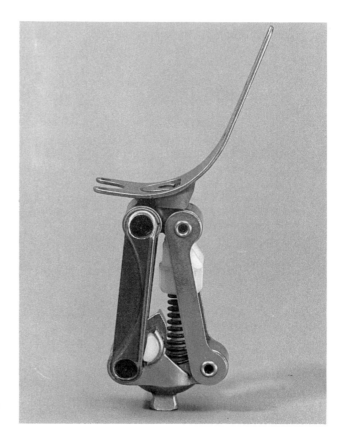

Fig. 24.3 Otto Bock modular polycentric knee.

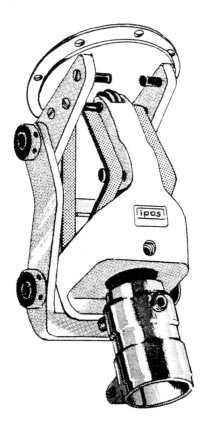

Fig. 24.4 IPOS–Balgrist knee.

References

Radcliffe C. W. (1957) Biomechanical design of an improved leg prosthesis. Berkeley, Ca: University of California. Institute of Engineering Research. Biomechanics Laboratory. (National Research Council. Prosthetics Research Board. Series 11, Issue 33.)

Radcliffe C. W. (1970) Prosthetic-knee mechanisms for above-knee amputees. In *Prosthetic and Orthotic Practice* (ed. Murdoch G.), pp. 225–249. London: Edward Arnold.

25

Biological Mechanisms as Potential Sources of Feedback and Control in Prostheses: Possible Applications

D.S. CHILDRESS

Introduction

Man is a user of tools and machines. Many of these tools, particularly those used in certain sports (e.g. tennis, squash), are used almost as if they were part of the human body itself. They are used without thinking of them. Other devices are more detached but are often controlled with much skill and finesse (e.g. automobiles, aircraft, helicopters). The human operators of these devices become attuned to their machines. This is partly the result of experience (nurture) and partly the result of the structure of the machines and of the operators and of the way they interact (nature).

The science of ergonomics (human factors) has grown up, at least partly, around study of human–machine interaction. One objective is to arrange for the human and the machine to work efficiently together so as not to create too much mental load or stress on the operator: stress that could lead to fatigue and errors. An important aspect of human–machine interaction has to do with design of control interfaces (manipulandums, etc.) and the provision and utilization of appropriate feedback signals. For example, it is much easier to drive an automobile through a steering wheel than through a computer keyboard. While it can be done both ways, one method is inherently more natural. In prosthetics, control can take on many forms; it is necessary to find the modes that are most natural.

Many machines are like habilitation or rehabilitation aids, in that they assist us in doing something we would otherwise find difficult or impossible. These devices often extend our physical capabilities or enhance our sensory abilities. They enable us to fly or to lift enormous loads. It is interesting that most of these machines are designed to be controlled by the hands and/or feet, although voice-controlled machines are beginning to alter this picture.

Prostheses are machines, and the user of a prosthesis can be considered as a human operator of the prosthesis. When the human–prosthesis system operates another machine we have a human operator within a human operator. And the 'inside' operator must usually control the prosthesis without use of hands or feet. Therefore, the operator of a prosthesis is a little different from the typical human–

197

machine systems that scientists have studied.

Because we use our limbs so freely and almost without thinking of them, it seems logical that designers should try to build prostheses such that they too are freely responsive to the will of the user. Some prostheses do seem to respond in natural and reflexive ways; however, many do not. The purpose of this chapter is to take a broad look at biological mechanisms that influence prosthesis control and to consider why some approaches may be better than others.

Empiricism and theory: towards a science of prosthetics

When most sciences begin, they are primarily empirical in nature. What is known is mainly known through experimental trials and practical studies. If a field develops into a science, this experimental information results in theories that unify what it known from experimental work. Important relationships become known as laws. Theory is valuable because it can make predictions concerning what is not known, and these predictions can be tested. If the tests are positive the theory is strengthened. Ultimately, the theories that develop in a field of study form a theoretical framework. This framework can then be used for practical design (e.g. aircraft, bridges) without the design itself being empirical. The theoretical framework thus accelerates and simplifies the design process, and makes it practical and cost-effective as well.

Prosthetics is a field still based largely on experience; perhaps it will always be so. On the other hand, a theoretical structure should be sought that will yield a 'prosthetics science' to guide surgery, prescription, and design.

Past and current control concepts of clinical practice

No attempt is made to identify all concepts; only those that have been of substantial use to amputees and those that relate to the remainder of this chapter are listed. They are:

1 Krukenberg procedure (a surgical procedure making large functional 'fingers' of the radius and ulna and maintaining natural skin sensation — particularly important to blind, bilateral, long below-elbow amputees).

2 Tunnel cineplasty (a surgical procedure that permits muscle force to be brought outside of the body — excellent control for the below-elbow amputee using biceps cineplasty for control of the terminal device).

3 Bowden cable-operated prosthesis (powered through body movement this control method has been particularly successful in upper limb prosthetics).

4 Extension prostheses (a body joint controls the position of the prosthesis which is basically an extension of the limb remnant — examples are the familiar PTB-type below-knee prosthesis and the below-elbow myoelectric prosthesis that is self-suspended).

5 Forced pendular prostheses (above-knee and hip disarticulation prostheses, with

or without joint damping).

6 Externally powered prostheses:

(a) Upper limb prostheses that are velocity-controlled through switches or through myoelectric signals.

(b) Upper limb prostheses controlled by position servomechanisms as originally proposed by Professor David Simpson (1968) at the University of Edinburgh.

These prosthesis control approaches may be divided into two groups: (1) those in which the biological system has substantial natural knowledge of what the prosthesis is doing, and (2) those in which the biological system has limited natural knowledge of what the prosthesis is doing. If these methods are examined closely, the better approaches will be seen to convey direct information to the operator about what the prosthesis is doing, and the best methods convey this information through the body's own mechanisms, particularly the body's own joint proprioceptors and skin sensors.

A theory of control

The theory proposed suggests that the forces, proprioception, and sensation of the body's joints provide the best form of biological control for prostheses. The author refers to this as *Simpson's theory,* because Simpson (1974) first articulated it as a control approach in his work on extended physiological proprioception (e.p.p.). The concept, of course, appears in part or in whole in several kinds of prostheses. The theory may be stated as follows:

'The most natural and most subconscious control of a prosthesis can be achieved through use of the body's own joints as control inputs in which joint position corresponds to prosthesis position, joint velocity corresponds to prosthesis velocity, and joint force corresponds to prosthesis force.'

The statement of this theory may not be in its most general, elegant, or complete form, but it is a reasonable beginning.

Theories that are good theories (i.e. theories worth spending one's time on) have, according to Weinberg (1981), the attributes of simplicity and naturalness. A good theory is also often in agreement with data, although this is not a sufficient or necessary condition for a good theory. A good theory may not always be right, but, as Weinberg has pointed out, it is not wrong to take a viewpoint because one does not have time to examine all theories and one must attach oneself to some spearhead if one is going to be able to push forward the frontier of science.

The theory suggested holds optimally for the PTB-type prosthesis, where the knee can control the prosthesis and can also give the body information about prosthesis position, velocity, and applied forces. It is believed that this accounts, in great measure, for the wide success of this prosthesis. The theory also applies to the Krukenberg procedure, to some extent to the tunnel cineplasty technique, in part to the Bowden cable-controlled prostheses (an often forgotten reason for their success), to the self-suspended below-elbow myoelectric prosthesis, and to the control concept of e.p.p.

What does the theory predict? It predicts that above-knee amputees may perform better in some sense without an artificial knee joint. We know this to be true when above-knee amputees participate in sports (e.g. basketball or hunting), because they frequently lock their knees to provide movement with more speed and assurance. Of course, this is at the expense of cosmetic ambulation. Also, effective sports prostheses for the above-elbow amputee are often designed without an elbow. Seliktar and Kenedi (1976) have investigated the idea of kneeless walking. The theory suggests further investigations along these lines.

There is physiological evidence that the brain controls motor functions without working directly in terms of muscle–joint configurations. Bernstein (1967) has argued cogently that control of human extremities is accomplished in some spatial sense rather than through specific muscle–joint schemata. A person is able to write his name at a blackboard with shoulder muscles in approximately the same way he writes it on a note pad using finger muscles. Therefore, we might expect control of a prosthesis through a shoulder joint to be as good as through an elbow or wrist joint. Doubler and Childress (1984a) showed this to be true for pursuit tracking tasks. Consequently, there is evidence to assume we may optimistically expect good control of prostheses from muscles and joints not normally involved in a movement as typically performed by the non-amputee. The prostheses developed in Scotland by Simpson (1974), using the e.p.p. approach, support this contention.

In extended physiological proprioception, feedback information is provided directly through the control interface (as with automotive power steering). This kind of feedback appears to be very useful in human–machine systems. Childress (1980) has designated this as a feedback classification. If an amputee cannot use this form of input (e.g. in the case of bilateral intrascapulothoracic amputations), and cannot obtain feedback through the interface, it may be necessary to provide supplemental feedback. A corollary of the theory presented would suggest the supplemental feedback be arranged so that pressure in the prosthesis is interpreted as pressure on the body, so that place of the prosthesis is represented by place mapping on the individual, and so that velocity of prosthesis movement gives an actual velocity indication to the user.

Pendular-type prostheses

Above-knee and some hip disarticulation amputees walk with a certain degree of adeptness without complete knowledge of prosthetic joint behaviour. This mobility also may have biological roots. Mochon and McMahon (1980) have proposed a ballistic model for walking in which many aspects of gait are modelled by passive pendular properties of body segments. In their view, muscles primarily play a role in the establishment of initial conditions for the swing phase of gait. Walking on passive, jointed prostheses may therefore be akin to regular non-amputee gait in which muscles play relatively minor roles and in which energy is transmitted to body segments across joints. Indeed, the hip disarticulation amputee who ambulates well makes a strong case for the ballistic walking model, just by the very act of walking.

Surgical–technical design collaboration

The existence of modern surgical procedures suggests a new look be taken at the surgical modification of limbs from the viewpoint of biological control of prostheses. The microsurgery techniques of hand surgeons, vascular surgeons, and neuro-surgeons enhance today's opportunities for improved prosthesis control through co-operation between surgeons, prosthetists, and prosthesis designers.

It is felt that tunnel cineplasty, perhaps microtunnel cineplasty, linked with e.p.p.-type servomechanisms could benefit many amputees. One disadvantage of tunnel cineplasty control of prostheses was that the muscle forces (except for the biceps) were frequently too low to be used effectively. Tunnel cineplastic servos eliminate the force problem while maintaining the output and feedback characteristics of this control mode. New surgical techniques may also be able to eliminate or improve problems associated with keeping tunnels clean and not infected.

Tunnel cineplastic servos offer the advantage of myoelectric control (i.e. local control) with the addition of feedback information through muscle, tendon, and skin concerning force, velocity, and position. They could be used effectively for the partial-hand amputee and the below-elbow amputee, as well as for higher level arm amputations. They might also be applicable for the above-knee amputee where motion would be primarily passive and by transfer of energy through the knee joint from the thigh segment. The cineplastic servo could tune or modify the motion as well as provide feedback about position and velocity. These cineplastic servos would likely take the form suggested by Gow *et al.* (1983) and by Doubler and Childress (1984b). This control approach is illustrated in Fig. 25.1.

Fig. 25.1 Diagram of cineplastic servo concept for prosthesis control. A position servomechanism constructed so that the muscle senses, through the control cable, the position and velocity of the variable under control (power-assisted pulling).

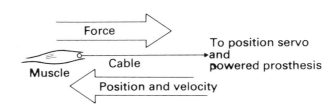

There exist many other possibilities for surgical and technological collaboration on prosthetic control issues. These include muscle transfers, the Van Nes rotation-plasty in limb salvage resections, and muscle divisions for myoelectric or cineplastic use. Scott and Tucker (1968) have considered various surgical techniques that might augment myoelectric control. Marquardt (1980), of course, has been a leader in surgical techniques to assist prosthesis control.

Control through residual muscle contraction

The fact that muscles can be voluntarily contracted makes them prime candidates for prosthesis control input. Besides tunnel cineplasty, the methods used for detection of muscle contraction are: (1) muscle bulge, (2) mechanical impedance change of contracting muscle, (3) electrical impedance change in contracting muscle, (4) electromyography, and (5) acoustic myography.

Muscle contraction can generally be somewhat naturally related to prehension, and this may be called the myoprehension principle. This principle suggests that muscles even quite remote from the hand relate to the act of gripping. One can test this very easily by strong clenching of the fist.

Muscles directly related to the lost function (e.g. biceps to elbow flexion) can be used to control the function in somewhat natural ways. Myoelectric control of the hand and of the elbow has been successfully applied in prosthetics; however, the lack of effective natural feedback in myoelectrically controlled prostheses remains a weakness of this control mode.

Neuroelectric control

Neuroelectric control offers much potential for multiple control channels and multiple sensory channels. Chronic nerve recording and stimulation appears possible. Attractive as this approach seems, it does not seem to be at as high a level of development today as myoelectric control was some 20 years ago. Therefore, neuroelectric control applications, in practice, seem to be several years away.

Conclusion

The way we interface persons with prostheses can profoundly influence human–prosthesis performance, and the proper use of the body's own biological mechanisms appears to be an important method for bringing about performance improvements. In order to make more rapid advancement, a prosthetics science is needed through which work can proceed in an organized manner. It is hoped that such a science will permit effective evaluation of control and design concepts without always requiring that they be empirically tried by amputees. After all, prosthetics design should be similar to design in other fields, and where would bridge building be if every design had to actually be built in order to find out if it would work.

References

Bernstein N. (1967) *The Co-ordination and Regulation of Movements,* p. 54. London: Pergamon Press Ltd.

Childress D. S. (1980) Closed-loop control in prosthetic systems: historical perspective. *Annals of Biomedical Engineering* **8**, 293–303.

Doubler J. A. & Childress D. S. (1984a) An analysis of extended physiological proprioception as a prosthesis-control technique. *Journal of Rehabilitation Research and Development* **21**, 5–18.

Doubler J. A. & Childress D. S. (1984b) Design and evaluation of a prosthesis control system based on the concept of extended physiological proprioception. *Journal of Rehabilitation Research and Development* **21**, 19–31.

Gow D. J., Dick T. D., Draper E. R. C., London I. R. & Smith P. (1983) The physiologically appropriate control of an electrically powered hand prosthesis. Paper presented at ISPO IV World Congress, London, by Bioengineering Unit, Princess Margaret Rose Hospital, Edinburgh, Scotland.

Marquardt E. (1980) The operative treatment of congenital limb malformation — part I. *Prosthetics and Orthotics International* **4**, 135–144.

Mochon S. & McMahon T. A. (1980) Ballistic walking. *Journal of Biomechanics* **13**, 49–57.

Scott R. N. & Tucker F. R. (1968) Surgical implications of myoelectric control. *Clinical Orthopaedics* **61**, 248–260.

Seliktar R. & Kenedi R. M. (1976) A kneeless leg prosthesis for the elderly amputee, advanced version. *Bulletin of Prosthetics Research* **10–25**, 97–119.

Simpson D. C. (1968) An externally powered prosthesis for the complete arm. In *Basic Problems of Prehension, Movement and Control of Artificial Limbs* Proceedings of Symposium **183:35**, 11–17. London: Institute of Mechanical Engineers.

Simpson D. C. (1974) The choice of control system for the multimovement prosthesis: extended physiological proprioception. In *The Control of Upper-Extremity Prostheses and Orthoses* (eds Herberts P., Kadefors R., Magnusson R. & Petersen I.), pp. 146–150. Springfield, Illinois: Charles C. Thomas.

Weinberg S. (1981) From a lecture given at Northwestern University, Evanston, Illinois.

HINDQUARTER/HIP DISARTICULATION

26

Tumour Pathology, Chemotherapy, Radiotherapy, and Surgical Options in the Treatment of Malignant Bone Tumours in the Region of the Hip

S.J. ARNOTT

Primary malignant bone tumours are rare, accounting for just over 1% of all malignancies. Conversely, the skeleton is one of the most frequent sites of metastatic disease. The most common primary malignant tumour of bone is osteosarcoma, followed by chondrosarcoma, Ewing sarcoma, and giant cell tumour. All others are extremely rare (Dahlin 1957).

Management of Ewing tumour

Ewing tumour is a disease about which there has been considerable controversy since the time when it was first described. Initially there was great doubt as to whether it was indeed a true primary tumour of bone or whether it represented an expression of metastatic disease from neuroblastoma. There is, however, now no doubt that Ewing sarcoma is a true tumour of bone arising in childhood, being rare over the age of 15 years. Apart from the controversies which have arisen regarding the true histological nature of this tumour, there have been, and still are, controversies regarding its method of management. The principal areas of controversy have concerned the extent of surgery, if any, which should be performed; the extent of radiotherapy and the dose which should be employed; and the influence of chemotherapy and the agents which should be used.

It was quite evident in the early 1940s that Ewing tumours were highly radiosensitive. However, in spite of the initial rapid response of the primary tumour following irradiation, local recurrence was common, and widespread metastatic disease both to the lungs and to other bones resulted in overall survival rates of less than 10%. These poor results encouraged the use of amputation as the primary method of treatment at this time. However, in the late 1940s increasing doses of radiotherapy began to be employed, and these undoubtedly led to improvements in local tumour control (Fernandez *et al.* 1974). Unfortunately metastatic disease was still a significant problem, and survival rates remained low. It was not until the late 1960s and early 70s, when chemotherapy began to be employed, that local tumour control rates increased substantially, and at the same time survival improved (Pomeroy & Johnson 1975). This improvement was seen particularly in the treatment of patients with limb tumours. However, control of centrally placed primary tumours, especially those arising in the pelvis, continued to be a problem, and this is indeed still the case today.

With the improving efficacy of radiotherapy and chemotherapy, there has been a gradual tendency to employ surgery to a lesser degree. Certainly in the more commonly occurring limb tumours surgery is now used mainly to obtain histological confirmation of the diagnosis. In patients with Ewing sarcoma there are, however, a number of important principles regarding the technique of biopsy which must be followed. The incision should be as short as possible, and should be placed within probable irradiation portals. The biopsy should be taken from a site where soft tissue is interposed between skin and tumour, otherwise there may be problems following the administration of radiotherapy and chemotherapy. Cortical bone removal should be avoided, as this may lead to subsequent pathological fracture.

Following an appreciation that high-dose radiotherapy was needed in spite of the radiosensitivity of this tumour, sophisticated techniques of radiotherapy treatment planning have been developed in order that the highest doses may be restricted to the site of the primary tumour. Initially the whole involved bone needs to be irradiated to moderate dose levels, following which treatment is coned down onto the primary tumour-bearing area and the dose increased to the highest level (Tefft et al. 1978). When the lower limb is being irradiated, circumferential treatment of the limb must be avoided in order to prevent the problem of lymphoedema. For lesions arising in the pelvis, not only does the whole ilium need to be included initially, but also the sacrum in its entirety because of the pattern of spread within the bone. Following a period of four weeks' radiotherapy, shrinkage of the fields may be carried out, excluding the sacrum, but it is rarely possible to avoid irradiating substantial volumes of the ilium itself. This has an important bearing on any surgery which may be subsequently contemplated, particularly since all of these patients will have had adjuvant cytotoxic chemotherapy, which in many cases will enhance the radiation effects on the normal tissues.

Undoubtedly the introduction of cytotoxic chemotherapy has contributed substantially to the improved survival rates which are now achieved in patients with Ewing sarcoma. However, there has been controversy concerning which drugs should be employed. The drugs which have been shown to be most effective in this disease are cyclophosphamide, vincristine and actinomycin D. More recently adriamycin has been introduced, but this drug produces substantially increased toxicity. For some time there was considerable debate as to whether it was necessary to employ adriamycin, but a study carried out by the Ewing's Sarcoma Intergroup in the United States demonstrated quite conclusively that those regimens which incorporated adriamycin were associated with not only a reduced incidence of metastatic disease but also an increased disease-free survival rate (Perez et al. 1981). Indeed the regimens incorporating adriamycin were superior not only to those which included only cyclophosphamide, vincristine and actinomycin D, but also those in which whole-lung irradiation was added to this combination of drugs. Thus, with the use of radiotherapy and chemotherapy it is now possible to achieve disease-free survival rates in excess of 70% in patients with Ewing sarcoma arising in the limbs. Therefore, it is reasonable to continue to adopt the policy that in tumours arising, for example, in the lower limbs the principal role for surgery should remain that of obtaining a biopsy and histological confirmation of the diagnosis. However, treatment by this method for tumours arising in the pelvis is much less satisfactory, and survival rates only of the order of 20% are achieved. Whilst metastatic disease remains a problem, undoubtedly local recurrence occurs with a much higher frequency in pelvic tumours than in peripherally situated lesions. Enthusiastic surgeons have therefore more recently been attempting surgical techniques similar to those employed in pelvic osteosarcoma, and possibly the time has now come for a re-evaluation of the role of surgery with prosthetic replacement in Ewing sarcoma arising in the pelvis.

Management of osteosarcoma

Osteosarcoma is also a tumour arising in young people, the greatest incidence being in the 10–25 years age group. However, it should not be forgotten that, while the incidence falls thereafter to lower levels, it does not fall to zero, and cases of osteosarcoma may therefore be found sporadically in patients of older age. There is, of course, the rise in incidence in patients over the age of 60 due to the association of osteosarcoma with Paget disease. Whilst any bone may be involved by osteosarcoma, the vast majority of such tumours arise around the knee. About 90% arise in long bones, the most common site being the lower end of the femur (Lichtenstein 1977). However, occasionally a sarcoma will arise in a vertebra or the iliac bone. In a long bone the metaphysis is usually affected, but infrequently the tumour may arise more in the mid-shaft region. On rare occasions the tumour may be multicentric.

There have been many changes in the management of patients with osteosarcoma during the past 30 years. However, it is not yet clear which is the optimum approach, and there are still many unanswered questions. The traditional management in the United Kingdom, until relatively recently, was that of the 'Cade' approach (Cade 1955). Basically this consisted of giving patients radical radiotherapy to the primary tumour and then observing them at frequent intervals thereafter, searching during this period for the development of pulmonary metastases. Should the patient remain metastasis-free after an interval of between six and nine months, amputation was carried out. This approach was based on the knowledge that the vast majority of patients would inevitably develop pulmonary metastases, usually within nine months of diagnosis, and that it was therefore inhumane to carry out what would be an unnecessary amputation for most patients (Marcove et al. 1970). A subsequent review of British patients referred to major orthopaedic centres in the United Kingdom seemed to confirm that delayed amputation preceded by radical radiotherapy was at least as effective as immediate amputation (Sweetnam *et al.* 1971). However, this review also indicated that subsequent amputation might be required even in the presence of metastases for painful local tumour recurrence or pathological fracture, and indeed the un-controlled primary tumour arising in patients who had been so heavily irradiated caused many surgical problems. A further difficulty associated with this approach to treatment was the problem of persuading patients who were making apparently good progress to have a subsequent amputation. A further interesting finding of this study was that it highlighted the fact that younger patients, and those with sarcomas arising in Paget disease, have the poorest survival.

It was therefore not surprising when in the early 1970s, following enthusiastic reports of the value of chemotherapy, the Cade technique was abandoned. One of the first reports indicating the effectiveness of chemotherapy was by Jaffe (1972), which initially described the effectiveness of methotrexate in patients with metastatic disease. Subsequently this drug regimen was used in an adjuvant fashion at the time of primary management (Jaffe *et al.* 1974). In this latest study high doses of methotrexate were advocated, as it was implied that low doses were ineffective. Primary amputation was recommended for all patients, as it was alleged that any tumour poorly controlled by radiotherapy might act as a focus for the development of drug-resistant cells. Further reports began to appear at about the same time which demonstrated the effectiveness of other drugs such as adriamycin (Cortes *et al.* 1974) and combinations of drugs consisting of cyclophosphamide, vincristine, melphalan and adriamycin (Sutow *et al.* 1975). However, in all these studies comparisons were made with historical controls, and the results were reported prematurely. This led initially to great optimism regarding the effectiveness of adjuvant chemotherapy, but also some degree of confusion concerning whether the apparent improvement in survival was really due to the use of adjuvant chemotherapy.

In the mid-1970s this confusion was heightened by two further studies. One was carried out by the Medical Research Council comparing the effectiveness of relatively low-dose methotrexate combined with vincristine with the same combination of drugs combined with adriamycin. Nearly 200 patients were included in this study. No obvious difference between the two chemotherapy regimens in terms of either survival or the incidence of metastases was discovered, and the results in many respects seemed similar to what one might have expected from amputation alone. A second report describing a trial carried out at the Mayo Clinic also suggested that there was no improvement from the use of adjuvant chemotherapy, and that for a variety of reasons survival rates in patients managed by primary surgery alone had improved over the years without the use of adjuvant cytotoxic chemotherapy (Taylor *et al.* 1978, Edmonson *et al.* 1980). A number of other studies performed at this time similarly failed to demonstrate any benefit from the use of adjuvant cytotoxic chemotherapy. Several reasons may be considered to account for this. One explanation might be that the natural history of the disease was changing, although there was little evidence of this. Alternatively, variations in patient selection could have influenced the results reported by specialist centres. In addition, the introduction of sophisticated screening techniques for metastases would have now excluded some patients who would have been included in historical studies. Further, more aggressive salvage treatment for metastases, including multiple thoracotomies, was by now being widely adopted. Certainly, the increased public awareness of this disease meant that patients were being referred at an earlier stage, with tumours which were less locally advanced, and which, as a result, might have been associated with a lower frequency of metastases.

However, undoubtedly chemotherapeutic agents had been demonstrated to be effective in patients with metastatic disease, and further studies continued to be carried out. Importantly, in the late 1970s alternative approaches to management began to be investigated. These included a move away from primary amputation as the treatment of choice towards attempts at limb conservation if at all possible. These approaches included the use of pre-operative chemotherapy in order to make limb salvage surgery possible. One of the first exponents of this technique was Rosen (Rosen et al. 1976) in the Memorial Hospital in New York, who over the years developed chemotherapeutic regimens of increasing aggression. His T4 and T7 protocols which appeared in the 1970s were reported as showing improved survival (Rosen et al. 1979). However, the latest T10 protocol has been associated with the best survival of all (Rosen et al. 1982). The principle behind this approach is that pre-operative chemotherapy is given, after which limb salvage surgery is performed. During the period of chemotherapy a specific endoprosthesis is fashioned. At the time of surgery the degree of tumour destruction in the specimen is assessed and subsequent chemotherapy is tailored according to this response. If the response has been good the patient continues with the same chemotherapy regimen, but if the response is poor an additional drug, cisplatin, is introduced. The latest reports of this study have indicated quite outstanding survival figures. Unfortunately at no other centre in the world have such good results been obtained, and there has been much controversy concerning the validity of the Memorial results (Lange & Levine 1982). However, if one examines the results which are now obtained from many different international centres, it can be seen that long-term disease-free survival is being achieved in approximately 50% of patients compared to around 20% in historical series. One important recent randomized trial carried out by the Multi-Institutional Osteosarcoma Group has confirmed this expected survival of 50% (Link et al. 1985). This was a moderately large series of 156 patients comparing the use of initial front-line chemotherapy followed by conservation surgery with the use of cytotoxic chemotherapy if and when metastases developed. The two-year relapse-free survival in patients who received front-line chemotherapy was 56%, compared with only 18% in those patients in whom cytotoxic chemotherapy was delayed. For those patients who refused any cytotoxic chemotherapy the survival was poorer, being only of the order of 10%. A large number of studies are now being conducted throughout the world investigating the use of adjuvant cytotoxic chemotherapy given pre-operatively together with conservation surgery if at all possible. The aims of these studies have been to investigate the effectiveness of cytotoxic chemotherapy together with the question of how long it is necessary to administer chemotherapy. All of the regimens used in osteosarcoma are highly toxic and expensive, and it would be of considerable benefit if the chemotherapy programmes could be curtailed as much as possible. For example, this is one of the aims of a current multicentre European investigation of patients with osteosarcoma (European Osteosarcoma Intergroup 1983).

Conclusion

As a result of the many developments which have occurred in the management of osteosarcoma, the place of radiotherapy remains unclear, except in certain well-defined situations. There can be no doubt that irradiation of the primary tumour is of value in the presence of metastatic disease, although the possible use of surgery must not be forgotten. In certain anatomical sites, surgery for the primary tumour may not be a feasible proposition, for example when tumours arise in the vertebrae. Undoubtedly, however, for the majority of patients the approach should be that of cytotoxic chemotherapy given pre-operatively followed by surgery, which should be conservative in type if at all possible.

Thus, in the two types of bone tumours where chemotherapy and radiotherapy have made a large impact, one of the principal benefits associated with treatment has been the avoidance of amputation for many patients. While for a Ewing tumour the emphasis is on chemotherapy and radiotherapy, the use of surgery, particularly in pelvic tumours, requires re-evaluation. Radiotherapy now has little place in the management of patients with osteosarcoma. High-dose pre-operative chemotherapy is the treatment of choice, followed by surgery with conservation of the limb whenever possible. The use of these high-dose chemotherapy regimens does not, in the vast majority of patients, cause additional problems related to the insertion of the prosthesis or with wound healing.

References

Cade S. (1955) Osteogenic sarcoma: a study based on 133 patients. *Journal of the Royal College of Surgeons of Edinburgh* 1, 79–111.
Cortes E. P., Holland J. F., Wang J. J., Sinks L. F., Blom J., Senn H., Bank A. & Glidewell O. (1974) Amputation and adriamycin in primary osteosarcoma. *New England Journal of Medicine* 219, 990–1000.
Dahlin D. C. (1957) *Bone Tumors*. Springfield, Illinois: Charles C. Thomas.
Edmonson J. H., Green S. J., Ivins J. C., Gilchrist G. S., Cregan E. T., Pritchard D. J., Smithson W. A. & Dahlin D. C. (1980) Methotrexate as adjuvant treatment for primary osteosarcoma (Letter). *New England Journal of Medicine* 303, 642–643.
European Osteosarcoma Intergroup Protocol 80831 (1983) Randomised pilot study to assess the

tolerability and efficacy of two drug combinations in patients with osteosarcoma. Brussels.

Fernandez C. H., Lindberg R. D., Sutow W. W. & Samuels M. L. (1974) Localised Ewing's sarcoma — treatment and results. *Cancer* **34**, 143–148.

Jaffe N. (1972) Recent advances in the chemotherapy of metastatic osteogenic sarcoma. *Cancer* **30**, 1627–1631.

Jaffe N., Frei E. (III)., Traggis D. & Bishop Y. (1974) Adjuvant methotrexate and citrovorum-factor treatment of osteogenic sarcoma. *New England Journal of Medicine* **291**, 994–997.

Lange B. & Levine A. S. (1982) Is it ethical not to conduct a prospectively controlled trial of adjuvant chemotherapy in osteosarcoma? *Cancer Treatment Reports* **66**, 1699–1704.

Lichtenstein L. (1977) *Bone Tumors*, 5th edition. St. Louis: C. V. Mosby Co.

Link M., Goorin A. & Miser A. (1985) The role of adjuvant chemotherapy in the treatment of oseteosarcoma of the extremity: preliminary results of the multi-institutional osteosarcoma study *Proceedings of the American Society of Clinical Oncology.*

Marcove R. C., Mike V., Hajek J. V., Levin A. G. & Hutter R. V. P. (1970) Osteogenic sarcoma under the age of twenty-one. A review of one hundred and forty five operative cases. *Journal of Bone and Joint Surgery* **52A**, 411–423.

Pomeroy T. C. & Johnson R. E. (1975) Prognostic factors for survival in Ewing's sarcoma. *American Journal of Roentgenology, Radium Therapy and Nuclear Medicine* **132(3)**, 598–606.

Perez C. A., Tefft M., Nesbit M., Burgert E. O., Vietti T., Kissane J., Pritchard D. J. & Gehan E. A. (1981) The role of radiation therapy in the management of non-metastatic Ewing's sarcoma of bone: report of the intergroup Ewing's sarcoma study. *International Journal of Radiation Oncology, Biology and Physics* **7(2)**, 141–149.

Rosen G., Murphy M. L., Huvos A. G., Guiterrez M. & Marcove R. D. (1976) Chemotherapy, en bloc resection and prosthetic bone replacement in the treatment of osteogenic sarcoma. *Cancer* **37**, 1–11.

Rosen G., Marcove R. C., Caparros B., Nirenberg A., Kosloff C. & Huvos A. G. (1979) Primary osteogenic sarcoma: the rationale for pre-operative chemotherapy and delayed surgery. *Cancer* **43**, 2163–2177.

Rosen G., Caparros B., Huvos A. G., Kosloff C., Nirenberg A., Cacacio A., Marcove R. C., Lane J. M., Mehta D. & Urban C. (1982). Pre-operative chemotherapy for osteogenic sarcoma: selection of post-operative adjuvant chemotherapy based on the response of the primary tumor to pre-operative chemotherapy. *Cancer,* **49**, 1221–1230.

Sutow W. W., Sullivan M. P. & Fernbach D. J. (1975) Adjuvant chemotherapy in primary treatment of osteogenic sarcoma: A south-west oncology group study. *Cancer* **36**, 1598–1602.

Sweetnam R., Knowelden J. & Seddon H. (1971) Bone sarcoma: treatment by irradiation, amputation or a combination of the two. *British Medical Journal* **2**, 363–366.

Taylor W. F., Ivins J. C., Dahlin D. C., Edmonson J. H. & Pritchard D. J. (1978) Trends and variability in survival from osteosarcoma. *Mayo Clinic Proceedings* **53**, 695–700.

Tefft M., Razek A., Perez C., Burgert E. O., Gehan E. A., Griffin T., Kissane J., Vietti T. & Nesbit M. (1978) Local control and survival related to radiation dose and volume and to chemotherapy in non-metastatic Ewing's sarcoma of pelvic bones. *International Journal of Radiation Oncology, Biology and Physics* **4(5–6)**, 367–372.

27

Interferon Treatment of Primary Osteosarcoma

U. NILSONNE

Introduction

A clinical trial with interferon as adjuvant treatment of osteosarcoma was begun in 1971 in the Karolinska Hospital, Stockholm. At that time interferon was known only as an antiviral substance which is produced by any cell infected by viruses. Thus interferon may be defined as a physiological substance belonging to the immune defence of an organism: chemically interferon is a glycoprotein of low molecular weight.

There are several hypotheses that viruses might be carcinogenic. In the case of osteosarcoma it has been possible to induce osteosarcoma-like tumours in the hamster and the rat using certain viruses. Electron microscopy of human osteosarcoma has revealed particles which have been interpreted as viruses. Thus it was considered that if osteosarcoma has something to do with a virus infection it would be justifiable to perform a trial with interferon as adjuvant therapy, particularly in view of the poor prognosis.

Clinical trial and results

Human leucocyte interferon produced in Professor Kari Cantell's laboratories, Helsinki, was used in the trial. However, it is now known that many types of interferon exist: the α-interferon is the leucocyte type; β-interferon is produced by, for example, fibroblasts and γ-interferon from cells immunologically active. With recombinant DNA technology it should soon be possible to produce interferon of all types in large quantities and at a relatively low cost. Since 1971 60 cases of classical osteosarcoma have been treated with interferon as adjuvant therapy. The series is not randomized; it is a consecutive series of all cases of osteosarcoma in the Karolinska Hospital not having metastases at the time of diagnosis. The treatment consisted of surgical removal of the tumour, mainly by amputation, but in some cases by wide local resection. Interferon has been the only adjuvant treatment; neither chemotherapy nor irradiation has been used. Interferon was given for 18 months in a dose of 3 000 000 interferon units daily or every second

214

day as an intramuscular injection. There were no side-effects of clinical importance, and in no case did the treatment have to be interrupted.

The present five-year survival is about 50% as compared to 18% in the historical controls. For the concurrent controls, namely osteosarcoma patients treated elsewhere than in the Karolinska Hospital and without interferon, the survival rate for patients treated with chemotherapy is also about 50%. In 18 cases local tumour resection and some form of reconstruction was performed. In four of these cases local recurrence necessitated a later amputation.

During the course of the clinical trial, Dr Hans Strander, who is internationally well known in interferon research, showed that interferon does not only have an antiviral effect. He was able to demonstrate that in *in-vitro* systems of osteosarcoma cell lines interferon has a very marked inhibitory effect on cell division, thus blocking the growth of osteosarcoma cells. He was also able to show that interferon stimulated the activity of the lymphocytes styled 'natural killer cells', which have an antitumoral effect. However, the mechanisms in the antitumoral activity of interferons are not well known.

Effect of interferon on transplanted osteosarcoma

Human tumours can now be studied after transplantation to athymic nude mice. As these experimental animals do not reject allogenic grafts the transplanted tumour has a capacity to grow with unchanged characteristics in the new host. Such a system has been used to study the effect of interferon on transplanted human osteosarcoma. Interferon given to the nude mice caused slowing down of the growth of the tumour. However, the sensitivity of the tumour to interferon varied from slowing down to total cessation of growth. It can also be demonstrated that after interruption of interferon treatment the tumour regains the ability to grow. Further, the effect of interferon is related to dose. Thus, a lower dose of interferon might only reduce the growth rate of the tumour, whereas a higher dose may bring growth to a standstill.

These experiments show that interferon has a significant influence on transplanted human osteosarcoma. The effect seems to be cytostatic rather than cytotoxic and is also apparently dose-related. It is not yet possible to be precise as to what clinical conclusions can be drawn from these observations. Probably it would be desirable to increase the interferon doses so far used and perhaps also prolong the duration of treatment. It is not yet known if this can be performed without undesired side-effects.

Summary

Experimental evidence has been provided that interferon may block the growth of osteosarcoma cells. In the clinical trial conducted at the Karolinska Hospital the five-year survival is of the order of 50%, a figure comparable with most series where chemotherapy has been used. The choice between amputation and local tumour resection requires to be refined and more precise criteria developed.

Further reading

Brosjo O., Bauer H. C., Brostrom L. A., Nilsonne U., Nilsonn O. S., Reinholt F. P., Strander H. & Tribukait B. (1985) Influence of human alpha-interferon on four human osteosarcoma xenografts in nude mice. *Cancer Research* **45 (11Pt. 2),** 5598–5602.

Hofman V., Groscurth P., Morant R., Cserhati M., Honegger H. P. & von Hochstetter A. (1985) Effects of leukocyte interferon (*E. coli*) on human bone sarcoma growth *in vitro* and in the nude mouse. *European Journal of Cancer and Clinical Oncology* **21(7),** 859–863.

Strander H. A. (1986) Interferon in the treatment of human neoplasm. *Advanced Cancer Research* **46,** 1–265.

28

Skeletal Biomechanics Following Radical Excision

J.P. PAUL & S.E. SOLOMONIDIS

Introduction

The loading of the pelvis due to muscular forces in standing or walking has been little studied for the normal individual. Goel and Svensson (1977) undertook a mathematical analysis of the forces on the pelvis in a normal individual based on cadaveric measurements, making a series of assumptions related to the forces transmitted by particular muscles and ligaments, and considering only the frontal view in one-legged standing. Because of the assumptions made, their results can be treated as order of magnitude data only. Fig. 28.1 is a modification of Figure 2 of their manuscript to show the system from which the significant forces were determined. The forces at the hip joint and in the corresponding musculature are not shown, since the 'free body' used is pelvis plus leg. The significant forces are the sacroiliac joint force and the tensions in the iliolumbar ligament, the sacroiliac ligament, the sacrospinous ligament, and the symphysis pubis. The hemipelvis can therefore be seen to be effectively a beam supported at the sacroiliac joint and at the symphysis pubis, and loaded by the hip joint force and by the tensions in the appropriate ligaments. Therefore, any components introduced to replace excised bony structure on the pelvis must have an intrinsic strength and provision for attachment to the pelvis sufficient to carry these loads in bending.

Effect of excision of part of femur

In the case of radical excision of a substantial part of the head and shaft of the femur, the usual consequence is the elimination or the reduction to very small values of the forces transmitted to the femur by the muscles normally having origin or insertion there. Since it has been shown clearly by Paul (1967), Morrison (1968), and Proctor and Paul (1981) that the major part of the force developed at any joint in the leg is due to muscular action, the patient receiving a long bone replacement will, necessarily, transmit a smaller amount of force at the joint in question. It may be assumed, however, that the two joint muscles, for instance between pelvis and shank, may still be effective, so that the relief of joint loading may not be of the magnitude which might be expected. The other effect of absence of muscular tension is that the skeletal implant requires to transmit all of the load due to bending developed, for instance, by the offset of hip joint force from the axis of the shaft of femur corresponding to the length of the femoral neck. However, in the absence of any known biomechanical analysis of the gait of such patients, it is not possible to predict with any certainty whether this would increase or reduce the stressing of the implant relative to those inserted in the more normal circumstance of degenerative joint disease.

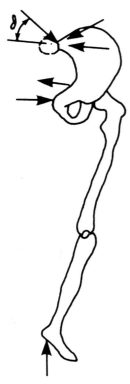

Fig. 28.1 Forces on the pelvis in one-legged standing. Adapted from Goel & Svensson (1977).

Effect of amputation

Where complete ablation is undertaken at the level of the proximal femur or at hip disarticulation level, substantial changes are introduced in the transmission of load to the remaining pelvis on the amputated side. There have been a few studies of the locomotion of such patients in which biomechanical data have been assessed, allowing the calculation of the loads transmitted at the prosthesis–socket interface and consequently at the socket–trunk interface (Solomonidis *et al.* 1977, Solomonidis & Berme 1978).

Unpublished data from S. E. Solomonidis are the basis for Fig. 28.2, showing the temporal factors relating to gait of a patient with a hip disarticulation prosthesis. The contrast between the durations of swing and stance phases for the prosthesis and the sound leg are immediately obvious. It is interesting to note that whereas the total time spent in double support, i.e. approximately 24% of the gait cycle, relates closely to that for normal individuals walking at moderate speed, there is a gross inequality between the two periods of double support, with that following heel contact on the prosthetic side being very much shorter than the other period. This appears to correspond to the major problem experienced by this type of amputee, i.e. finding enough time to accelerate his limb forward sufficiently rapidly to achieve ground contact before toe-off of the sound leg.

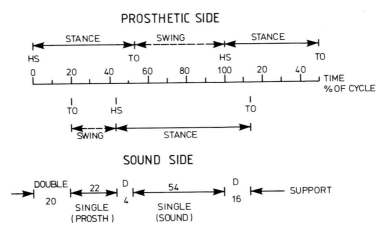

Fig. 28.2 Timing of events in the cycle of walking in a straight line on a level surface for an amputee with a hip disarticulation prosthesis.

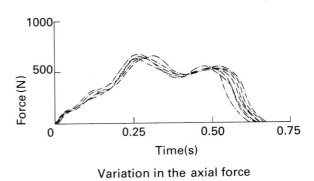

Fig. 28.3 Longitudinal force component on the shank of the prosthesis for several cycles of level straight-line walking by a hip disarticulation amputee. Adapted from Solomonidis & Berme (1978).

Variation in the axial force

It will be noted that the stride indicated and the one following are somewhat dissimilar in temporal factors. This phenomenon is better illustrated in Fig. 28.3, from Solomonidis and Berme (1978), where the differences in time of occurrence of maximum axial force for a number of steps from one disarticulation amputee are shown. These authors reported the results of tests conducted on three patients following disarticulation amputation in which a pylon force transducer (Berme *et al.* 1975) was incorporated into the shank of the prosthesis. This transducer measured six quantities corresponding to the three components of force about reference axes of the transducer and the moment about these axes. From the curves of flexion/extension moment at the prosthetic and contralateral side reported by these authors, it is possible to produce Fig. 28.4, which shows the variation with time of the hip moment in flexion and extension, indicating a comparison between the prosthetic and the sound side curves in respect of shape, magnitude, and duration. For the sound side, these moments will be transmitted by tension in the flexor or extensor muscles, whereas on the prosthetic side they must be transmitted to the socket by loads developed in the flexion limiter or extension bumper in association with the joint force. The transmission of these socket forces to the trunk of the patient will be through the substantial abdominal and posterior surfaces of contact between socket and trunk. The force transmitted at the prosthetic hip joint will largely be transmitted through the ischium to the pelvis, corresponding to a significant change from the loading on the sound side. If the pelvis is intact on the amputated side, this loading will be transmitted to the sacroiliac joint, but may tend to give higher stresses in the pelvis on the operated side than would load transmission through the acetabulum. During the walking cycle the abduction/adduction moments transmitted at the hip by the prosthesis would tend to cause tilting of the socket on the trunk as viewed from the front. The values of these moments reported by Solomonidis and Berme are very variable between test subjects, but the maximum values are of the same order of magnitude as the moments transmitted in normal individuals and correspond to the longitudinal prosthetic load being offset from the centre of mass of the body. Such moments will be easily transmitted in a well-fitted socket by variation in interface pressure on the sides of the prosthesis.

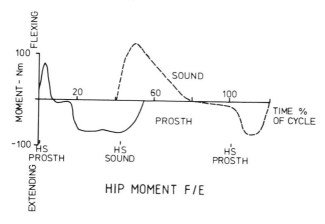

Fig. 28.4 Flexion–extension moments at the prosthetic and contralateral hips of a hip disarticulation amputee walking in a straight line on a level surface.

Conclusion

It is seen then that in the pelvis of patients suffering radical surgery, these stresses may exceed those in the pelvises of normal individuals, and therefore considerable evidence of bony resorption would not be expected provided the patients maintained a reasonable level of activity.

References

Berme N., Lawes P., Solomonidis S. & Paul J. P. (1975) A shorter pylon transducer for measurement of prosthetic forces and moments during amputee gait. *Engineering in Medicine* **4(4)**, 6–8.

Goel V. K. & Svensson N. L. (1977) Forces on the pelvis. *Journal of Biomechanics* **10(3)**, 195–200.

Morrison J. B. (1968) Bioengineering analysis of force actions transmitted by the knee joint. *Biomedical Engineering* **3**, 164–170.

Paul J. P. (1967) Forces transmitted by joints in the human body. *Proceedings of the Institute of Mechanical Engineers* **(3J)**, 8–15.

Proctor P. & Paul J. P. (1981) Ankle joint biomechanics. *Journal of Biomechanics* **15 (9)**, 627–634.

Solomonidis S. E. & Berme N. (1978) Locomotion of the hip disarticulation amputee. *Engineering in Medicine* **7 (1)**, 17–20.

Solomonidis S. E., Loughran A. J., Taylor J. & Paul J. P. (1977) Biomechanics of the hip disarticulation prosthesis. *Prosthetics and Orthotics International* **1**, 13–18.

29

Design of Prosthetic Implants (in Relation to the Hip)

J.T. SCALES

Introduction

Amputation is psychologically, physically and financially an undesirable operation which, in the majority of cases in which it is performed, is the only clinically acceptable procedure. There is, however, a small group of potential amputees, variously estimated at between 0.5 and 2.5%, for whom limb preservation using a custom-made endoprosthesis is now a possible and preferred treatment. Paradoxically, the evolution of the Stanmore Limb Preservation Programme started with an amputation. A boy aged 12 years whose entire left leg was affected with fibrous dysplasia (Seddon & Scales 1949) was in 1949 given a proximal femoral replacement hand-carved in low molecular weight polyethylene* (Fig. 29.1). This made possible a mid-thigh amputation rather than a disarticulation at the hip joint. The patient, now aged 48 years, has led an active life working as a foreman tool-maker and is on his 'feet' most of the day. He also does his own inside and outside house maintenance.

Between July 1949 and 31st March 1985, 643 temporary and permanent endoprostheses have been designed and made by the Department of Biomedical Engineering at Stanmore and used in 615 patients with conditions affecting the upper limb, pelvis and lower limb (Table 29.1). In 11 of the patients a temporary implant was subsequently replaced with a permanent one. Seven of the patients had two major implants; in ten patients there has been revision of a permanent implant because of local recurrence, mechanical failure of the implant, or loosening. The conditions treated between 1949 and 1985 are shown in Table 29.2. The progress of the patients has been followed up either personally by the author or by the surgeons involved or their successors. This review deals with some of the design features of the 217 endoprostheses used in the treatment of conditions of the pelvis and proximal femur.

*'Alkathene', made by Imperial Chemical Industries PLC, Plastics Division, Welwyn Garden City, Herts.

222

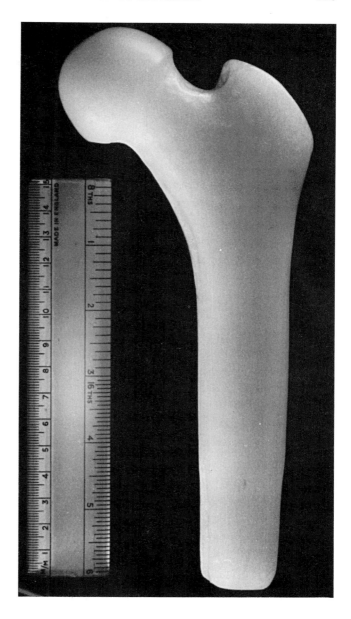

Fig. 29.1 Hand-carved polyethylene femoral replacement.

General considerations in the design of endoprostheses

The bones can transmit forces of considerable magnitude. It has been estimated that in Olympic high jumping the load on the hip joint can reach 12 times body weight and on the knee joint 24 times body weight (Smith 1975). Fortunately the intermittent loading on an endoprosthesis is considerably less and of the order of

Table 29.1 Prostheses inserted — sites (including 11 temporary prostheses).

	to 31.3.85
Hemipelvis and hip	10
Total femur, hip and knee	13
Proximal femur and hip	194
Mid-shaft of femur	7
Distal femur and knee	231
Distal femur, knee and proximal tibia	3
Proximal tibia and knee	78
Distal tibia and ankle	2
Total humerus and elbow	12
Proximal humerus	74
Distal humerus	17
Distal radius	2
Total	643

1–3 times body weight through the hip joint and 2–4 times body weight at the knee joint, although accidental loadings may be higher. The fluctuating load will be applied 1.0–2.5 million times per year. A permanent implant used in a young patient may be required to function for upwards of 70 years without planned maintenance in a hostile environment containing 0.9% sodium chloride and other reactive chemicals at 37 °C. Most endoprostheses replace a joint. The bearing surfaces of these artificial joints degrade or wear with the production of products that may cause a local foreign body response or systemic effects such as, for example, sensitivity to metallic elements. In the long term the soft tissues rubbing on the non-articulating parts of a prosthesis can produce abrasion products that contribute

Table 29.2 Conditions treated — cases.

	to 31.3.85
Bone tumours and destructive lesions of bone	496
Trauma, with or without failed surgery	21
Degenerative and developmental lesions, with or without failed surgery	115
Total	632

to a reactive tissue or systemic response. In the adult the prosthesis can be considered to be a passive device that attempts to restore a defect and the function of the limb by acting as a hinged distance piece mechanically stabilized in the remaining bone. In the child a more complex situation prevails in that the device in a long bone must be active and enable growth in length of the limb to keep pace with that of the remaining limb. This presents a complex problem since the growth of bone is a three-dimensional phenomenon with, for example, changes in the spatial relationship of the marrow cavity of a long bone.

The design of custom-made endoprostheses is determined by the site of the lesion, the pathological condition, the extent of bone involvement and the need to allow for a salvage procedure, i.e. revision or amputation, should there be a failure of the fixation of the prosthesis in the bone, recurrent dislocation of the hip joint, mechanical failure of a component, infection, local recurrence of disease or skin breakdown. It is not always possible to determine from radiological and other investigations prior to operation the extent of involvement of bone and soft tissues by a disease process such as osteosarcoma or chondrosarcoma. Patients should be warned that the final decision as to whether amputation or prosthetic replacement is the appropriate treatment can in some cases only be taken at operation. Further, they should appreciate that, while limb preservation using a prosthesis offers considerable advantages as regards the quality of life compared with amputation, there is a possibility of certain complications that may ultimately lead to a more extensive procedure than if amputation had been the primary treatment. The design of custom-made prostheses requires both clinical and measurement radiographs. Clinical radiographs are needed since the definition of measurement radiographs may not be adequate to determine the extent of a lesion. The making of measurement radiographs is a critical step in the design and ultimate performance of the endoprosthesis. Prostheses are expensive to manufacture, and the greater the length of a partial bone replacement the more critical becomes the determination of dimensions of the remaining part of the bone if secure long-term fixation is to be achieved.

Prostheses for the pelvis

Lesions of the pelvic bones, if of limited extent, i.e those which do not involve the medial third of the ilium, can sometimes be treated by excision of the lesion and endoprosthetic replacement. It is impossible from anteroposterior and lateral radiographs to make a satisfactory pelvic replacement. To date a two-stage procedure using a temporary hand-moulded acrylic bone–cement spacer which maintains the relationship of the femur and pelvis has been the method of choice. The pelvis is a hoop under tension. The loss of integrity of the hoop following removal of the acetabulum cannot be made good by a prosthesis which can only be attached to the remaining portion of the ilium, approximately a third of which must be left for attachment of what is essentially an acetabular element. It has been found that in the course of time the remaining portion of the ilium may hinge backwards on the sacroiliac joint, and thus an arthrodesis of this articulation may be required early in the post-operative period. It is the immediate hingeing and loss of the hoop structure of the pelvis that makes fixation to any remaining part of the pubis or ischium on the same side of the pelvis or the opposite side unsatisfactory. After resection of the tumour a bone–cement cast of the transected surface of the ilium is taken. Included in the cast are Steinmann pins, which are inserted in the position in the remaining ilium to be occupied by the definitive fixation rods. When the casting has hardened, the pins are removed to enable the cast to be withdrawn. By this means the correct orientation and relation of the holes in the prosthesis through which will pass the iliac fixation rods can be established. Using the acrylic cast of the transected surface and a positive replica cast of the bone removed (Fig. 29.2a), a metal prosthesis (Fig. 29.2b) can be prepared which will abut correctly on the transected surface of the ilium and allow the intramedullary rods to be inserted in the predetermined position. The rods are held captive by cementing an high-density polyethylene (HDP) cup in the metal acetabulum.

For a one-stage procedure an identical size model of the pelvis must be constructed using CT scans and a hot-wire pantograph technique. By stacking together sheets of polystyrene foam of the thickness of the CT scan slices from which the 'actual size' image of the bone has been cut out, a negative cast of the pelvis is formed. From this is prepared a positive cast of the pelvis using plaster of Paris or other suitable casting material. The proposed resection can then be carried out, enabling a replacement with appropriate means of fixation to be designed and made. At operation the proposed plane and site of transection must be achieved if the prosthesis is to fit and function satisfactorily. The author prefers the two-stage procedure.

Prostheses for the femur — procedure for taking measurement radiographs

The design and manufacture of a custom-made femoral prosthesis requires true anteroposterior and mediolateral measurement radiographs which should include the acetabulum, femur and tibia with ankle joint of both lower limbs. Radiographs should be made with a 'long' cassette, ideally 100 cm x 45 cm. If several overlapping films have to be taken, the patient must be maintained in the same position. Whenever possible these views should be taken with the patient standing and the film marked as such.

Measurement scale

A radio-opaque graduated scale is used with each radiograph, placed alongside, parallel to, and in the same plane as the bone being X-rayed, i.e. alongside the

(a)

(b)

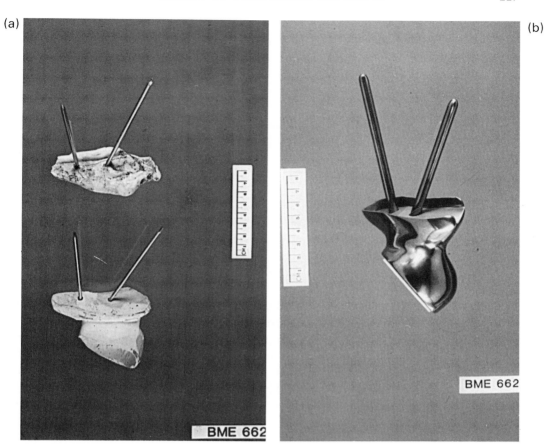

Fig. 29.2 (a) Top, acrylic cast of cut surface of ilium with Steinmann pins. Bottom, plaster cast of specimen with Steinmann pins in position, face of cast having been prepared from acrylic cast. (b) Finished titanium prosthesis showing fixation rods and cut surface of prosthesis that abuts on ilium. The tray is filled with bone cement.

femur for the hip or knee joint. As an insurance against misplacement or obscurity of the scale, the anode/film distance (AFD) and the object/film distance (OFD) should be noted. The object/film distance should be measured from both the proximal and distal 'landmarks' of the bone, e.g. the greater trochanter and one of the condyles of the femur, as the distances may not be identical. From these measurements the percentage enlargement can be calculated.

Views required for an upper femoral replacement:

1 *Standard lower limb film.* This view can only be attempted if a 100 cm cassette is available. (Small patients fit on 90 cm.) The film should include both lower limbs, from the femoral heads to the bottom of the feet. The patient should stand in the AP position, feet sufficiently far apart from an imaginary line from the centre of

the head of the femur to pass vertically through the lateral malleolus. The femoral condyles must be in the true AP position, i.e. when each condyle is at the same distance from the film, irrespective of the position of the patella. A radio-opaque plumb line should hang in front of the cassette. Patients with unequal leg lengths should have a block placed under the short leg to level the pelvis. This fact must be noted on the film, including thickness of the block. If graduated screens are not available, a graduated aluminium wedge placed on the tube eliminates exposure problems between the ankles and the hips.

2 *Turning laterals of each lower femur.*   Again the graduated scale is used. The femoral condyles must be lateral. The other leg must be swung away to show as much hip as possible. This film is to show the bowing of the femur and is important to enable accurate contouring of the intramedullary stem.

3 *Coned views of head and neck of femur.* If a coned AP view of the head and neck of each femur is required, the film is placed in true AP position with the patient supine and the leg internally rotated about 20°. The rotation may only be possible on the normal limb. Each limb should be X-rayed separately and with a graduated scale centred over the neck of the femur. The plane of the scale should be in the midline of the acetabulum. Coned stereo views may be required in cases where the normal anatomy of the head is distorted, e.g. following osteotomy, fracture, or congenital dislocation of the hip. If long cassettes are not available, in order to show the entire bone and its articulations two views of each bone (hip down and knee up) in both AP and lateral positions are required, with the graduated scale on each film. Rotation of the limb between films should not be allowed.

Designing the femoral prosthesis

In the case of the femur, if there is doubt about the extent of bone involvement the prosthesis must be capable of being adapted to replace the whole of the bone. R.B., a male patient born October 1926, first noticed aching in his right thigh in March 1972. He was referred to the Royal Orthopaedic Hospital, Birmingham, in March 1975, when a radiograph showed a lesion involving the proximal half of the right femur; its extent could not be determined (Fig. 29.3a). A diagnosis of chondrosarcoma was confirmed by biopsy. A prosthesis was designed (Fig. 29.3b) which could replace the proximal 26 cm of the right femur and the hip joint or the whole femur with hip and knee joints. On 17th April 1975, a proximal femoral replacement was attempted. Frozen sections of marrow at the transection site demonstrated chondrosarcoma. The remainder of the femur and the knee joint were therefore removed and the total femur prosthesis, a self-retaining RCH 100* acetabular cup and a hinged knee prosthesis were used. The acetabular cup and

---

*Trade name of ultra high molecular weight polyethylene made by Ruhrchemia A. G., Oberhausen-Holten, West Germany.

tibial component were fixed in the bone with acrylic bone cement. The patient was fully active without walking aids and was back at work as a building worker by October 1975. A radiograph of 10th April 1984, shows his present condition (Fig. 29.3b). The acetabular and tibial fixations are secure. He does his own gardening and climbs ladders when decorating and carrying out home repairs.

(a)   (b)   (c)

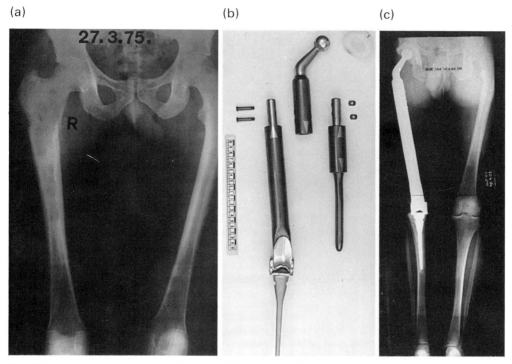

Fig. 29.3 (a) Chondrosarcoma of right femur. (b) Interchangeable components for partial and total femoral prostheses. (c) Radiograph showing condition nine years after operation.

The fixation of the prosthesis in the diaphysis of the bone should be entirely intramedullary. Extramedullary methods of fixation involving plates, screws or bolts compromise the entire blood supply of the bone and lead to bone necrosis and fracture of the fixation. The stem of the prosthesis should be polished, of D shape cross-section, and contoured to fit the marrow cavity, allowing minimal clearance at that part of the marrow cavity of minimum anteroposterior and mediolateral dimensions. Generally, the transection site of the bone should be 5 cm distant from the limit of the lesion as judged from NMR, CT and/or isotope scans. The distance of the transection site from the limit of the lesion may have to be reduced by up to 3 cm if the fixation is likely to be jeopardized. The length of stem of a prosthesis should ideally be not less than 14 cm, although at times shorter stems have been used in the distal femur and performed satisfactorily.

The intramedullary stem of a proximal femoral component must be bolted to the shaft of the prosthesis so that, if recurrent dislocation at the hip does occur because of loss of tissue, the prosthesis can be replaced without disturbing the intramedullary fixation.

(a)   (b)

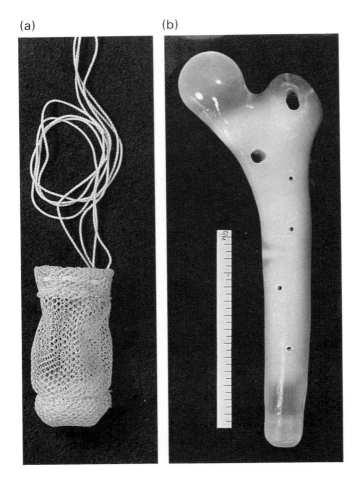

Fig. 29.4 (a) 'Sock' of lock-knit polyester bobbin net with draw cord. (b) Acrylic prosthesis with holes for attachment of tissues.

No provision is made for the attachment of tissues to pelvic or femoral prostheses. Experience has shown that, if either local or general attachments to prostheses are attempted, either the tissues pull away from the attachment or, if general apposition to the shaft is achieved by sewing tissues to a polyester net covering, limitation of movement occurs. Further, if an implant becomes infected and net attachment methods have been used, it is often difficult to remove net that has become incorporated into soft tissues. There is one application, however, where a non-stretch lock-knit polyester bobbin net is useful. If a prosthesis is used following a disarticulation procedure with amputation through the thigh, retraction of the tissues from over the end of the prosthesis can be prevented by using a 'sock' of net (Fig. 29.4a). The end of the prosthesis should be protected by 8–10 layers of net sewn into the base of the sock. The sock is held in place by a draw cord tightened in a groove around the shaft of the prosthesis. The tissues are brought together and sewn to the net pad over the end of the prosthesis. Repair tissue invades the net and holds the muscles in place as well as protecting the skin from tension and impact injury that might otherwise lead to skin necrosis.

The following case illustrates the advantages of the procedure. A 21-year-old male patient, R.S., with polyostotic fibrous dysplasia was referred to the late Mr H. Jackson Burrows at the Royal National Orthopaedic Hospital (RNOH) in 1951 after a series of pathological fractures of the left femur. A mid-thigh amputation was performed, the remaining femur being replaced with an acrylic proximal femoral prosthesis made with holes for attachment of muscles (Fig. 29.4b). After two years, necrosis of the skin occurred over the distal end of the prosthesis, the muscles having retracted. The acrylic stump was shortened by a further 4.5 cm and covered with a polyester sock of the type shown in Fig. 29.4a held in place by the draw cord secured in a groove made 5 cm from the end of the prosthesis. There has been no further trouble from the acrylic stump in the ensuing 24 years.

Prosthetic replacement in children presents a major problem in that limb growth may be severely retarded by the removal of one or both epiphyses when a long bone is replaced. The first extending prosthesis, with a screw mechanism, was used in 1976 at the Royal Orthopaedic Hospital, Birmingham, to replace the distal femur of a girl aged ten years. Since that time a further 31 prostheses with an extension mechanism have been used in child bone tumour patients, although only one of these was for the proximal femur (Fig. 29.5). It consists of a femoral head and shaft of titanium alloy type TA1, the shaft having a sliding member that is prevented from rotating and carries an intramedullary stem cemented into the femur. Inside the stem unit is a piston driven distally by the injection of tungsten carbide ball-bearings, increasing the length of the prosthesis. From time to time ball-bearings can be injected into the prosthetic shaft through a small incision, using a special introducer tube. One ball lengthens the prosthesis by 6.35 mm. The femoral component articulates with an HDP Stanmore-type acetabular cup. Fig. 29.5 shows a post-operative radiograph with deliberate increase in length of left limb to allow for some growth of the right limb before the need to extend the prosthesis. This sometimes removes the need for leg lengthening during the period the patient is recovering from cytotoxic therapy.

A problem more commonly encountered at the other end of the age spectrum is that of replacing the proximal half of the femur, for example for a failed total hip replacement, where fracture of the distal shaft of the femur is associated with shortening of the limb. Because of the obliquity of a fracture the site of transection of the distal part of the femoral shaft may be such that there is insufficient bone stock left to provide a reliable fixation. When this is the case a total femur and knee joint prosthesis is required. It is not possible to determine prior to operation

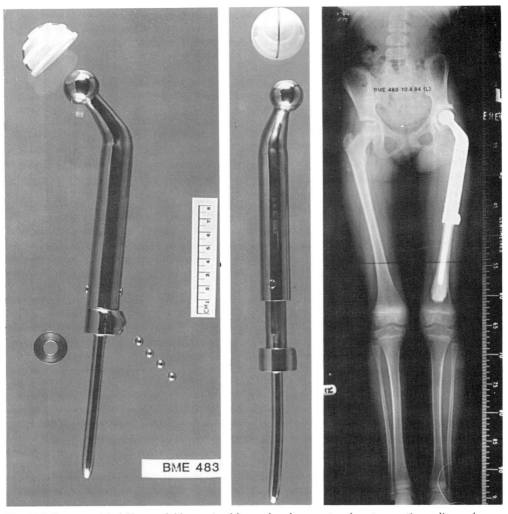

Fig. 29.5 Stanmore Mark II extendable proximal femoral replacement and post-operative radiograph.

whether equality of limb length can be achieved. For such a case an adjustable total femoral prosthesis is designed. Using dimensions obtained from radiographs of the opposite limb as well as the affected limb, the required extension can be calculated. Fig. 29.6 shows a prosthesis used in treating a patient of 80 years of age with severe osteoporosis, who had a failed left total hip replacement with a history of infection and an ununited spiral fracture of the distal shaft of the femur. In a younger patient the need to preserve the knee would have influenced the design of the prosthesis so that if at operation it was found possible to secure a reasonable fixation in the distal fragment of the femur, the prosthesis could be used without a knee joint. In a case where shortening has occurred, fine adjustment of the length of the prosthesis must be possible to ensure that the correct tissue tensions are achieved to reduce the risk of subsequent dislocation. The prosthesis consists of a proximal element with a slotted stem which slides inside the distal part of the prosthesis (Fig. 29.6). This carries an oblong key to prevent rotation of one part of the prosthesis on the other. To obtain the correct length the tibial component of the knee joint is cemented into the tibia and the appropriate size of cup cemented into the acetabulum. When the bone cement is hard the prosthesis is asssembled and the hip reduced. Traction is applied to the limb to obtain the desired tension in the tissues. The prosthesis is inserted and held in position while

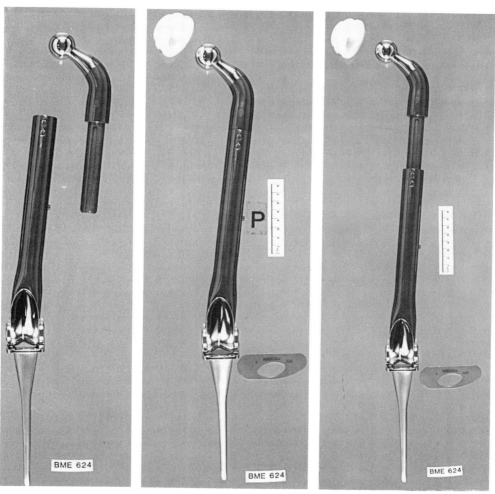

Fig. 29.6 Adjustable Stanmore total femoral prosthesis. Cement is introduced through port, P. Tibial component used with a plateau plate.

a creamy mix of acrylic bone cement is injected through the threaded port, P. When the correct amount of cement has been injected the port is closed with a threaded plug. Experience has confirmed the need to design the prosthesis with the largest diameter of femoral head that can be used with the appropriate size of acetabular cup. Ideally a 32 mm internal diameter cup should be used. Even if the patient has a securely anchored 22 mm internal diameter cup, this should be replaced with a cup of larger internal diameter if the risk of subsequent dislocation is to be materially reduced.

Materials for the manufacture of prostheses

Most prostheses are fabricated from a number of components and all the materials used must be biologically acceptable. In a few patients the constituent elements of both cobalt–chromium–molybdenum and stainless steel alloys can induce a state of lymphocyte-mediated hypersensitivity (Elves *et al.* 1975). Patients should be patch-tested using the metals in question before manufacture of a prosthesis. There are no clinical reports of problems with commercially pure grades of titanium (T1–T5) or titanium alloy containing 6% aluminium and 4% vanadium (TA1). No clinical complications have occurred when these materials have been used in combination with cobalt–chromium–molybdenum alloys of the compositions specified in BS 3531 Part 2, 1980, Table 1. Stainless steel alloy of the type specified in the same standard, Table 1, composition B, is suitable for the manufacture of one-piece prostheses. The mechanical properties of forged stainless steel for highly stressed parts of the prosthesis such as the intramedullary stem require that the stem be of adequate cross-section for the fatigue load it may have to sustain. Stainless steel prostheses must be made from one piece of metal if the risk of fretting corrosion in the long term is to be avoided.

Conclusion

Experience with Stanmore-designed custom-made prostheses since 1949 indicates that this form of treatment for limb preservation is, if the cases are properly selected, a clinically reliable procedure. It is, however, advisable that patients are treated at centres where adequate clinical experience and support facilities for this form of treatment are available.

Acknowledgements

The extensive experience of the Department of Biomedical Engineering at Stanmore with the design, manufacture and clinical use of major bone and joint replacement prostheses has only been possible because of the collaboration of many surgeons in various hospitals, but especially in the Royal National Orthopaedic Hospital, Stanmore (Mr H. B. S. Kemp, Mr J. N. Wilson), the Royal Orthopaedic Hospital,

Birmingham (Mr R. S. Sneath), and The Middlesex Hospital (Mr D. R. Sweetnam). I am indebted to the staff of the Department of Biomedical Engineering, in particular Dr K. W. J. Wright, Mr R. H. Ansell and Mr R. H. Child. I also wish to acknowledge the considerable help given by a number of companies, especially O.E.C. Orthopaedic, now Biomet Ltd, Bridgend, and I.M.I. Titanium Ltd, Birmingham, and also the Department of Health and Social Security, London, which has in various ways funded much of the work.

References

Elves M. W., Wilson J. N., Scales J. T. & Kemp H. B . S. K. (1975) Incidence of metal sensitivity in patients with total joint replacements. *British Medical Journal* **4 (5993)**, 376–378.

Seddon H. J. & Scales J. T. (1949) A polythene substitute for the upper two thirds of the shaft of the femur. *Lancet* **ii**, 795–796.

Smith A. J. (1975) Estimates of muscle and joint forces at the knee and ankle during a running activity. *Journal of Human Movement Studies* **1**, 78–86.

30

Prostheses for the Hip Disarticulation and Hemipelvectomy

A.W. McQUIRK

Introduction

With very few exceptions, the limb of choice would be made using components designed to the principles of the Canadian hip disarticulation prosthesis, which has now been universally accepted. In recent years many variations and innovations in design of components have taken place, particularly in stride length limiters, built-in alignment devices at the hip joint, lightweight modular systems, and one-piece cosmesis, all of which have contributed to greater patient acceptance and improved prosthetic function. It is essential that simple criteria are used to define the prosthetic application, these being (1) comfort, (2) function, and (3) cosmesis, and they should be considered in that order.

When one speaks of comfort one thinks of the socket, and to obtain a socket it is necessary first to take a cast of the amputation stump. One must consider what is required of the socket before explaining the method used to take the cast. The socket should provide the following functions: (1) suspension, (2) weight-bearing, (3) lateral containment. In modern prosthetic application suspension is integral to the socket design and the framework of the skeleton can be used to satisfy this requirement using both iliac crests. For weight-bearing the ischial tuberosity and gluteal region are used. Therefore, in the design of the socket the largest possible weight-bearing area is obtained. Lateral containment is required so that correct suspension, weight-bearing, stability and alignment may be maintained. The method of casting described here encompasses those design criteria. A close-woven elastic stretch stockinette is pulled over the body (Fig. 30.4). This stockinette contains and compresses the soft tissues and gives a good outline contour of the body shape. If the patient is obese then a double-strength elasticated stockinette should be used, thus providing greater compression of the soft tissues and producing a shape closer to the socket design than would otherwise be the case.

Casting method for hip disarticulation

The cast is taken in three phases to obtain the functions required of the socket.

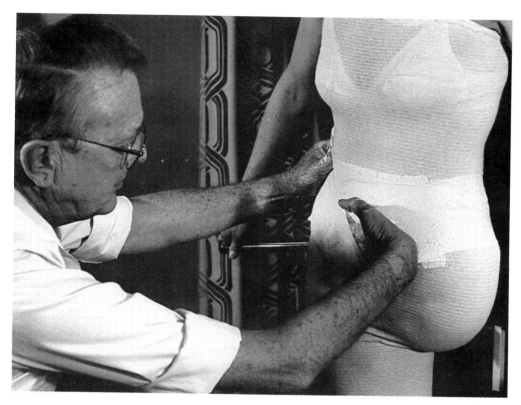

Fig. 30.1 First phase of the casting procedure. The bandage is folded over the hand and taken diagonally upwards and over the iliac crest on the other side.

The first phase of the casting procedure is designed to obtain suspension, and for this 15 cm plaster bandages are used. Bandaging is begun over both iliac crests starting level on the anterior abdominal wall over the iliac crest on one side, completely around the posterior aspect and forward over the opposite iliac crest, then downward diagonally, the bandage being held with the flat of the hand. The bandage is folded over the hand and taken diagonally upwards and over the iliac crest on the other side (Fig. 30.1). This procedure is continued using two bandages, carefully controlling the tension when passing over the iliac crests. Two very important points: the bandages must be very wet, and they must be applied with speed. Moreover, the wrap must not encroach on the lower rib cage and the bandage should finish at a level 3 cm distal to the anterior superior iliac spine. While the cast is still wet the prosthetist improves the identification of the bony anatomy with his hands, the first finger of each hand being pressed inwards and diagonally downwards on the proximal curve of each iliac crest, the thumbs lying flat on the lower abdomen, and the web of the first finger and thumb located over the anterior superior spine, the other three fingers of each hand meanwhile lying lightly over the iliac area. A firm and steady pressure is applied until the plaster is dry (Fig. 30.2).

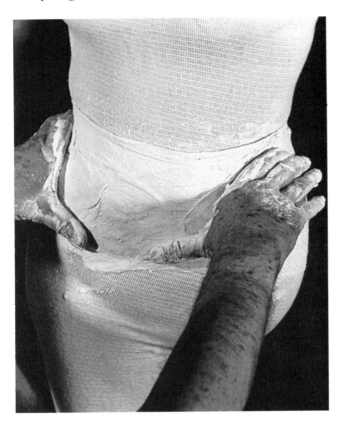

Fig. 30.2 Identification of the bony anatomy. Pressure is applied until the plaster is dry.

The second phase is the forming of the weight-bearing section of the cast which will give a faithful reproduction of the anatomy for the socket requiring the minimum of modification. This can only be done with the full body weight applied during this phase of the plaster wrap. To obtain this a casting rig has been designed (Fig. 30.3), which has an adjustable platform to obtain the correct height. On this platform is placed an anterior block with its posterior surface cut at an angle of 50° which, when applied to the wet plaster wrap, produces the correct surface to be reproduced in the socket for the hip joint attachment. This block needs to be set with external rotation of 5°. Under weight-bearing the soft tissue tends to displace and leave the bone structure more prominent. It is important to obtain an even pressure over the largest possible weight-bearing area. Attached to the anterior block on the rig is a 20 cm wide strong rubber strap which passes distally under the stump, passing through an adjustment fitted to the top of the posterior block. This produces a hammock sling into which the patient sits compressing and controlling the soft tissue. *Note*: This block is shaped so that it does not come into

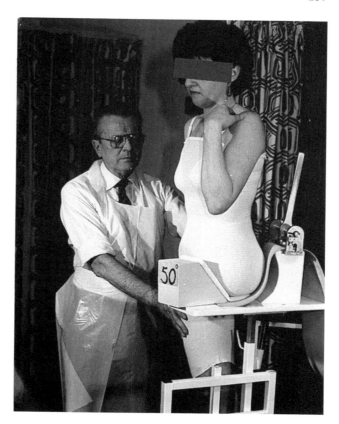

Fig. 30.3 Casting rig for the second phase of the casting procedure.

contact with the stump (Fig. 30.4). Finally a check is made to ensure the correct height of the rig so that when the patient's full body weight is applied the iliac crests are level. The platform is then removed and a plaster slab using six layers of 15 cm plaster bandage is applied starting perpendicularly from the anterior proximal brim of the first phase of the cast downwards and under the amputation side keeping the edge of the plaster slab up against the thigh of the sound limb then upwards to the posterior proximal brim of the first phase of the cast. Again this phase must be completed with speed and the plaster slab must be very wet. At this stage the casting rig platform is replaced under the stump and the patient's full body weight applied whilst the plaster is still wet. If any puckering appears, lift the plaster away from the anterior and posterior proximal brim and pull by hand proximally, pressing back firmly to the first phase of the cast.

Third phase. Up till now the soft tissues on the distal lateral side of the amputation stump have not received attention; 15 cm plaster bandages are again used and the wet bandages are pulled firmly over this lateral portion so that the soft tissues are firmly and evenly compressed. To maintain the tension an advantage has already

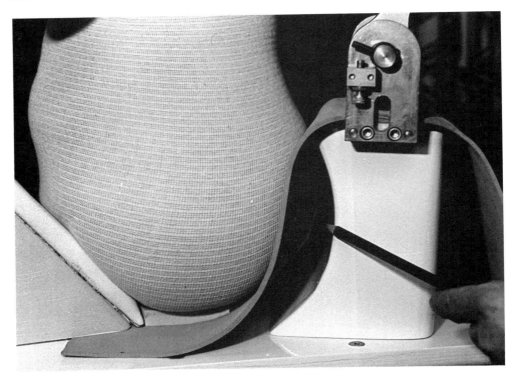

Fig. 30.4 The patient sits in the hammock sling formed by the rubber strap. Note that the posterior block is shaped so that it does not contact the stump.

been established with the first phase of the cast which is dry and hard; accordingly the wet bandage can be taken diagonally upwards over the iliac crest on the sound side ensuring a firm anchorage. The full cast is now complete.

Before the cast is removed the trim lines are checked — a line 12 mm above the anterior inguinal crease and 12 mm superior to the trochanter continued posteriorly. When the completed cast is dry, reference lines should be marked on the lateral and anterior surfaces. The anterior line should indicate the midline of the amputation 'stump', which inclines inwards and downwards 2° towards the centre weight line. The lateral line should be marked downwards from the midline and inclined 2° anteriorly at the base. It is important to check the patient sitting with the cast still applied (Fig. 30.5). The cast is removed by cutting from the distal edge to the proximal edge anteriorly on the non-amputation side. When the cast is removed the form of the ischial tuberosity and surrounding weight-bearing area and the iliac crests are easily identified. From the negative cast the positive plaster model on which the socket is fabricated is made. The amount of rectification which is required to the positive model should be minimal and should consist only of cleaning and smoothing. It is important that the reference lines are transferred on to the positive model.

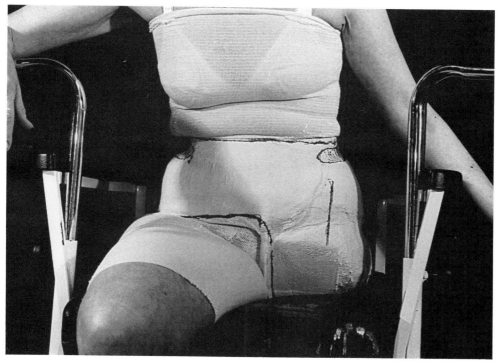

Fig. 30.5 The patient is checked seated with the cast still applied.

Casting technique for hemipelvectomy

Those criteria and functional requirements already laid down for the hip disarticulation prosthesis still hold true. As far as the suspension role of the cast is concerned there remains only the iliac crest on the sound limb side. On the amputation side suspension depends on where the posterior pelvic section has taken place; the more of the posterior part of the ilium that is left the better the prospect of achieving suspension on the amputation side. In many cases it is possible to obtain some suspension by moulding over the remaining ilium and below the rib cage. Therefore, *the first phase* of the casting procedure for the hemipelvectomy may be carried out exactly as for the hip disarticulation.

The second phase of the cast construction is the fashioning of the weight-bearing area, and here the problem becomes greater. With the complete removal of the ischial tuberosity the only potential weight-bearing region that is left on the amputation side is provided by compression of the soft tissue, which may result in the proximal brim of the socket impinging on the lower rib cage with consequent discomfort. Moreover as this soft tissue compression can be anything up to 5 cm in circumference the prosthesis has to be made that amount longer, which gives it a very bad appearance when sitting. Therefore an attempt is made to use the posterior ischial tuberosity on the sound limb to obtain some force transference. To be effective, however, this transverse bearing must be built in at the casting stage. Thus the second phase of casting should be carried out in a similar manner to that of the hip disarticulation but with the following important modifications:

1 The adjustable platform must be shaped to include the transverse bearing so that it will fit intimately around the proximal posteromedial aspect of the thigh of the sound limb.

2 When applying the wet plaster bandages, the line from the proximal anterior brim is followed down under the medial aspect of the base of the amputation 'stump' and posteriorly round the sound limb, allowing 2.5 cm of the bandage to be flat on the posteromedial thigh of the sound limb. Thereafter the bandage is applied to follow around and up to the proximal brim on the lateral sound side, level with the posterior edge of the trochanter. It is important that the anterior block as described in the casting method for hip disarticulation is still used, so as to obtain an angled interface ready to accept the hip joint. It is recognized that this utilization of the contralateral ischium for support is at variance with the practice in other centres (Lyquist 1958, Hampton 1965), but the results have proved very effective.

Static alignment

Anterior aspect

Once the casting stage is complete a solid positive plaster model can be obtained on which to fabricate the socket. Success or failure will depend not so much on the material used for the socket but more on the accuracy of the positive model. Sockets can be made of various materials including leather, plastic laminate, polypropylene or a combination of these materials with, for example, soft sections of silicone. If the design of the socket is correct it should effectively 'lock on' to the patient and there should be no proximal/distal movement in the socket. If such movement is present then the patient will get a 'hammering' effect at the ischial tuberosity which will produce discomfort in time. The prosthesis has to be attached to the socket by means of a hip joint, and the positioning of this joint is vital. Many functions are centred around the joint. If the hip joint is set too far distally this will impede the sitting position.

If the joint is set too far proximally then the thigh-piece of the prosthesis will be too long in the sitting position and extend the knee beyond that of the sound limb. From experience it has been found that the best position for the joint in the anterodistal area viewed from the medial aspect will require the axis of the joint to be located on a line 2.5 cm above the ischial tuberosity. It should be displaced laterally. This is obtained by dividing equally mediolaterally the angular surface which is produced in the casting. In setting the midline of the joint 12–25 mm laterally, the axis should be inclined 2°. When viewed from the anterior aspect, the thigh should incline medially at the distal end, e.g. when using a modular system the thigh tube will present the same angled appearance as that of the natural femur. In the walking phase the patient will naturally raise the hip on the amputation side; the joint will then be horizontal.

In the vertical axis the joint should be externally rotated 5° to the line of progression. In walking during swing phase the patient always internally rotates the pelvis, thus bringing the joint back into the line of progression.

Lateral aspect

Viewed from the lateral aspect the static alignment of the prosthesis is most important. A vertical line dropped through the ischial tuberosity and the ankle joint should pass 6 mm anterior to the knee centre. This arrangement will ensure that the knee is stable at all times throughout single support on the prosthesis but may result in somewhat sluggish knee flexion when swing is initiated. Correct alignment of the socket with respect to the thigh section when the hip joint is fully extended is achieved by a positive stop between the anterior inferior aspect of the socket and the posterior proximal aspect of the thigh. As a result of the anterior positioning of the hip joint the thigh section requires to be angled posteriorly from the hip to achieve the required position of the knee joint.

Dynamic alignment

To obtain fine tuning of the individual patient's gait it must be possible to carry out alignment alterations; this facility is provided in systems that are now available. It is important to have alignment potential at the hip joint to alter slightly the angles as described in static alignment. Further alignment potential is provided by the incorporation of an alignment device just above the knee. It is important to check alignment of the hip joint and knee joint in combination continually, not only during walking, but also when the limb is in the sitting position. Again it is important to remember that the rubber stop between the hip joint and socket is a vital part of the static and dynamic alignment.

Stride limiter mechanism

It was found in the very early stages of fitting the Canadian-type hip disarticulation prosthesis that, if a controlled amount of flexion of the hip joint was obtained which positively limited the stride length, the patient had a greater sense of security and a much more relaxed gait. Accordingly over the years a number of hip joints which provide for adjustable stride length have been designed. This allows the clinic team, including the patient, the opportunity to obtain the optimal stride length for a more functional, cosmetic, and economic gait. It also enables the patient to vary the cadence to some extent, independent of the natural frequency of the prosthesis.

This chapter describes a procedure for dealing with a very small but vital group of amputees. The following passage from Van der Waarde (1984) is quoted, as it is felt to be of great significance.

'Weight of prosthesis — the average weight of the hip disarticulation prosthesis varies from four to nine kilograms — depending on the additional optional extras in the prosthesis — which is generally deemed acceptable. The use of torque absorbers, 4-bar linkage hip and knee joints, and multi-axial feet all add significantly to the overall weight. The selection of lighter materials for the components as well as for the socket is great importance.'

The author considers 9 kg completely unacceptable and the target should be the 4 kg prosthesis.

Finally, due acknowledgement is made to McLaurin (1957) for the original development of the Canadian hip prosthesis. The experience gained in fitting the prosthesis as described here is based solely on a rigid adherence to the basic principles derived from this work.

References

Hampton F. (1965) A hemipelvectomy prosthesis. *Prosthetics International* **2 (2)**, 3–24.
Lyquist E. (1958) Canadian-type plastic socket for a hemipelvectomy. *Artificial Limbs* **5 (2)**, 130–132.
McLaurin C. (1957) The evolution of the Canadian-type hip disarticulation prosthesis. *Artificial Limbs* **4 (2)**, 22–28.
Van der Waarde T. (1984) Ottawa experience with hip disarticulation prosthesis. *Orthotics and Prosthetics* **38 (1)**, 29–35.

31

Kinematic Aspects of the Canadian Hip Disarticulation Prosthesis: Preliminary Results

R.L. VAN VORHIS & D.S. CHILDRESS

Introduction

The gait of one person wearing a Canadian hip disarticulation prosthesis has been studied and the kinematic performance of the prosthesis during ambulation examined. The experimental data, supplemented with mathematical models, have allowed us to examine (1) the pendular properties of the prosthesis, (2) the kinematic and gait differences associated with using a hydraulic knee mechanism or a constant-friction knee unit, and (3) the problem of ground clearance of the prosthesis during swing.

Objective characterization of motion of the hip disarticulation prosthesis during gait has not been extensively addressed in the literature on prosthesis performance. This lack of information on hip disarticulation prosthesis behaviour is probably related to the relatively small number of persons fitted with these prostheses. The authors think this lack of information has inhibited progress in hip disarticulation prosthesis development. McLaurin (1957) described the evolution of the Canadian hip disarticulation prosthesis, and Radcliffe (1957) and McLaurin (1969) have examined the biomechanics of this prosthesis. Foort (1957) and Hampton (1964) have described the construction of this prosthesis and examined its clinical application. Winter (1980) has presented data relating to the energetics of ambulation on a hip disarticulation prosthesis.

Methods

A long-time user (23 years) of a Canadian hip disarticulation prosthesis volunteered to be a subject for the study. This subject, a remarkable walker, had worn a prosthesis with a constant-friction knee joint for a number of years before switching to the use of a hydraulic mechanism (Dupaco). She had two prostheses that she could use interchangeably. One of these limbs was used to construct another leg (duplicating the thigh and shank) for her with a constant-friction knee mechanism and with the same alignment as her regular prosthesis. This leg could be attached to her regular prosthetic socket for experimental tests. She had no trouble adapting

245

to this prosthesis because of her previous experience with constant-friction swing phase control.

Mass centres of the limb segments were determined through balance beam measurements. Inertia was determined by measuring the natural frequency of oscillation of the limb segment about its proximal joint axis. Tachometers were mounted to the prosthesis at the knee and hip joints to obtain angular velocities. These signals were integrated to obtain angular position. Electrical pressure switches were placed on the prosthesis at the toe and heel and at the knee and hip joints as 'event indicators' (toe-off, heel-strike, movement of thigh segment from hip extension stop, and full knee extension respectively). Toe and heel switches were also placed on the shoe of the non-amputated limb.

Walking speed was determined by measuring step length and step duration. Felt discs, saturated with ink and applied to the shoe heels, were used to mark the floor for step length determination. A lightweight, flexible cable connected the subject to the instrumentation and recording apparatus (tape recorder). It caused minimal interference with ambulation. Orientations of the prosthetic limb segments in space were determined photographically at specific times of the gait cycle. The subject walked in dim light, viewed by a polaroid camera with the lens open. The 'event switches' were used to trigger a strobe light at the appropriate event time (e.g. at toe-off or at initiation of thigh movement away from the extension stop).

Results

Motion analysis showed that the prosthesis with the constant-friction knee could basically be described by simple pendulum models, albeit *not* passive pendulums driven only by gravity. After toe-off, the thigh section remained in its fully extended position against the extension stop while the shank segment moved about its joint like a pendulum with distributed mass (compound pendulum). When the shank moves into the knee extension stop, a collision results, accompanied by small oscillations. After the collision the thigh and shank sections move together about the hip as another (longer) compound pendulum. Energy of the collison of the shank and thigh promotes movement of the thigh from the extension stop (thigh flexion). The prosthesis with the constant-friction knee unit, at the time of initial hip flexion, is shown in Fig. 31.1a. Notice that the knee is fully extended.

With hydraulic damping at the knee, the limb swings as a double pendulum. Fig. 31.1b shows the prosthesis at the moment the thigh section begins to move from the extension stop. The shank supplies energy to the thigh through the hydraulic mechanism; therefore, hip and knee joint rotation occur simultaneously.

Angle–angle diagrams (hip versus knee) for gait using the two kinds of swing phase control are shown in Fig. 31.2 along with the diagram for typical non-amputee gait. Neither swing phase control helps the amputee emulate non-amputee motion very well, but the hydraulic mechanism appears to give a result more in keeping with the typical non-amputee pattern. Data showed that the gait pattern with hydraulic knee damping was more balanced between the prosthetic and non-amputed side (i.e. step duration and step length were more closely matched). Also, with the hydraulic unit, mean walking speed at the normal walking rate was about 12% greater than with the constant-friction component.

(a)   (b)

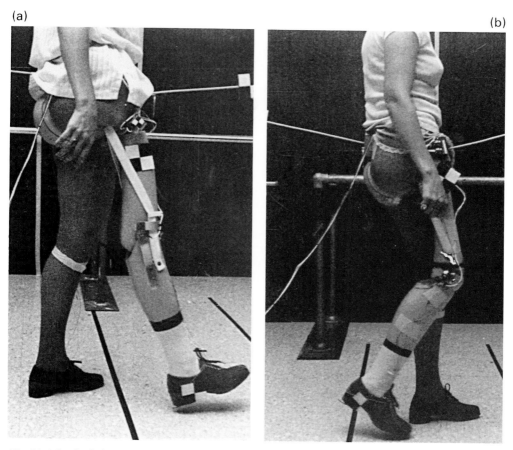

Fig. 31.1 Strobed photographs of amputee. (a) Walking on hip disarticulation prosthesis with constant-friction knee swing phase control. The strobe occurs at the onset of hip joint flexion, when the thigh segment begins to move from the hip extension stop. Note that the knee is fully extended at this instant. (b) Same amputee walking on hip disarticulation prosthesis with hydraulic knee swing phase control. The strobe occurs at onset of hip flexion. Note degree of knee flexion at this instant.

Mathematical models of the prostheses were constructed for the limbs with the two kinds of swing phase control. Both were solved for the swing phase situation using the measured initial conditions of the joints (position and velocity) at the beginning of shank extension and assuming gravity as the only external force applied. The hydraulic mechanism was modelled assuming a linear relationship between force and extension of the damper. In both models the time of swing predicted was considerably longer than the observed swing time during actual gait.

Ground clearance was about the same in the limb with the hydraulic knee as in the limb with the constant-friction knee. This was surprising at first because conventional wisdom indicates that foot clearance can be aided by hip and knee flexion. Analysis showed that this is true only if there is substantial knee flexion (e.g. 60°) and that small knee flexion, as obtained in the prosthesis with the hydraulic knee, was actually detrimental to floor clearance because of the geometry of the shank and foot.

(a)

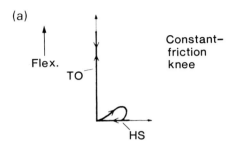

(b)

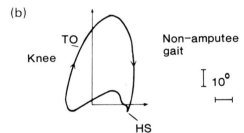

(c)

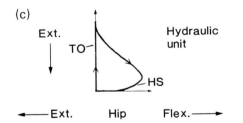

Fig. 31.2 Angle–angle diagrams (hip joint angle versus knee joint angle). (a) Hip disarticulation prosthesis during walking using a constant-friction knee. (b) represents non-amputee gait. (c) Hip disarticulation prosthesis during walking using a hydraulic knee mechanism.

Discussion

Although only once case was studied, the data and models indicate that a hydraulic knee mechanism in a hip disarticulation prosthesis can produce gait patterns that are more anthropomorphic than if the constant-friction knee is used. This advantage must be weighed against greater cost, greater complexity, and greater weight of the hydraulic knee. It may be that walking speed is increased through use of a hydraulic knee, but this would need to be determined through testing a larger subject sample. The subject in the study preferred the prosthesis with the hydraulic knee. The models of the swing limb had a swing time longer than the observed swing time. This is in agreement with McMahon's (1984) results for non-amputee gait. It indicates that the user of the prosthesis is able to transmit energy to the limb through the hip joint. The mechanism for this transfer has not been precisely characterized and needs further study.

Mochon and McMahon (1980) have shown that ballistic walking models can be used to characterize human gait reasonably well. In their model initial conditions set the ballistic course. The fact that a hip disarticulation amputee, like the subject in the study, can ambulate so well on a completely passive limb supports the concept of the ballistic walking model.

The prosthesis with the constant-friction knee experiences a collision during each cycle of gait, whereas the limb with the hydraulic unit has a smooth extension of the shank. Nevertheless, the collision between the shank and thigh provides feedback to the user in the form of vibration, which indicates that the knee is at or near its fully extended position. This feedback may help some amputees to walk with more confidence.

Foot clearance of the floor is an important problem for users of hip disarticulation prostheses. Many prosthetists construct the prostheses for these users 1–2 cm short to facilitate foot clearance of the walking surface. The studies described show that the toe is a primary culprit in clearance problems and that dorsal flexion of the foot, as with the Anglesey leg or the Hydra-Cadence leg, might be helpful to the amputee because less elevation of the prosthetic hip would be necessary for clearance of the walking surface, thus reducing energy requirements.

References

Foort J. (1957) Construction and fitting of the Canadian-type hip disarticulation prosthesis. *Artificial Limbs* **4(2)**, 39–51.

Hampton F. (1964) A hemipelvectomy prosthesis. *Artificial Limbs* **8(1)**, 3–27.

McLaurin C. A. (1957) The evolution of the Canadian-type hip disarticulation prosthesis. *Artificial Limbs* **4(2)**, 22–28.

McLaurin C. A. (1969) The Canadian hip disarticulation prosthesis. In *Prosthetic and Orthotic Practice* (ed. Murdoch G.), pp. 285–304. London: Edward Arnold Ltd. (1970).

McMahon T. A. (1984) *Muscles, Reflexes, and Locomotion,* p. 203. Princeton, N. J.: Princeton University Press.

Mochon S. & McMahon T. A. (1980) Ballistic walking. *Journal of Biomechanics* **13**, 49–57.

Radcliffe C. W. (1957) The biomechanics of the Canadian-type hip-disarticulation prosthesis. *Artificial Limbs* **4(2)**, 29–38.

Winter D. A. (1980) *Waterloo Biomechanics, Part 2.* Application of biomechanics package to the assessment of prosthetic and orthotic gait. Proceedings of an International Conference on Rehabilitation Engineering, Toronto. pp. 291–294.

32

Rehabilitation of the
Hip Disarticulation Amputee

T.J. DONNELLY

Most hip disarticulation amputees are found in the younger age groups, thereby reducing some of the problems found with many amputees, e.g. exercise tolerance and energy expenditure. One study on the subject of the hip disarticulation amputee found that the energy cost per unit distance (work) was 80–125% greater than in normal subjects (Nowroozi et al. 1983).

Preprosthetic phase

In most cases little time is available for physiotherapy prior to operation, and therefore most preparation for prosthetic fitting takes place post-operatively. As there is no standard type of temporary prosthesis available as at other levels, efforts are concentrated on those muscle groups which will have extra loads placed upon them when using a Canadian-type prosthesis. The muscles principally involved are the trunk extensors and flexors, and the abductors of the contralateral hip. The muscles of the sound limb have to be maintained, as do those of the upper limbs, as they are important in transfers at the early stages. Balance exercises are taught as soon as is practicable, starting with sitting balance and progressing to standing. The patient is taught to walk with elbow crutches or with a walking frame.

On delivery of the prosthesis

The patient should have a well-healed stump before fitting begins. Thereafter instruction in putting the limb on as part of normal dressing practice is instituted, and the need for good stump hygiene is emphasized. Some patients will wear the socket next to the skin, but many will wear pants to absorb sweat. It should be explained that, due to unaccustomed surfaces being loaded, some discomfort over the first week or two may be experienced. The patient should be made aware of the extra exercise requirements and reassured that those physical demands are in keeping with the level of amputation and are not the result of his shortcomings.

The patient is taught the operation of the knee joint and how to rise from and sit down on chairs. Weight-bearing is begun between parallel bars with lateral transference of weight from the sound limb and off again. The patient is taught to hip hike, then to step with the prosthesis, and moves on to forward transference of weight, rocking his weight onto the prosthesis and off. The patient's confidence in the prosthesis grows as he realizes that the limb will support his weight safely and in reasonable comfort.

Balance exercises are maintained with the patient standing with the hands off the bars, weight-bearing on both legs, rocking from the sound limb on to the prosthesis and back. Resistance is applied to the pelvis in as many situations as possible with the patient instructed 'don't let me push you; don't let me pull you', etc.

Co-ordination exercises are initiated to improve control of the prosthesis to include stepping with the prosthesis and placing the foot on various marks on the floor. Repetition of this type of exercise will allow the patient very quickly to make use of the proprioceptive input from other sites such as the pressure on the lower abdomen in flexion and on lower lumbar spine and sacrum in extension.

Walking training

When the patient can confidently bear weight on the prosthesis and step with the sound limb, walking can begin. First the patient hip hitches or hikes and, by a lumbar flexion flick, the prosthesis swings through. By design the line of gravity passes anterior to the knee which is thus stabilized in extension at heel-strike through to foot-flat, the sound limb being at toe-off.

The weight passes over the prosthesis to full weight-bearing at mid-stance, and thence until the hip comes into full extension, coinciding with heel-strike on the sound side. Prosthetic knee flexion proceeds until at mid-stance the knee swings through to decelerate before heel-strike again. The cycle being complete, the patient gains speed, and certain problems become apparent; these are due to inevitable irresolvable differences between normal gait and that of the hip disarticulation amputee. To swing the prosthesis through, the patient must hip hike, and then vault with the sound limb in order to gain the time necessary for the longer swing phase; thus there is always a difference in step timing. The patient may also laterally flex to the sound side during swing phase of the prosthesis; this is to be discouraged. The use of mirrors at this stage should be considered, giving the patient the chance to correct without altering his posture by looking down. This is to be encouraged, as the patient is persuaded to feel what is happening rather than looking down at the prosthesis, causing flexion and impairing the swing action. Attention is also paid to heel-strike and achieving an even step length.

When the patient can walk comfortably and smoothly in the bars then walking with sticks is begun. It should be emphasized that the sticks are an aid to balance and are not for weight-bearing. The patient is taught a three-point gait:
1 Place the sticks forward, using a wide base.
2 Place the prosthetic foot between the sticks.

3 Bring the sound limb through and place the foot in front of the prosthetic foot.
The cycle begins again. The patient is instructed never to have the sticks and both feet in the same line, as this is unstable. The patient will next progress to free walking outside the parallel bars. Each time the patient advances to the next stage of gait training, the new technique is taught within the bars, as it is important that the patient should have no fear of falling when attempting anything new. When the three-point gait has been safely adopted, a two-point gait can be introduced; in most cases this does not require to be taught as patients will usually adopt this pattern themselves. The essential difference in the gait is that both sticks and the prosthesis are moved through together. This is a more fluent gait, and the patient gains speed and confidence and soon progresses to using one stick held in the opposite hand from the prosthetic side. In this way continuity of the reciprocal arm swing is maintained, improving balance and discouraging the patient from weight-bearing through the stick. When this is achieved, functional activities are taught.

Stairs. The first attempts should be on a staircase with a handrail. The physiotherapist remains on the lower steps during both ascending and descending to arrest any fall. Ascending, the patient places the sound limb on the upper step then brings up the stick and prosthesis together. Descending, the patient lowers the prosthesis and stick to the lower step first. The lifting and lowering of body weight as performed by the sound limb as a reciprocal stair-climbing gait is not achievable.

Inclines. The patient can manage low-grade inclines with his normal reciprocal gait but on steeper slopes resorts to the same technique as for stairs.

Surfaces. Varying surfaces can be used to improve the patient's control of the prosthesis, beginning with carpet and progressing through tarmac, grass, gravel, and sand to ensure the patient has the confidence to tackle these conditions when met.

Obstacles. Obstacle courses can be used to effect in confronting the patient with many differing problems in a short space of time. Almost anything can be used, the only limit being imagination. Stairs, carpets, bollards, hoops, boxes, sandbags, swing doors, all can be used to test the patient's balance and co-ordination and to improve the patient's manoeuvring in confined spaces. While appreciating that not every situation can be foreseen, most of the common difficulties can be simulated.

Protection in falling is difficult to teach, and practice is contraindicated when a wound or osteoporosis is present. It is more often described to the patient than practised. In falling forwards, any walking aid is discarded and hands placed forward to break the fall; nothing else is practical, it is what patients do! The risk of a Colles or clavicular fracture is weighed against more serious injury to face or head. On falling backwards, if the patient has the presence of mind to flex the trunk, he may land on the 'buttocks' and, of course, on the socket, which will be uncomfortable certainly, but preferable to an occipital fracture.

Rising from a fall unaided should be taught by lowering the patient to the floor, to a sitting position. First a check is made as to the whereabouts of the stick if any, and the patient rolls over onto the prone position and then onto hands and knees. If indoors, the patient can crawl to a suitable piece of furniture, kneel on the prosthesis and use the sound limb to rise to standing. If outdoors, the stick can be retrieved by crawling, the patient again kneels on the prosthesis and raises himself by the sound limb and pressure on the stick to assist the ascent to regain a stable, balanced position.

Ideally, the home environment is assessed and problems highlighted, e.g. stairs requiring handrails, high doorsteps, edges of rugs, etc. Aids may be required such as handrails in toilet, bathseats, raised toilet seats, etc. With the technology available, most will be able to drive a car. All treatment, aids, advice and encouragment are aimed at the patient achieving maximum mobility and independence.

Reference

Nowroozi F., Salvandelli M. L. & Gerber L. H. (1983) Energy expenditure in hip disarticulation and hemipelvectomy amputees. *Archives of Physical Medicine and Rehabilitation* **64**, 300–303.

33

Prosthetic Care and Rehabilitation in Hip Disarticulation, Hemipelvectomy and Hemicorporectomy

H. SCHMIDL

Introduction

The prosthetic management of patients after hip disarticulation or hemipelvectomy requires certain conditions, making it necessary to view the problem as a whole and not solely from a technical standpoint. The segment of the body removed in the case of such an amputation comprises nearly 1/5 of the human body. This segment, now to be artificially replaced, has a decisive function involving not only the amputee's static balance but also the dynamic process of motion. As a consequence of the amputation, a loss in mass of about 20% occurs, resulting in the body's centre of gravity being displaced upwards and towards the remaining and supporting leg. This in turn affects the stability and the harmony of individual movements. This change in the centre of gravity has a disturbing effect on the dynamic process of walking with respect to the prosthesis, especially during heel-strike and later in the stance phase when rolling over the ball of the artificial foot. By means of careful encompassing of the residual pelvis via the pelvic socket design a stable equilibrium with the prosthesis can be provided only by taking into consideration the position of the centre of gravity which is influenced by the body height, weight, and somatic type, and in the long term the condition of the remaining muscles, posture and age. It is clear from this that the position and especially the path of the centre of gravity in motion will vary with each amputee.

After hip disarticulation or hemipelvectomy, stabilization and control of the prosthesis are significantly influenced by the shape of the pelvic 'stump' and the anchoring of the musculature.

Although it seems that amputation techniques for hip disarticulation were available in the middle of the eighteenth century, it was not until about 150 years later that the first hemipelvectomy was performed. The description of the amputation technique was published by Girard in 1895. Amputation more distally in the leg had been performed for several thousand years, but the possibilities for procedures in the pelvic region were not realized until comparatively recent times, presumably due to problems with control of haemorrhage and blood replacement. More proximal surgical intervention is clearly even more difficult, e.g.

hemicorporectomy (Fig. 33.1) was performed successfully for the first time at Minneapolis in 1961 (Aust & Absolon 1962). Accordingly experience with the prosthetic fitting techniques at these high levels of amputation has been relatively short.

In the past 50 years an increasing number of amputations in the pelvic area have been seen, mainly performed for neoplasm. More recently, however, traumatic amputations in the pelvic area have also increased, occasionally due to industrial injuries, but mainly due to traffic accidents, among which motor-cycle accidents rank first. In looking at the patients who have been fitted in Budrio, a large increase of high-level amputations can be noted. There were only 106 amputees in the year 1975, but by 1984 the number had risen to 274, of which more than 70% were hemipelvectomies.

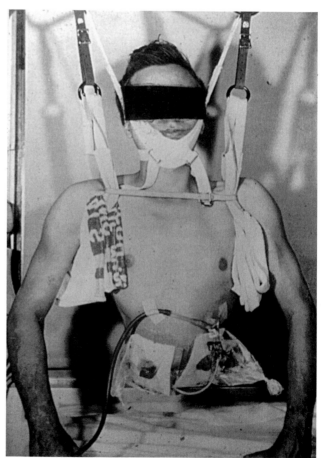

Fig. 33.1 Hemicorporectomy.

Design criteria

The physical restoration of these people is not only a technical problem as, in addition to the functional defect, the patient suffers from psychological trauma. Accordingly the principles of design of the prosthesis must ensure functional restoration and also recognize the need to restore the outward appearance. Hence the following are the design criteria:

Value in use.

Comfortable socket.

Static and functional alignment.

Cosmesis.

Studies and experience in the field of rehabilitation of amputees for many years and the application of the above criteria have resulted in prostheses providing more successful rehabilitation.

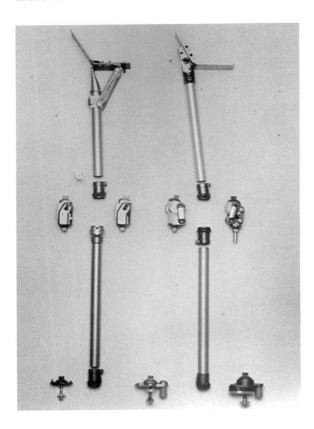

Fig. 33.2 Modular prosthetic system used for hip disarticulation and hemipelvectomy.

Value in use

The development of modular prosthetic systems has significantly improved the value in use of the prostheses as a result of better function, brought about by interchangeable components and easily changed segment lengths. A balanced equilibrium of forces between stump musculature, the centre of gravity of the body mass and the body supporting point can be obtained, thus ensuring less effort in walking with the prosthesis. This is especially important as an amputation in the pelvic area requires a relatively high energy output during walking with the prosthesis, and therefore systems which need less energy are of great value.

Optimum fitting comprises the use of a system (Fig. 33.2) ensuring an individual prosthetic design by means of interchangeability of the functional parts, viz. the foot, knee and hip joint components and the torsion adaptor.

Comfortable socket

Special attention should be paid to the fabrication of the socket as it represents the connecting element between body and prosthesis and furthermore provides for the transfer of force actions in standing and walking and permits control of the mechanical functions of the prosthesis. The weight-bearing potential, stability and the suspension each have an important influence on the connection between the pelvic 'stump' and pelvic socket and on the prosthesis itself.

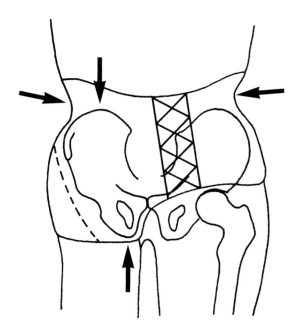

Fig. 33.3 Hip disarticulation — the socket is carefully shaped around the ischium, the iliac crests and the sacrum.

There is, of course, a difference in the body supporting point between the hip disarticulation and hemipelvectomy. In the case of hip disarticulation a body supporting point is available in the form of the ischium (Fig. 33.3), which if properly evaluated provides a stable equilibrium, but only if the suspension of the pelvic socket at the same time prevents significant movement between stump and socket. This can be achieved without difficulty as the pelvic stump is held in position in the pelvic socket by means of careful shaping around the ischium, both iliac crests and the sacrum. The silastic sacrum pad (Fig. 33.4) laminated into the pelvic socket not only serves the purpose of preventing rotation between pelvis and socket but at the same time plays an important part in the control of movement of the prosthesis.

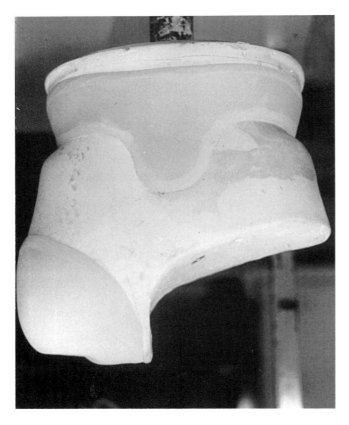

Fig. 33.4 Silastic sacrum pad prevents rotation of the pelvis in the socket and assists in control of movement of the prosthesis.

In the case of *hemipelvectomy* the situation is completely different (Fig. 33.5), as the bony structure is not available and for this reason body support must be looked for in the soft tissue areas, taking into special consideration the structural nature of the pelvic 'stump'. Unstable muscle substance and soft tissue at the amputation side nearly always prevent the establishment of a stable equilibrium between prosthesis and stump. Stabilization and weight-bearing points on the amputation side are the lateral pelvic 'stump' area and the lower thoracic area, and on the opposite side the area of the upper iliac crest. In special cases the socket brim must be extended to the lower costal arch on the contralateral side (Fig. 33.6). The weight-bearing potential and the stability of the pelvic socket are especially influenced by the clasp-like pelvic fixation and the sacrum pad, which also stabilizes the spine. Hemipelvectomy procedures often entail exteriorization of lower bowel or ureters, thus causing even more problems in the fabrication of the pelvic socket. In these cases a trial socket is nearly always indicated.

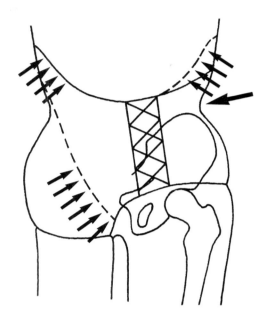

Fig. 33.5 Hemipelvectomy — weight-bearing and stabilization areas.

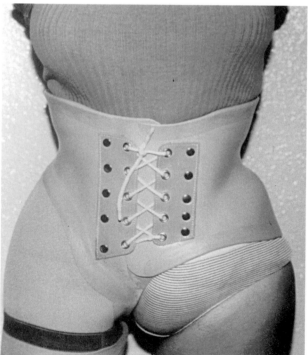

Fig. 33.6 In some cases the brim of the hemipelvectomy socket must extend into the lower costal arch on the contralateral side (*see also* Fig. 33.5).

An important point to consider is the quality of lateral support, which if poor will not allow prosthetic fitting after a hemipelvectomy. Even after hip disarticulation the lateral support substantially influences the total stability of the pelvic prosthesis. In both cases, however, the position and characteristics of the artificial hip joint play an important role.

Static and functional alignment

The next criterion comprises the static alignment on which the functional value is dependent. The connecting element between pelvic socket and prosthesis is the hip joint, which simultaneously suspends and provides movement for the whole prosthesis.

During gait the prosthesis is controlled by movement of the pelvis acting through the socket and thence via the hip joint, and so the hip joint can be considered the

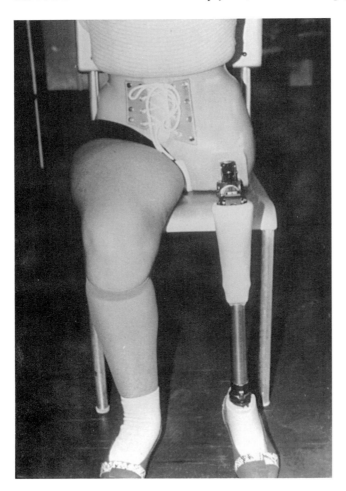

Fig. 33.7 The Otto Bock 7E7 hip joint in the normal sitting position.

main element of the prosthesis. Therefore it is necessary that the hip joint is provided with the characteristic properties which are required for optimum fitting. These are inward and outward rotation, and abduction and adduction as well as flexion and extension of the pelvic socket. The 7E7 hip joint of the Otto Bock modular system not only offers the above characteristics but also permits optimum horizontal levelling of the pelvic socket and as a result allows a normal sitting position (Fig. 33.7). The hip joint position is individually assessed and should be 50% of the distance from the body centre to the lateral pelvic wall. In special circumstances, and mainly in hemipelvectomies, this position can be laterally displaced by 10 mm in order to improve lateral stability (Fig. 33.8).

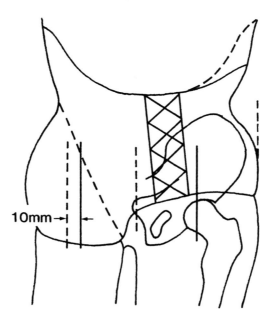

Fig. 33.8 Hip joint position.

A modular system facilitates the fabrication of artificial limbs with a higher rehabilitation value, provided the design criteria are met and meticulously applied. Whatever construction technique is employed, accurate assessment of the individual body centre of gravity is essential. This is expressed in ensuring that both static and dynamic weight-bearing lines are drawn on casts and sockets. The benefit of modular assembly systems is in the provision for rapid changes in the nature and spatial configuration of components.

Static alignment of a prosthesis after hip disarticulation or hemipelvectomy begins when the plaster cast is taken (Fig. 33.9). This requires that to obtain the plaster mould the patient is placed in the correct posture, bearing in mind the body supporting point and the frontal and lateral weight-bearing lines. An incorrect position of the body always prevents optimum static alignment. The respective functional elements of the prosthesis are fixed in the Otto Bock alignment apparatus having regard to the heel height and the various hip, knee and foot components, which due to their properties have special alignment characteristics and values.

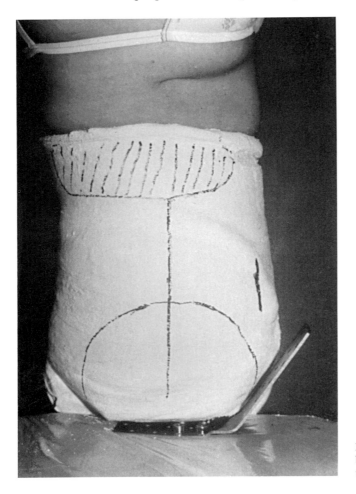

Fig. 33.9 Static alignment begins when the plaster cast is taken.

The weight-bearing line differs from one individual to another, and is calculated in the balancing apparatus. During the alignment procedure the components must be adjusted correspondingly. The alignment apparatus also ensures parallel concordance of hip, knee and foot axes, thus ensuring correct and dynamic action of the prosthesis. The newly developed functional element 4R56 of the Otto Bock Modular System also permits static alignment to be accurately performed even in patients of smaller stature after pelvic amputation as it includes an angular adjustment of 10°.

Special mention should be made of the torsion adaptor for pelvic prostheses. This provides dynamic pelvic rotation of the prosthesis, which is much appreciated by the amputee and produces a far better gait pattern. Furthermore there is a marked reduction of shear forces and energy expenditure.

The result of an accurately performed static alignment is optimal prosthetic function which may be defined as a correctly dynamic gait pattern without the assistance of a cane.

Cosmesis

People losing 1/5 of their body substance need an integrated comprehensive rehabilitation in addition to restoration of function by a prosthesis. Even in this context it can be seen again and again that the cosmetic appearance of the prosthesis has an important influence on the restoration of the amputee (Fig. 33.10). The final result undoubtedly will be a negative one if the prosthesis, even if it functions well, does not offer a good cosmetic appearance. Indeed, if the cosmesis is bad

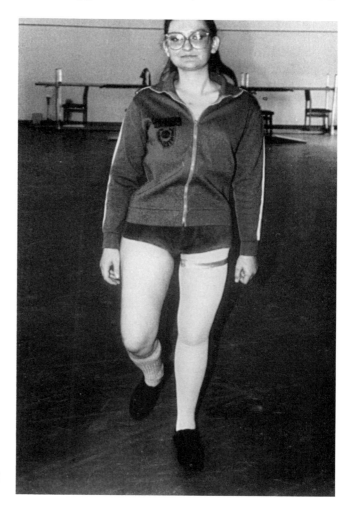

Fig. 33.10 Cosmetic appearance has an important influence on the restoration of the amputee.

the amputee may refuse the prosthesis however well it functions. A modular system provides the possibility of fully restoring the outward appearance of the amputee. Walking training as part of the rehabilitation programme is not only necessary, but if performed to a recognized protocol ensures an optimal alignment and gait with the prosthesis (Fig. 33.11).

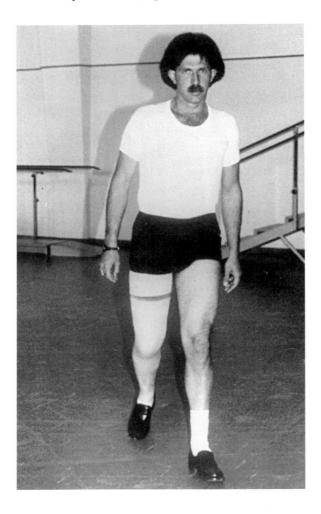

Fig. 33.11 Walking training helps to ensure optimum alignment and prosthetic gait.

Fitting problems — bilateral hip disarticulation and hemicorporectomy

The situation, however, is more complicated in the case of a bilateral hip disarticulation, or even more so in a hemicorporectomy. In the first case the pelvic socket and the static alignment include characteristics which are identical with the unilateral hip disarticulation. It is advisable to use a torsion adaptor, thus offering the possibility of obtaining a good dynamic phasic movement by means of rotation in connection with the separate sockets (Fig. 33.12).

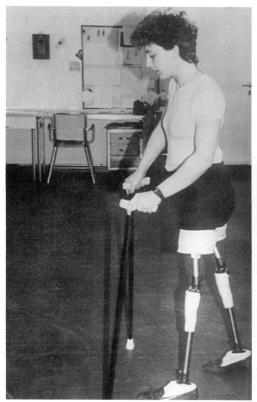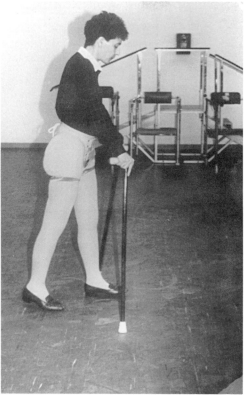

Fig. 33.12 Bilateral hip disarticulation.

Fitting presents severe problems in the case of a hemicorporectomy (Fig. 33.13). The case illustrated is a traumatic one at the level of the lower third part of the pelvis, the distal part of the residual trunk being covered by skin grafts. As a consequence the patient could not even adopt a sitting position without an orthopaedic device. By application of a very soft silicone padding in the pelvic socket and thoracic support it proved possible to enable the patient first to adopt a sitting position and then to walk with modular prostheses. This, however, was only possible by incorporating two torsion adaptors (Fig. 33.14) with a 40° rotation. The amputee now walks by means of a four-point gait with the assistance of crutches (Fig. 33.15).

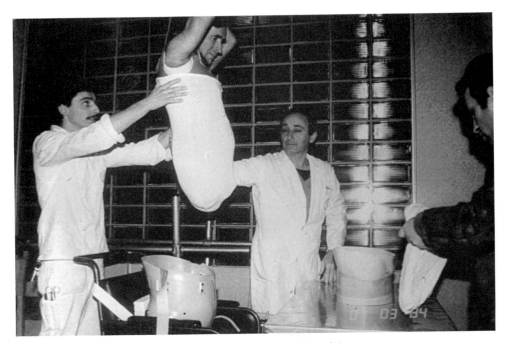

Fig. 33.13 Hemicorporectomy at the level of the lower third of the pelvis.

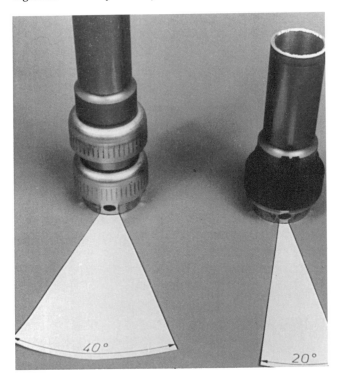

Fig. 33.14 Torque adaptors.

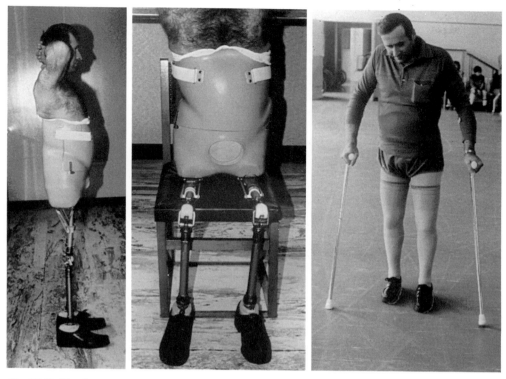

Fig. 33.15 Hemicorporectomy patient standing, sitting and walking with crutches.

Conclusion

In prosthetic fitting and rehabilitation of unilateral and bilateral amputees in the pelvic area it should be emphasized that each individual presents as a fitting with individual problems. The problems in question can only be solved if all criteria are satisfied. An important factor for optimum fitting is good co-operation of the rehabilitation team, in which the surgeon must be included. Last, but not least, it is essential to develop human contact with the patients which, with reference to fitting of this kind, must be close and carefully analysed. If there is a clear understanding for the feeling and the personality of the amputee to be fitted then, and only then, will the final result of prosthetic fitting and functional rehabilitation be satisfactory.

Reference

Aust J. K. & Absolon K. B. (1962) A successful lumbo-sacral amputation: hemicorporectomy. *Surgery* **52(5)**, 756–759.

Further reading

Dankmyer C. H. & Doshi R. (1981) Prosthetic management of adult hemicorporectomy and bilateral hip disarticulation amputee. *Orthotics and Prosthetics* **35(4)**, 11–18.

Girard C. (1895) Disarticulation de l'os iliaque pour sarcome. *Congres Franc Chirurgie* **9**, 823–827.

Horvath E. Uber die dynamische Belastungslinie im sogenannten Standbein. Otto Bock-Technische Information — 3500 -09.78.

Kramer H. & Waigand H. (1968) Technische Versorgung von Dismelie Kindern mit Huftexartikulationsprothesen. *Orthopädie-Technik* **20**, 331–332.

Madden M. (1986) The flexible socket system as applied to the hip disarticulation amputee. *Orthotics and Prosthetics* **39(4)**, 44–47.

Mulby W. C. & Radcliffe C. W. (1960) An ankle-rotation device for prostheses (UC-B Ankle Rotator Model Q74A) Technical Report 37. Biomechanics Laboratory, University of California: San Fransisco and Berkeley.

Ockenfels P. A. (1968) Management and construction procedure of bilateral split-bucket type hip disarticulation prosthesis. *Orthotics and Prosthetics* **22(2)**.

Schmidl H. (1965) La protesizzazione nella disarticolazione di anca, nelle emipelvectomie e nelle emicorporectomie. Atti Congresso Nazionale FIOTO, Rome, 24–26 October, 1965.

Schmidl H. (1976) Versorgungsmoglichkeiten Bei Huftexartikulationen und Hemipelvectomien. *Orthopädie-Tecknik* **27**, 88–92.

Shurr D. G., Cook T. M., Buckwalter J. A. & Cooper R. R. (1983) Hip disarticulation: a prosthetic follow up. *Orthotics and Prosthetics* **37(3)**, 50–57.

University of California (1947) Fundamental studies of human locomotion and other information relating to the design of artificial limbs. Prosthetic Devices Research Project. Berkeley, 2 vols.

Van Tiel W. W. (1983) Justiereinheit fur die obere Achse einer Huft-Exartikulations-Prothes. (Alignment unit for the proximal part of a hip disarticulation prosthesis.) *Medizinisch Orthopädisch Technik* **103**, 153–156.

Van der Warrde T. (1984) Ottawa experience with hip disarticulation prosthesis. *Orthotics and Prosthetics* **38(1)**, 29–35.

Van der Warrde T. (1985) Konstruktionsvarianten der huftexartikulationsprothese. (Hip disarticulation prostheses design variations.) *Orthopädie Technik* **36**, 661–664.

Volkert R. (1985) Probleme in der Oberschenkel-und Beckenprothesen Versorgung. (Problems of prosthetic management after above-knee and hip disarticulation). *Orthopädie Technik* **36**, 68–73.

Waigand H. (1975) Neurtige-Prothesen bei Amelien beider unteren Extremitaten. *Orthopädie-Technik* **26**, 178–179.

CONGENITAL LIMB DEFICIENCY

34

Nomenclature and Classification in Congenital Limb Deficiency

H.J.B. DAY

Introduction

In the past the lack of any proper system of classification of congenital limb malformations was partly concealed by the use of Greek or Latin quasiscientific terms which merely described the anomaly. 'Brachyphalangia' doubtless sounded more impressive than 'short fingers'. Furthermore, as most clinical conditions were described by more than one of these terms, confusion abounded, and any attempt to compare incidence and the results of treatment was frustrated. It was therefore a great advance when Frantz and O'Rahilly published in 1961 a classification which, providing a comprehensive system of nomenclature, was rapidly adopted in the United States of America. However their system was not accepted so well in Europe because some of the terms used appeared to be contradictory. 'Hemimelia', literally half a limb, is appropriate to a loss equivalent to an elbow disarticulation, but the same term was proposed for a loss between shoulder and elbow. Furthermore the terms 'partial hemimelia' used for below-elbow loss, and 'paraxial hemimelia' for failure of formation of the radius or ulna merely increased the confusion.

In 1966 Burtch proposed a revision in which the word hemimelia was replaced by 'meromelia' (part limb), although the overall classification remained the same. Unfortunately instead of replacing the Frantz and O'Rahilly classification, Burtch's revision became an alternative. A third system used in the United States was proposed by Swanson in 1964 and is accepted by the American Hand Society. This is an overall classification which includes soft tissue as well as skeletal abnormalities and lists seven categories:

1 Failure of formation of parts.
2 Failure of differentiation of parts.
3 Duplication.
4 Overgrowth (gigantism).
5 Undergrowth (hypoplasia).
6 Congenital constriction band syndrome.
7 Generalized skeletal abnormalities.

In Germany a different set of terms, again based on Greek roots, was in common use including peromelia, ectromelia and dysmelia, which were not accepted in the United States. The only terms on which there was any general agreement were amelia and phocomelia. The latter is misused more than any other, in that all types of limb deficiency are commonly and regrettably referred to as phocomelia, whose meaning of 'seal limb' should restrict its use to cases where a hand is attached directly to the shoulder (or a foot to the pelvis). In 1969 Henkel and Willert produced a systematization of the German nomenclature based on a progression in the severity of the deficiency and using such terms as hypoplasia and aplasia. Unfortunately they also produced a somewhat contradictory phrase, 'partial aplasia'.

It was against this background that the International Society for Prosthetics and Orthotics set up a Working Group to propose a system of terminology which might be acceptable internationally. The Committee, under the chairmanship of the late Hector Kay, met first in Dundee in 1973 and quickly reached agreement on certain intentions and constraints:

1 The classification should be restricted to skeletal deficiencies, and therefore the majority of such cases would be examples of the 'failure of formation of parts' listed as the first category in the American Hand Society's classification.

2 The deficiencies would be described on anatomical and radiological bases only. No attempt would be made to classify in terms of embryology, aetiology, or epidemiology.

3 Classically derived terms such as hemimelia, peromelia, ectomelia, etc. should be avoided because of their lack of precision and the difficulty of translation into those languages which are not related to Latin and Greek. The new nomenclature should use simple precise words understandable in the English-speaking world and readily translated into all other languages.

The group then addressed itself to the original Frantz/O'Rahilly work which had proposed four basic categories of deficiency:

   Terminal transverse — in which the limb has developed normally in a proximo-distal direction to a particular level beyond which no skeletal elements exist.

   Terminal longitudinal — in which the pre-axial or post-axial bones together with the corresponding elements of hand or foot are absent.

   Intercalary transverse — in which a whole segment (or segments) is missing but the hand is present and is attached directly to the elbow or shoulder, or the equivalent in the lower limb.

   Intercalary longitudinal — in which the pre-axial or post-axial element is absent but the hand or foot is complete.

There was no disagreement with the classification of terminal transverse deficiencies in which the affected limb resembles an amputation stump, but doubt was expressed about the validity of intercalary deficiencies, in that all such cases have some abnormality of the hand or foot, either in structure or size, and can therefore never be said to be truly normal. All are therefore manifestations of a longitudinal failure, and it is the distribution and magnitude of this failure which determines the clinical appearance, as exemplified by the reduction series of Henkel and Willert. Such a progressive reduction provides a paradox in that the most severe longitudinal deficiency is one in which no skeletal element has formed — the true amelia, which has the appearance of a transverse deficiency. Indeed the latter would be the best designation for such a case.

It was decided, therefore, that only two categories would be needed, *transverse and longitudinal*. The former would include all those previously known as terminal transverse and which resembled amputation stumps. The presence of soft tissue finger or toe buds would not affect the inclusion of cases in this category. The *longitudinal* category would include all other cases. A scheme was then drawn up in which *transverse* deficiencies (Fig. 34.1) would be described by the level at which the limb terminated, using the words shoulder (pelvis), arm (thigh), forearm (leg), carpal (tarsal), metacarpal (metatarsal), phalangeal, together with a secondary descriptor to indicate the level of termination within that named segment — it being understood that all elements distal to that level are absent. In *longitudinal* deficiencies (Figs. 34.2 and 34.3) all bones affected would be named, as nouns, together with a secondary descriptor to indicate whether such a bone is totally or partially absent.

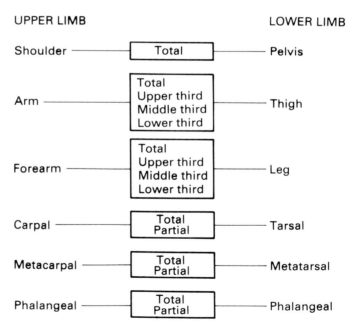

Fig. 34.1 Designation of levels of transverse deficiencies of upper and lower limbs.

Note. Total absence of the shoulder or hemipelvis (and all distal elements) is a transverse deficiency. If only a portion of the shoulder or hemipelvis is absent, the deficiency is of the longitudinal type.

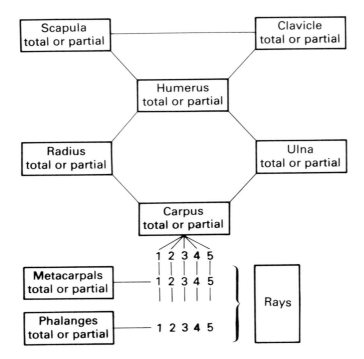

Fig. 34.2 Description of longitudinal deficiencies of the upper limb.

A trial of the system at 15 clinics in Europe and the U.S.A. during 1974 confirmed that the classification worked well, but some small refinements were agreed at a further meeting of the Committee in Montreux in 1974. Unfortunately, the first publication of the classification by Kay in 1974 (and another which did not appear until 1975) preceded this meeting and therefore does not include the refinements. Swanson published the final version in 1976, and this now forms the basis of a draft proposal to the International Standards Organization Technical Committee No. 168, and has also been incorporated in the Impairment Code of WHO.

International nomenclature for classification of skeletal limb deficiencies

First state whether the deficiency is transverse or longitudinal.

Transverse

1 State the side of the patient affected.
2 State the level of loss as in Fig. 34.1, it being understood that all skeletal elements distal to that level are absent.
3 For levels of loss in the carpal (tarsal), metacarpal (metatarsal) or phalangeal regions, the words total or partial are used as a second-order descriptor, e.g. carpal

total would indicate a wrist disarticulation type, whereas the presence of one row of the carpus would be described carpal partial.

4 Always put the level of loss first, followed by supplemental conditions, e.g. transverse, right, carpal partial, with hypoplasia of radius and ulna. (Note that both forearm bones are named as they may not be equally affected.)

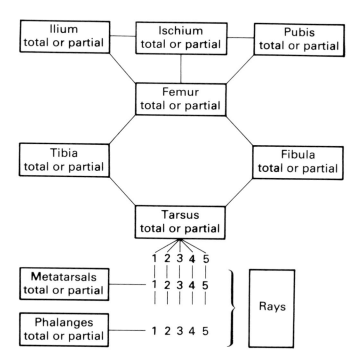

Fig. 34.3 Description of longitudinal deficiencies of the lower limb.

Longitudinal

1 State the side of the patient affected.

2 State the extent of deficiency of each bone as in Figs. 34.2 and 34.3 proceeding from the most proximal bone to the most distal, as follows:

(a) *Shoulder and pelvic girdles.* State which bones are totally absent and which are partially absent. In the event of partial absence identify and state the part of the bone which is absent.

(b) *Humerus, radius and ulna: femur, tibia and fibula.* State which bones are totally absent — state the approximate fraction of the bone which is absent and the position (proximal–distal) of the deficiency.

(c) *Carpus, tarsus.* State whether totally or partially absent (i.e. some carpal or tarsal bones are present). Further description of partial deficiencies by naming or enumerating individual bones may be added.

(d) *Metacarpals, metatarsals and phalanges.* State the number of digit(s) affected commencing from the radial or tibial side. State which *metacarpals* (metatarsals) are totally absent and which are partially absent. Further description of partial deficiencies by means of a fraction of loss and its position may be added. State which *phalanges* are totally absent and which are partially absent. Further description by naming the affected phalanx (i.e. proximal, intermediate, or distal) may be added.

Note. For brevity when referring collectively to a metacarpal or metatarsal and its corresponding phalanges the term 'ray' may be used.

3 State the presence of hypoplasia for any bone that has not been described as totally or partially absent.

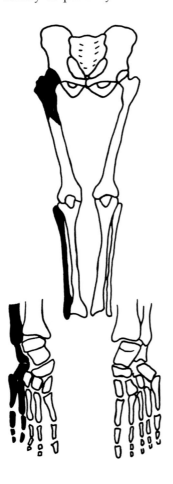

Fig. 34.4 Longitudinal, right, femur partial, proximal ⅓, fibula total, tarsus partial, rays 4 and 5 total.

The classification in use

The application of this system to cases of transverse deficiency is simple and produces a brief, accurate description, e.g. the common below-elbow level of loss is written as transverse forearm, upper ⅓, and might well be spoken of as a transverse upper forearm deficiency. The longitudinal deficiencies tend to be less succinct but provide an accurate account of the anatomy. The example shown in Fig. 34.4 would be described as longitudinal, right, femur partial, proximal ⅓, fibula total, tarsus partial, rays 4 and 5 total. It would be unrealistic to expect such a designation to be used in speech, when almost certainly such a case would be referred to as one of PFFD with absence of the fibula.

It is common for clinical records to include not only a word description but an outline drawing of the skeleton with the absent segments marked (Fig. 34.4). In the author's view this has the disadvantage of implying that the remaining bones are normal in shape and size, which is seldom the case, particularly in longitudinal deficiencies. A stylized representation is preferred (Fig. 34.5a) as not only can total or partial absences be shown, but any hypoplasia, angulation or synostosis of the remaining bones can be indicated together with various types of surgical intervention (Fig. 34.5b).

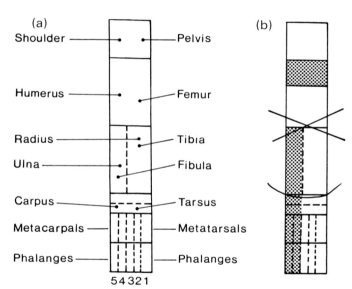

Fig. 34.5 (a) Stylized representation of limb. (b) Longitudinal, right, femur partial, proximal ⅓, fibula total, tarsus partial, rays 4 and 5 total. Knee has been arthrodesed and Syme amputation performed.

Summary

A system of classifying congenital skeletal limb deficiencies on an anatomical basis is described. All such deficiencies are considered to be *transverse* or *longitudinal*. The former resemble amputation stumps and the level of termination is named — no skeletal elements existing beyond this level. All other cases are *longitudinal* deficiencies in which all bones affected are named. Any bone not named is present and of normal form.

References

Burtch R. L. (1966) Nomenclature for congenital skeletal limb deficiencies, a revision of the Frantz and O'Rahilly classification. *Artificial Limbs* **10(1)**, 24–25.

Frantz C. H. & O'Rahilly R. (1961) Congenital skeletal limb deficiencies. *Journal of Bone and Joint Surgery* **43A**, 1202–1224.

Henkel H. L. & Willert H. G. (1969) Dysmelia, a classification and a pattern of malformation of congenital limb deficiencies. *Journal of Bone and Joint Surgery* **51B**, 399–414.

Kay H. W. (1974) A proposed international terminology for the classification of congenital limb deficiencies. *Inter-Clinic Information Bulletin* **13,7**, 1–16.

Kay H. W. (1975) The proposed international terminology for the classification of congenital limb deficiencies, the recommendations of a working group of the International Society for Prosthetics and Orthotics, London. Spastics International Medical Publications in association with W. Heinemann Medical Books Ltd. and J. B. Lippincott Co.

Swanson A. B. (1964) A classification for congenital malformations of the hand. *New Jersey Bulletin, Academy of Medicine* **10**, 166–169.

Swanson A. B. (1976) A classification for congenital limb malformations. *The Journal of Hand Surgery* **1(1)**, 8–22.

35

Surgical Management of Lower Limb Deficiencies

L.M. KRUGER

Introduction

Surgical management of lower limb deficiencies is best undertaken only in a centre which is accustomed to treating such deficiencies. It is not only the surgery but a knowledge of the life history of a particular limb deficiency, and the growth characteristics of the child, and in particular of the long bones, which is important. It is not enough to think in terms of the child at age one or two, it is important to know what the child is going to be on attaining maturity and to plan the surgical approach to the lower limb so that all surgical intervention can be accomplished at one sitting with a view of what the end result will be in adult life. Primary consideration should be given to functional restoration, and this is perceived in childhood as the child taking part in all normal activities, including tennis, skiing, baseball, etc.

Management philosophy

In earlier years the philosophy of management of lower limb deficiencies was simply the provision of such bracing or orthotic devices or orthoprostheses as were necessary to restore length and permit the child to get about. Such individuals certainly are viewed as 'cripples', and in our philosophy it is much more important to convert these limb deficiencies to true amputation, which can be appropriately fitted with modern prosthetic devices so that the child is viewed as a whole individual from infancy into adult life. This view is important for the child's own psychological development, as well as for relationships with others, schooling, and the ultimate vocational decisions in adult life.

It is important to recognize physiological differences between the child and the adult, and these primarily relate to growth, although psychological differences are important as well. With regard to growth, one must always attempt to retain all epiphyses in surgical intervention in the infant. For example, if there is a very short below-knee stump and this can be preserved, growth of the proximal tibial epiphysis will eventually lead to a sufficiently long below-knee stump for a good below-knee fitting. Under no circumstances should a knee joint be sacrificed unless absolutely necessary. Even split-thickness grafting over a tibial stump is preferable to knee disarticulation or above-knee amputation.

Transtibial amputation under eight or ten years of age should never be undertaken because of the high incidence of 'spiking'. It is preferable, whenever amputation of a lower limb is necessary, to perform either a Syme-type amputation (disarticulation at the ankle joint), or a modified Boyd amputation, fusing the os calcis to the distal tibia. The latter is to be reserved for the older child, in whom possible damage to the distal tibial epiphysis will not be important. In the younger child, the Syme ankle disarticulation is the procedure of choice, leaving the cartilage intact. Transtibial amputation should not be undertaken and, if for some reason it is absolutely necessary, as in the amputations of patients with proximal femoral focal deficiency (PFFD), then stump capping after the fashion of Marquardt (1981) should be considered.

In the partial transverse deficiency of a lower limb, prosthetic fitting is usually possible without any surgical intervention. On occasion spiking may occur even in these congenital deficiencies, as shown by Pellicore *et al.* (1974), and then revision and/or stump capping may be necessary. For the patient with bilateral below-knee level amputation, prosthetic fitting is usually possible without any surgical intervention.

For the patient with above-knee and below-knee amputations, the author prefers to fit the children with 'stubbies' prior to going to articulated limbs. When the child has attained good balance and is walking, the stubbies may be lengthened and shortly thereafter articulated limbs may be fitted.

In the bilateral above-knee transverse deficiencies, again it is preferable to start the child in 'stubbies', elongate the stubbies so that the child develops good trunk balance, and then proceed to articulated limbs.

For the child who has a complete amelia of a single lower limb, prosthetic fitting without surgical intervention is accomplished, but the phocomelias or complete longitudinal deficiency of the femur, tibia, and fibula leave a foot attached at pelvic level. In past years it was thought that perhaps it was best to maintain this, that it would ultimately find some function in converting a disarticulation type of fitting into an above-knee fitting. This is not the case, and it is just as well to remove this foot early in life and to proceed with a disarticulation fitting.

Tibial deficiencies

Partial longitudinal deficiency of the tibia can usually be diagnosed at birth, since there is clinical evidence of a knee joint. It is not necessarily the case that ossification of the retained proximal fragment of the tibia will be noted at birth by X-ray. Ossification will frequently be delayed. This delay may confuse the diagnosis if one relies solely on the X-ray, since ossification may be delayed even until as late as four to five years of age. In such instances, if one suspects that there is a knee joint, arthrography should delineate the presence of the cartilaginous anlage of the proximal tibia. In such cases, amputation should be deferred. If the proximal tibial fragment is short, then tibiofibular synostosis is indicated in order to have a good, long below-knee stump. Fusion of os calcis to the distal fibula, or disarticulation at the ankle, is then carried out, and the child is fitted as a below-knee amputee.

Complete longitudinal deficiency of the tibia is currently treated by disarticulation at knee level. In the past, as far back as 1904, fusions of the fibula to the femur, and of the os calcis to the fibula, were carried out. However, length discrepancy ultimately necessitated amputation. Brown (1971) described his technique of implanting the fibula beneath the distal femur, but the criteria necessary for a successful Brown procedure are such that it is now recognized that this procedure will rarely be successful. Brown postulated that if there is a good quadriceps extensor mechanism, including a patella, if the fibula is not proximal to the distal femoral epiphysis, and if the child can be treated prior to one year of age, it is possible to apply skeletal traction for four weeks and then implant the fibula in the intracondylar notch of the distal femur and reconstruct the extensor mechanism, attaching it to the fibula and fixing the fibula to the femur with two wires. This is later followed by a disarticulation of the foot from the distal fibula or fusion of the os calcis to the fibula and transtarsal amputation, thus creating a below-knee situation. Failure of this procedure with recurrent knee flexion deformity has caused most surgeons to abandon it. The author has reverted to the disarticulation at knee level with prosthetic fitting between one year and 1½ years, or as soon as the child is standing on the normal foot in the unilateral case, or cruising on the knees in the bilateral case. It is important to recognize that longitudinal deficiency of the fibula may be accompanied by other anomalies and not infrequently is genetically transmitted.

In the multiple limb deficiencies, where longitudinal deficiency of the tibia may be associated with PFFD, with contralateral deficiency of the fibula, or with any combination of lower limb deficiencies, decision-making is the key to successful management of the child. In many instances it will be necessary to do reconstructive surgery. Multiple surgical procedures have been abandoned as they keep the child in the hospital for long periods of time in bracing and unusual prostheses. It is felt that if one knows the life history of the limb deficiency, one should plan for a single operative procedure which will permit the child to remain in his normal environment, to attend school with his peers, and to develop with such prosthetic devices as are necessary. As a result of this, the author resorts to early amputation when it is realized this may be the ultimate outcome.

Longitudinal deficiency of the fibula

Longitudinal deficiency of the fibula is perhaps the most frequently encountered long bone deficiency. As with all other limb deficiencies, it is important to recognize that it is not simply the absence of a single long bone, but a complete limb deficiency with deficit in the skin, as evidenced by dimpling of the skin over the remaining tibia. There is a deficiency in the tibia itself which is frequently kyphoscoliotic (anteriorly bowed); there is frequently abnormality of the distal tibial epiphysis; there is usually valgus of the knee with underdevelopment of the lateral femoral condyle and perhaps no tibial spines or cruciate ligaments; there is usually abnormality of the tarsus; and there may be absence of one or more of the lateral rays of the foot, causing significant foot deformity.

When a child is born with 5 cm or more of length discrepancy, equalization of leg length in adult life will be nearly impossible, and it is considered that this discrepancy at birth is an indication for early amputation and prosthetic restoration. Additional indications include the severe foot deformity. Even if leg length can be maintained, a two-rayed or a single-rayed foot is extremely difficult for the patient to manage, shoe wear is almost impossible, and the foot deformity poses a psychological hazard. It is considered that severe deformity of the foot is likewise an indication for amputation.

Experience has shown that length discrepancy is progressive, and that those children with a normal or essentially normal tibia frequently have the greatest foot deformity, whereas those with an essentially normal foot have a very short tibia, or associated PFFD and femoral shortening. Experience has shown that the large majority of children with a unilateral longitudinal deficiency of the fibula come to Syme disarticulation and prosthetic restoration.

In the bilateral case, if the tibia is straight, and if there is a reasonably good foot, this foot can be brought plantigrade and the patient can retain his normal feet. If, on the other hand, the feet are severely deformed, it is again probably best to resort to either Syme or Boyd amputation and prosthetic restoration. Similarly, in the early years, we paid no attention to the remaining tibia if we could get the foot plantigrade. In adult life many of these people were extremely short, and resented this fact, and on at least one occasion the patient came back in later life to request amputation of his feet and prosthetic restoration of height. The length of the tibia is monitored, and where the tibia is 50% of the length of the femur or less progressive discrepancy is anticipated. These patients are much better off with early ablation of the foot and prosthetic restoration. This maintains their height with their peers as they enter school. It does not interfere with function. Children who have had Syme or Boyd amputations take part in all sports activities, including basketball, football, baseball, skiing, and tennis.

In 58 children with unilateral longitudinal deficiency of the fibula, 44 have been amputated. All are independent. In no instance has a Boyd or Syme amputation required revision, and all carry out full normal activities and do not consider themselves at all restricted. Ten of the 14 not amputated should have been amputated. Additionally, five patients with bilateral deficiencies have been amputated and fitted with Syme-type prostheses with excellent results. The height of at least three who have not been amputated is such that they are extremely short when compared to their peers, and this poses a psychological problem. These patients would be much better off with the loss of the foot and restoration of height by prostheses. Hospital records show that as early as 1934 amputation was used as definitive treatment for longitudinal deficiency of the fibula and this practice continues today. Many children once grown up have returned with their own families to show that they have normal children. None has been unhappy with this approach to treatment.

On at least two occasions children have been seen with longitudinal deficiency of the fibula treated elsewhere in an effort to maintain the foot. In one instance a 15-year-old with unilateral deficiency of the fibula had undergone attempts at leg-lengthening, which resulted in a deep infection and non-union, and she remained on crutches from age three until age 15, at which time, instead of Syme-type amputation, she required above-knee amputation and then was able to walk without crutches for the first time in her life. In another instance where an effort was made to reconstruct the leg, a compartment syndrome occurred, the child lost all musculature in the lower limb, and was then fitted with an orthoprosthesis in which the foot was incorporated into the prosthetic socket. Since he had a deficiency on the contralateral side as well, he had extreme difficult in walking, until reconstructive surgery and appropriate amputation was carried out. The conclusion is that if one knows the life history of longitudinal deficiency of the fibula, it is much better to consider amputation and prosthetic restoration early in life rather than to subject the patient to multiple attempts at reconstruction.

References

Brown F. W. (1971) The Brown operation for total hemimelia tibia. In *Symposium on Selected Lower Limb Anomalies: Surgical and Prosthetic Management* (ed. Aitken G. T.), pp. 20–28. Washington D.C.: National Academy of Sciences.

Marquardt E. (1981) The multiple limb deficient child. In *Atlas of Limb Prosthetics: Surgical and Prosthetic Principles* (American Academy of Orthopaedic Surgeons), pp. 601–608 St. Louis: C.V. Mosby.

Pellicore R. J., Sciora J., Lambert C. N. & Hamilton R. (1974) Incidence of bone overgrowth in the juvenile amputee population. *Inter-Clinic Information Bulletin* **13(15)**, 1–8.

36

The Van Nes Rotationplasty for Congenital Defects of the Femur

R. GILLESPIE

Introduction

The operative technique for combined fusion of the knee and rotationplasty of the limb in the management of congenital deficiency of the femur is presented. The technique described allows earlier definitive prosthetic fitting of a child with proximal femoral deficiency; it has reduced the number of operative procedures needed to obtain the optimal function from that deficient limb; and it has enabled these procedures to be performed at an earlier age. The technique differs from those previously described and represents a significant improvement in management of the patient with femoral deficiency.

The original description for increasing the function of a grossly shortened lower limb by rotating the extremity through 180° and using the ankle joint as a knee within a prosthesis has been attributed to Borggreve (1930). He described how a patient who had lost a large segment of the femur was treated by rotating the rest of the limb through the gap left by resection of the distal femur. This concept was further popularized by Van Nes (1950), who described three patients in whom he had performed similar procedures, rotating the limb through 180°. This article by Van Nes reveals that the rotation was performed through the femur in one case, through the femur and knee in two stages in the second case, and through the knee joint in the third case.

Since these original descriptions, rotating the limb through 180° has become known as the Van Nes rotationplasty. However, more recent descriptions (Kostuik *et al.* 1975, Kritter 1977) refer to the technique as a tibial rotationplasty. Kritter used a fibular strut to stabilize the tibial osteotomy, and in the series described by Kostuik *et al.* the tibial osteotomy was, in most cases, fixed with a plate and screws. Other methods of fixation have also been used including Kirschner wires, staples, and intramedullary rods.

The place of tibial rotationplasty or Van Nes rotationplasty in the management of a patient with a unilateral proximal focal femoral deficiency (Fig. 36.1) has been established. However, subsequent derotation of the limb following operation has, in some patients, led to disappointing results, requiring either revision rotationplasty or Syme amputation. Other patients have developed a ball-and-socket ankle joint; this compensates for a moderate amount of derotation by increasing the range of movement in the subtalar joint of the foot within the prosthesis, thereby maintaining a useful extremity.

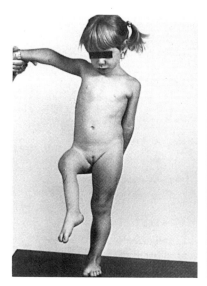 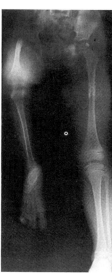

Fig. 36.1 A three-year-old child with proximal focal femoral deficiency of the right leg.

It is felt that the tendency to derotate after a tibial rotationplasty is due to the action of muscles arising proximal, and inserted distal, to the oseotomy, and acting across open and growing epiphyseal plates. This spiral line of muscles imparts a torque force which, in the presence of open epiphyses, derotates the limb during growth. In the operative technique which is described, the rotation is performed through the knee at the time of knee fusion, thus eliminating the spiral component of the action of the leg muscles. It avoids the need for separate operative procedures to accomplish the fusion and the rotation; and it provides for earlier fitting of the definitive prosthesis.

Method

The patient is placed on the operating table and draped so that the affected limb is completely exposed from iliac crest to toes. The contralateral limb should be easily palpable through the drapes to allow estimation of the shortening required to bring the foot of the deficient limb level with the knee of the normal limb.

After routine preparation of the skin, an incision is made overlying the anterolateral aspect of the knee. This incision begins considerably proximal to the knee and extends distally along the line of the tibia (Fig. 36.2). The subcutaneous tissues are dissected to display the capsule of the knee and the patellar tendon. This tendon is divided and the capsule of the knee incised. By traction on the tendon, the patella and quadriceps mechanism are retracted proximally, thereby displaying the knee joint. The structure of the knee is then clearly visible; the deficiency of the cruciate ligaments, the lack of formation of the femoral condyles, the intercondylar notch, and tibial spines are all readily apparent. The dissection is continued both medially and laterally, dividing the collateral ligaments and the capsule of the knee.

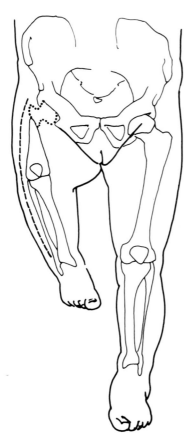

Fig. 36.2 Diagrammatic representation of proximal focal femoral deficiency. The cartilaginous proximal femur is shown as a dotted outline and the proposed incision is shown as a line of dashes.

Attention is then drawn to the medial aspect of the knee where, by careful dissection, the insertion of the adductor magnus is located, and the adductor hiatus with the neurovascular bundle is defined. In these children with very short limbs, the adductor magnus is inserted into the femur at an angle of approximately 80° to the femur as it comes directly from the pelvis; it does not, as in the normal individual, run almost parallel to the femur. That portion of the insertion of adductor magnus which is distal to the adductor hiatus and the femoral neurovascular bundle is detached and allowed to fall away from the femur, thus allowing further exposure of the femoral and popliteal arteries (Fig. 36.3). The attachments of the medial hamstrings are also divided.

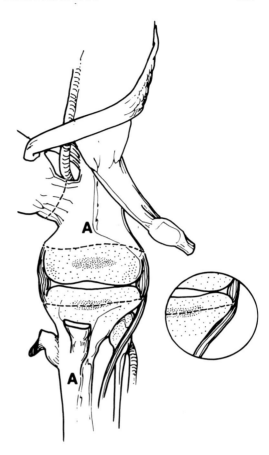

Fig. 36.3 Sartorius and quadriceps have been retracted to expose the adductor hiatus and femoral artery. The peroneal nerve is displayed in its usual location and with fibular hemimelia (inset). The proposed bone cuts are shown as dashes, with the ossific centres shaded. A, anterior.

Attention now focuses on the lateral aspect of the knee. Careful dissection in this region is necessary, particularly if there is an associated fibular hemimelia, in which case the peroneal component of the sciatic nerve lies adjacent to the proximal tibia rather than taking its normal course around the fibular neck (*see* inset, Fig. 36.3). Having located the peroneal nerve, the dissection is then continued proximally, tracing that nerve back to its junction with the sciatic nerve. Care is needed, as clearly damage to the peroneal nerve would negate any benefit deriving from performing the rotationplasty, since the foot would lack power to activate the prosthesis. Having located the neurovascular structures on both sides of the knee joint, they can safely be retracted away from the distal femur and the capsule can be divided all round the joint without danger. The origins of the medial and lateral heads of the gastrocnemius muscle are divided, and the knee is then entirely free of muscle and ligamentous attachments.

The next stage is to fuse the knee. The cartilage of the proximal tibia is removed down to the underlying ossific nucleus of the proximal tibial epiphysis; care is taken not to damage the epiphyseal plate. The distal femoral epiphyseal plate is located, and the entire distal femoral epiphysis is removed, including the epiphyseal plate. The level of division of the distal femur is governed by the overall length of the limb and by the length which is finally required.

An intramedullary rod is then inserted into the distal femur; it is brought out through the buttock and then pushed down through the proximal tibial epiphysis into the shaft of the tibia. The rotationplasty is performed through the knee fusion by rotating the limb as much as possible within the limits of the surrounding soft tissue. The tibial segment can usually be rotated more than 120°, and with care a full 180° of rotation at the level of the knee is possible. At this stage the femoral vessels should be palpated; they now lie anteromedial to the distal femur, having been freed from the confinements of the insertion of adductor magnus (Fig. 36.4a).

(a)   (b)

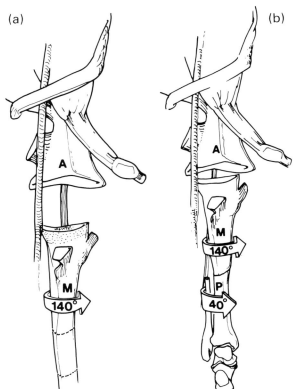

Fig. 36.4 (a) Portions of the distal femur and proximal tibia have been removed, allowing rotation of the proximal tibia. The femoral and popliteal arteries can rotate freely with the distal segment freed from the tether of the adductor magnus insertion. (b) The proximal tibial segment is rotated as much as possible and the remaining rotation required through the tibial shaft osteotomy. A, anterior; M, medial; P, posterior.

The incision is now continued distally along the line of the tibia. The tibia and fibula are exposed subperiosteally and fasciotomies of all compartments are performed. A section of bone is removed from the tibia and fibula should this be necessary to bring the foot up to the appropriate level (Fig. 36.4b). The foot is then placed in the desired position with respect to rotation and the intramedullary rod is driven down through the knee fusion and across the tibial osteotomy. Stability in both the sagittal and coronal planes is provided by the rod, and rotary stability is maintained by applying a hip spica cast incorporating the foot.

If after the operation swelling causes vascular embarrassment, the rod provides stability while the amount of rotation is reduced; when swelling subsides the desired amount of rotation can be regained (Fig. 36.5). This safety valve was not available in patients whose limbs were fixed with plate and screws.

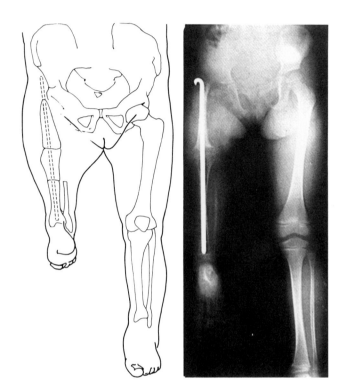

Fig. 36.5 The intramedullary rod fixes both the fusion and the osteotomy, allowing good stability and simple instrumentation.

Discussion

Up to the time of writing, five patients with proximal focal femoral deficiency have undergone this type of rotationplasty. In all cases solid union at both levels was obtained by six weeks, allowing fitting of the prosthesis at that stage. When the prosthesis is fitted the children undergo training to encourage development of the gastrocnemius and to teach them how the reversed position of the foot can power the below-knee section of the modified prosthesis.

The author feels encouraged to continue with this technique, as early gait studies suggest that the efficiency of the muscles is greater now thay do not run in spiral fashion around the limb (as they did when mid-tibial osteotomy was used as the sole rotation point); they now afford better control and power of the lower portion of the prosthesis. Furthermore, to date there have been no neurovascular complications, and the osteotomies and wounds have all healed without difficulty.

The technique has been applied to patients as young as two years old, and can be performed without difficulty as long as the proximal tibial ossific nucleus (as seen on the preoperative radiographs) is large enough to predict a solid knee fusion. With early operation greater mobility of the foot and ankle joint is maintained because of the reduced time in an exension prosthesis (Fig. 36.6) and because the osteotomies heal more readily than in older children.

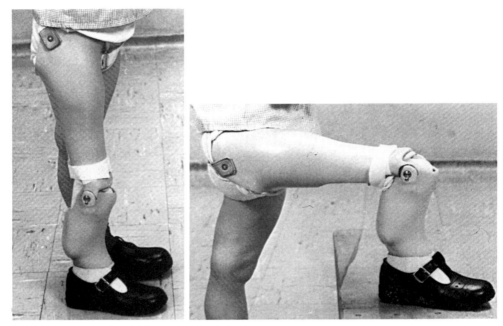

Fig. 36.6 Three-year-old child with right proximal focal femoral deficiency fitted with a modified below-knee prosthesis showing the flexion and extension of her new 'knee' joint.

The original paper by Van Nes suggests that he used techniques similar to those described in this chapter. However the surgical detail has not previously been published, and it is suggested that the technique described in this paper has many advantages over the tibial rotationplasties previously described.

References

Borggreve J. (1930) Kniegelenksersatz durch das in der Beinlangsachse um 180° gedrehte Fussgelenk. *Archive fuer Orthopaedische Und Unfallchirurgie* **28**, 175–178.

Kostuik J. P., Gillespie R., Hall J. E. & Hubbard S. (1975) Van Nes rotational osteotomy for treatment of proximal femoral focal deficiency and congenital short femur. *Journal of Bone and Joint Surgery* **57A**, 1039–1046.

Kritter A. E. (1977) Tibial rotation-plasty for proximal femoral focal deficiency. *Journal of Bone and Joint Surgery* **59A**, 927–934.

Van Nes C. P. (1950) Rotationplasty for congenital defects of the femur: making use of the ankle of the shortened limb to control the knee joint of a prosthesis. *Journal of Bone and Joint Surgery* **32B**, 12–16.

37

Prosthetic Management of Congenital Lower Limb Deficiency

H.J.B. DAY

Introduction

In cases of transverse deficiency of the lower limb a prosthesis will be needed unless the level of loss is very distal. The child with a longitudinal deficiency may require prosthetic care alone, or this may be combined with amputation or surgical reconstruction. Because of the necessity for length equalization and the problems of weight-bearing and stability, surgical correction of any of the major longitudinal deficiencies seldom obviates the need for a prosthesis or orthosis. The surgical procedure may, however, make it possible for the prosthesis or orthosis to be more functional and perhaps more aesthetically pleasing.

Although there is no point in providing a lower limb prosthesis until the child is ready to stand and walk, at perhaps 8–12 months, there is every need for early assessment to plan the management, and, if amputation or reconstruction is indicated, to develop a close collaboration between the surgeons and prosthetic specialist before any surgery is undertaken. Parents need to be informed, reassured, and have all their questions answered. They must be made aware that the programme has to be flexible, particularly for those children whose future joint development and length discrepancy may at first be matters of conjecture. They must understand that in the early years their child's interest will be to develop speed of walking rather than to acquire a good gait pattern. Supervision and training may produce a more elegant walk, leading to parental pleasure, but this is achieved only by an increase in energy expenditure by the child, who may then no longer be able to compete with his peers.

Transverse deficiencies

The prosthetic treatment of those with transverse deficiencies which resemble amputations and those longitudinal deficiencies which have been converted by amputation can be discussed together. The same prosthetic principles which are used for older patients must be applied, but it would, of course, be inappropriate to fit a one-year-old child who has a transverse thigh deficiency with an articulated prosthesis containing a knee swing phase control. It is more appropriate to make an ischial-bearing socket of plastic or metal and mount it on aluminium side bars above a simple foot. This provides a light effective prosthesis which can be lengthened with ease. Indeed, those with a level of loss at or above the knee can be maintained on this type of prosthesis for the first two or three years. A rather similar device in which a leather lacing ischial-bearing thigh corset is mounted on plain side bars can be used for those cases in which the level is in the upper half of the leg. Later some may need a prosthesis with a thigh corset and jointed side bars before changing to a PTB prosthesis. The desirability of this latter must be balanced against the risk of displacement of the lower femoral epiphysis. This risk is greatest, of course, in children who are very active, those who have short stumps, and in those dependent on a tight cuff suspension. Such a danger does not arise with a Syme amputation, which can be fitted with a total-contact socket rather earlier, as the stump is long and no cuff suspension is needed.

Longitudinal deficiencies

Longitudinal deficiencies which have not been converted by amputation usually present with shortening as well as deformity and foot defects, and it is the shortening which must be corrected first to allow the child to stand and walk. The required prosthesis is simple in design and consists of a light leather corset mounted on side bars at the correct height above a small prosthetic foot or shaped block. The child's foot can rest on a suitably padded cradle between the side bars and is maintained in position by a strap. At first, because the child wants to crawl as well as walk, minimal fastenings are used, and indeed the prosthesis will often be worn over clothes. Later, when the child is walking more, the foot should be contained in a soft leather bootee which will improve efficiency. By now the basic prescription requirements of the extension, or platform prosthesis, are becoming clear. The power, range and stability of the joints, together with the ability to bear weight, are the important factors. Partial weight relief can be provided by a thigh corset, whilst full relief will require ischial support. The provision of a corset and side bars should control lateral instability of the knee. If the range of movement or power of this joint is restricted, optional locks on the prosthetic knee joints may be required, whereas gross restriction of knee movement requires side bars without joints. The relationship of the various clinical factors with the prosthetic prescription was described and illustrated in tabular form (Fig. 37.1) by Day and Wright (1977), who described modern plastic prostheses to replace the traditional extension prosthesis with leather bootee, calf band, and lacing gaiters fastened to side steels.

For patients whose deficiency is distal to an effectively normal knee, a total-contact plastic socket mounted on a shank at the appropriate height above a prosthetic foot is satisfactory. The major problem is that the stage and size of the patient's foot, even in equinus, denies itself entry to the socket. An access trap, as in the Canadian Syme prosthesis (Foort 1956), positioned posteriorly allows

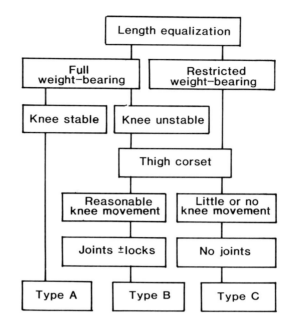

Fig. 37.1 Prescription scheme. The prescription must take into account the ability of the limb to bear weight, and the range of movement, power and stability of the joints.

entry, providing the foot is narrow as in longitudinal, fibula — total: tarsus — partial: rays 4 and 5 — total, deficiency (Fig. 37.2a). The aperture is closed with a rigid cover mounted on straps. A similar method can be used in cases of proximal femoral focal deficiency (PFFD) with absence of the fibula (Fig. 37.2b) (longitudinal, femur partial, proximal ⅓, fibula total, tarsus partial, rays 4 and 5 total), although in this case the knee is flexed and the socket extends proximally to provide ischial support. Occasionally in such cases an anterior position of the access trap is preferred. If the femur is markedly hypoplastic and the overall length discrepancy is great, the child is most likely to have had an arthrodesis of the knee with a Syme amputation, but occasionally such a course may be contraindicated or refused by the parents, in which case the short leg can be contained in a plastic socket, mounted on side bars and joints above a shin of plastic, wood, or metal.

The 'access trap' is not effective when the foot is of normal width and cannot enter the rigid socket unless the brim can be opened. This problem can be overcome in two ways, one of which involves replacing the front half of the socket by padded straps, which can be used only in a below-knee prosthesis and has the disadvantage of applying large forces via the limited area of the upper strap at heel-off. The alternative, and preferred, choice is to use a complete socket which has been split down the sides and the two halves hinged together at the toe, being held closed by straps. Such a socket can also be used for cases of PFFD when the socket is extended proximally to provide ischial bearing. In those who have had a 180° rotation osteotomy the foot is contained in a bootee in the shin. Stops may be needed on the side joints to limit the range of flexion. The conventional leather thigh corset may be replaced by a rigid plastic structure providing ischial support, whilst an elastic insert in one part of the periphery maintains a close fit.

(a)   (b)

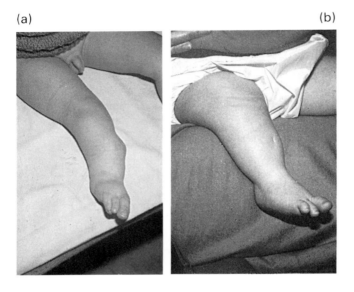

Fig. 37.2 (a) The narrow foot typical of fibular deficiency (longitudinal, fibula total, tarsus partial, rays 4 and 5 total) permits entry to a total-contact plastic socket via a posterior access trap. (b) A similar method can be used in cases of proximal femoral focal deficiency with absence of the fibula (longitudinal, femur partial, proximal ⅓, fibula total, tarsus partial, rays 4 and 5 total) — *see* text.

The more severe longitudinal deficiencies in which the foot is attached either directly to the buttock or via a very short segment provide individual problems about which it is difficult to generalize. However, a suitably shaped plastic socket, with or without an aperture for the foot, is mounted on a conventional limb structure. The child's foot may be very valuable both for suspension of the prosthesis and as a means of activation. Despite the absence of a joint between the pelvis and the 'leg', the latter is often capable of considerable power.

Those children with bilateral total absence of lower limbs will need sitting sockets to develop their balance at about six months. Later they may proceed via simple pylons to more elaborate prostheses, perhaps of the swivel walker type, but many opt eventually for a wheelchair life so that they can travel further and faster with less expenditure of effort. Such a decision can be taken only by the subject, who will weigh up the advantages and disadvantages as they perceive them. Indeed this decision has to be made by all who have limb deficiencies, and it is important that parents recognize that their child's wishes must be respected.

References

Day H. J. B. & Wright J. (1977) A system of extension prosthesis. *Prosthetics and Orthotics International* 1, 8–12.

Foort J. (1956) The Canadian Type Syme Prosthesis. Lower Extremity Amputee Research Project. University of California, Berkeley. Series II. Issue 30.

38

The Role of Surgery in the Arm and Hand

D.W. LAMB

Introduction

Congenital abnormalities of the upper limb and hand are common. They may affect one or both limbs and vary from a very minor deformity to those which are severe and complex. They are not infrequently associated with other skeletal abnormalities and with abnormalities of other systems, for example cardiac, gastrointestinal, urological, etc. There is no clear evidence of the incidence of these abnormalities around the world nor of their aetiology. Both of these factors are currently under review by the Committee on Congenital Abnormalities of the International Federation of Hand Societies. A concise classification is of importance, and most conditions, apart from the more bizarre, can be included in the classification sponsored by the International Federation. This is shown in Table 38.1 (Swanson *et al.* 1968).

Table 38.1 Classification of congenital abnormalities of the upper limb (recommended by the International Federation of Societies for Surgery of the Hand).

1 Failure of formation of parts
  1.1 Transverse
  1.2 Longitudinal

2 Failure of differentiation (separation) of parts

3 Duplication

4 Overgrowth (gigantism)

5 Undergrowth (hypoplasia)

6 Congenital constriction band syndrome

7 Generalized skeletal abnormalities

It is with the first group, namely the failures of development, that the author is mainly concerned for the purposes of this chapter, although surgery has an important role to play in many of the other groups. Failure of development was further considered by the subcommittee of the International Society for Prosthetics

and Orthotics (ISPO) under the Chairmanship of the late Hector Kay, which decided
that it could be subdivided into:

1 Terminal transverse absence.

2 Longitudinal absence (Kay 1975).

Surgery has little part in the management of terminal transverse absence; its
prosthetic management is dealt with later. Terminal transverse absence is always
a sporadic isolated defect without any inherited pattern, whereas longitudinal
deficiencies are not infrequently associated with syndromes which may be inherited
and associated with abnormalities of other systems.

The longitudinal group is often amenable to surgical treatment. The ISPO
classification is shown in Fig. 38.1. The more proximal deficiencies can seldom
benefit from surgery, unlike the distal group, which can be subdivided into:

1 Pre-axial or radial absence.

2 Central absence.

3 Post-axial or ulnar absence.

Each of these groups will be described, and indications for surgery and the choice
of methods that are available will be considered.

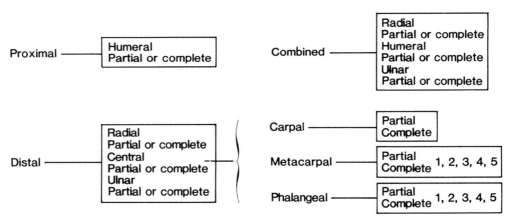

Fig. 38.1 Longitudinal absence.

Pre-axial or radial absence

This is a rare condition which may be present as:

1 Complete absence of the radius.

2 Partial absence of the radius.

3 Hypoplasia of the radius.

Complete absence is the most common of the three and leads to severe wrist
deformity. Not only is the radius absent, but usually the radial carpal bones and
often the thumb are missing or deficient (Fig. 38.2). It is the management of this
particular group which will be discussed.

The initial management is to try and prevent the development of a fixed deformity with soft tissue contractures, which may in turn lead to a secondary bowing of the ulna. A simple splint holding the wrist in the corrected position should be worn at night as soon as the child can tolerate this.

The later management will depend on the following factors:

1 Whether it is unilateral or bilateral.

2 The structure of the joints of the hand and its function.

3 Whether the elbow is stiff in extension.

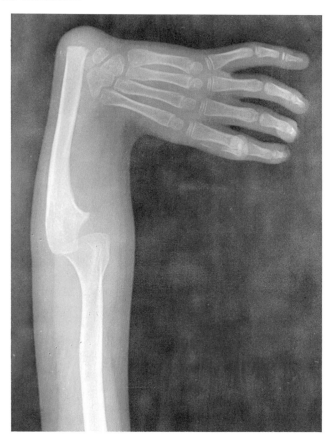

Fig. 38.2 Radiograph showing absence of radius, radial carpus and thumb.

1 In unilateral cases correction of the wrist deformity for cosmetic reasons is acceptable as there is normal function on the other side. In the bilateral case, the hand often functions quite well in the deviated position, but there is seldom complete independence in self-care activities, and this will depend very much on whether there is good active flexion of the elbow and the joints of the hand are not too stiff and deformed. However, the wrist deformity is an ugly one (Fig. 38.3) and if it can be corrected without detriment to function this is the policy to follow.

2 There is invariably restricted movement in the finger joints. The metacarpo-

phalangeal joints have limited flexion, and the proximal interphalangeal joints often have flexion contractures. The mechanical advantage of the flexor and extensor tendons is compromised by the radially displaced wrist, and if the wrist is straightened the advantages to hand function seem to outweigh any possible disadvantages.

3 The small child can get the radially deviated wrist to the mouth and the face without the necessity of elbow flexion, but as the child grows this becomes more and more difficult. A stiff extended elbow without at least 90° of active flexion is a definite contraindication to any operation to straighten the wrist.

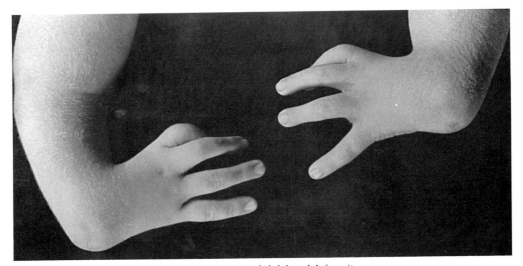

Fig. 38.3 Bilateral absence of the radius with typical club hand deformity.

Management (Lamb 1977)

Each individual child must be assessed carefully and a decision made based on the above factors. If it is decided that the wrist deformity should be corrected by operation the optimum time is somewhere about 9–12 months of age. Several operative procedures have been described and can be considered in three groups:

1 *Corrective osteotomy of the ulna.* This may produce some initial improvement in the appearance but inevitably relapse occurs during growth.

2 *Replacement of the missing bone by bone grafts.* The most promising method was that described by Starr with transfer of the upper fibula, which is reversed so that the growing epiphysis is at wrist level (Starr 1945). Unfortunately the epiphysis seldom grows, and this method has been largely abandoned. It has, however, been reintroduced using a vascularized free fibular graft. It is too early to know if this will be successful.

3 *Centralization of the carpus.* This method has proved to be the most satisfactory at present. It involves resection of sufficient of the central carpus to insert the lower end of the ulna. The fit should be neat and exact, with the lower end of the ulna inserted to a depth equal to its transverse diameter. The epiphysis must not be damaged and the dissection should be extraperiosteal. The position may then need to be maintained for a period with a Kirschner wire along the third or fourth metacarpal and up to the ulnar medullary cavity crossing the centre of the epiphysis.

To try and limit the recurrence of the deformity any muscle imbalance should be corrected. This may require transfer of the flexor carpi radialis to the dorsum of the wrist, and sometimes lengthening of superficial flexor tendons. Careful post-operative splintage and supervision is necessary to control any tendency to recurrence (Fig. 38.4).

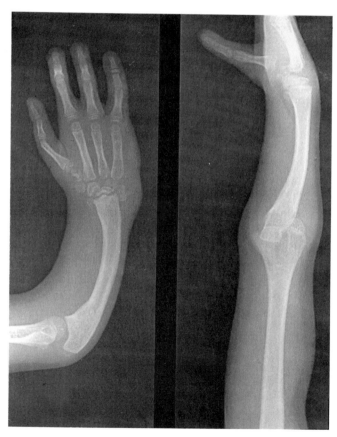

Fig. 38.4 Radiograph five years after centralization. Note lower ulna epiphysis still growing. Note also pollicization of index finger.

Buck-Gramcko (1985) has introduced a new operation of 'radialization'. Instead of inserting the lower ulna into the carpus he transfers it from the ulnar to the radial side of the developing carpal bones. It is too early to know if there is any similar tendency to recurrence following this procedure.

Most children with absent radius have either a four-fingered hand or a poorly developed 'floating' thumb. It is useless to try and improve the thumb by bone grafting and tendon insertion, and it is better to ablate the useless thumb and transpose the index finger into a thumb position (pollicization).

Following correction of the wrist deformity, the orientation of the hand and the type of prehension is usually changed from the ulnar side of the hand to the radial. It is important therefore to consider follow-up of centralization by pollicizing the index finger. The function and structure of the index finger are seldom normal, but usually good enough to provide a functioning thumb. The operation consists of shortening the index finger by removal of the proximal three-quarters of the metacarpal shaft with retention of the metacarpal head as a new trapezium. The head of the metacarpal has to be rotated so as to tighten up the volar structures to prevent an ugly hyperextension deformity developing. The ray is also rotated on its longitudinal axis through about 150° to bring the new thumb into its correct position. The operation embodies the following principles:

1 Transference of the neurovascular bundle as described by Littler (1953).

2 A suitable skin incision, such as that described by Barsky (1959), providing a volar-based skin-flap on the radial side of the hand which will form the new thumb web. The extension of the racquet incision at the base of the finger along the

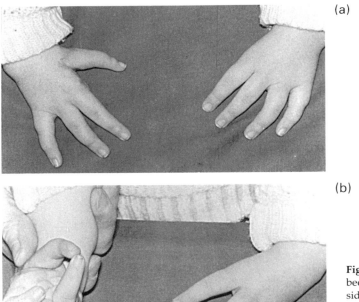

(a)

(b)

Fig. 38.5 (a) Pollicization has been carried out on the right side. Note the previous status of a similar four-fingered hand on the left side. (b) Ability to get good pulp to pulp prehension.

dorsum of the finger as described by Buck-Gramcko (1971) facilitates the next step of the operation, which is the reattachment of the first dorsal and first volar interossei muscles to the extensor tendon of the index finger at the old proximal interphalangeal joint. This will become the new metacarpophalangeal joint of the thumb and provide good stability and mobility of the new thumb.

This is a technically exacting operation as the radial digital vessels and nerve are often missing on the index finger and the vascular and nerve supply depends wholly upon an intact ulnar neurovascular bundle. Despite the often poor quality of the structures of the index finger, the functional rewards are often very helpful (Fig. 38.5).

Central absence

The aetiology is unknown and there are various types. Barsky (1964) separated them into two main groups:

1 The typical form (Fig. 38.6)

The central ray, and sometimes those of the index and ring finger, is missing, leaving a central V-shaped defect. The appearance is distressing but function is

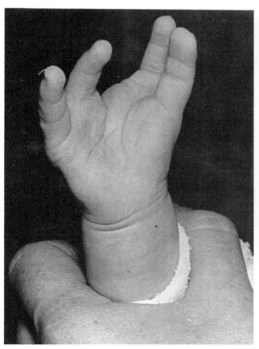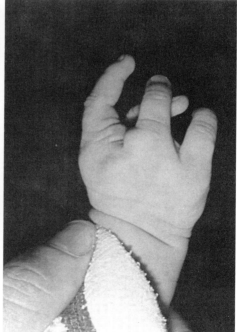

Fig. 38.6 Note central defect of middle ray, left hand.

usually good. It is usually bilateral, commonly associated with a similar foot deformity, and has an autosomal dominant inheritance.

Management. Surgery is usually only indicated for cosmetic reasons and function is unlikely to be improved. The cleft should be closed by approximating the adjacent metacarpals, and excess skin is excised. Sometimes the cleft is associated with a thumb/index web contracture, and in these circumstances the procedure described by Snow and Littler (1967) of transferring the redundant skin from the central cleft to deepen the thumb index web is recommended.

2 The atypical form

Barsky included in this type the central defect with more than one ray missing, but the author prefers to include in this group those central defects of the phalanges only, with metacarpals partially or totally present (Fig. 38.7). This group is usually

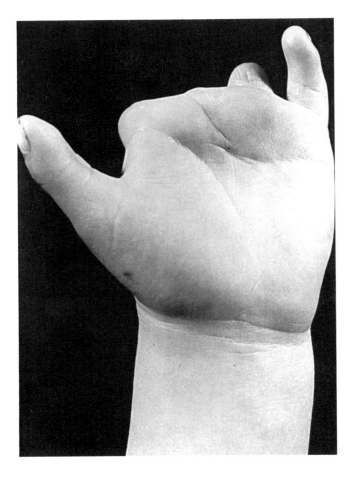

Fig. 38.7 Example of atypical type.

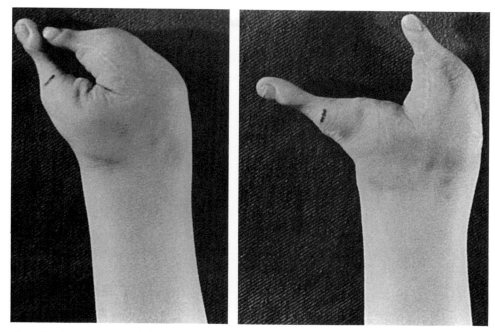

Fig. 38.8 Apposition of radial and ulnar components.

sporadic, has no familiar history and no foot involvement.

Management. There is usually obstruction by the central metacarpals of the ability to bring the thumb and little finger rays together for prehension. Surgery is carried out to allow pinch between thumb and little finger (Fig. 38.8).

Ulnar absence

This is uncommon and has three grades of severity:
1 Hypoplasia of the ulna
2 Absence of the distal ulna.
3 Complete absence of the ulna.
In all groups there may be some failure of development of the ulnar carpus, and in the more severe groups absence of the two ulnar hand rays. Thumb, index, and middle fingers are usually present, although seldom of normal development (Fig. 38.9).

Management

Hypoplasia seldom requires treatment. If the ulna seems to be progressively shortening relevant to the radius, this may be an indication to lengthen the ulna.

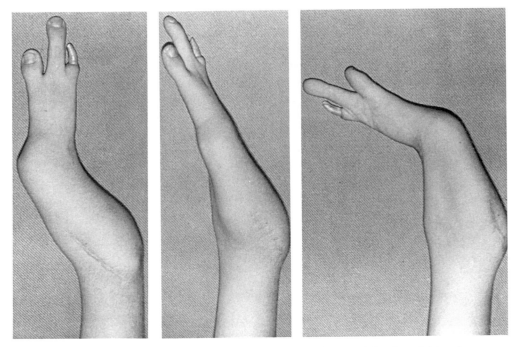

Fig. 38.9 Example of partial absence of ulna. Note the rather poor digits and the ulnar club hand deformity.

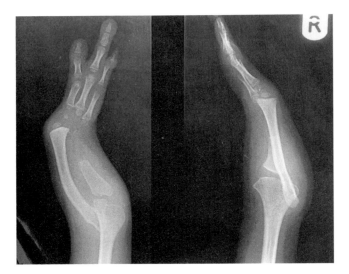

Fig. 38.10 Radiograph of partial absence ulna. Note upper third of ulna and dislocated radial head.

Partial absence is the most common type with the upper third of the ulna usually present. A fibrous anlage of the lower two-thirds of the ulna may be present and should be suspected if there is an increasing ulnar deformity of the hand during growth. The anlage should be resected.

Another deformity which may develop during growth is subluxation of the upper end of the radius. Initially this causes little problem and does not restrict elbow movement. However, as the radius grows displacement of the head may obstruct elbow movement and cause an unsightly swelling (Fig. 38.10). Resection of the upper radius may then be indicated. The most difficult decision to be made in this type is whether to construct a stable straight one-bone forearm, as described by Straub (1965). This has the disadvantage of losing any rotary movement of the forearm that may be present, but it may correct deformity and improve appearance. The procedure consists of resection of the upper third of radius and implantation of the lower two-thirds of the radius on the remaining upper third of the ulna.

In total absence of the ulna there is usually no useful surgical treatment. It is commonly associated with contractures of the elbow in a marked degree of flexion.

References

Barsky A. J. (1959) Congenital anomalies of the thumb. *Clinical Orthopaedics and Related Research* **15**, 96–110.

Barsky A. J. (1964) Cleft hand: classification, incidence and treatment. *Journal of Bone and Joint Surgery* **46A**, 1707–1720.

Buck-Gramcko D. (1971) Pollicization of the index finger. Method and results in aplasia and hypoplasia of the thumb. *Journal of Bone and Joint Surgery* **53A**, 1605–1617.

Buck-Gramcko D. (1985) Radialization as a new treatment for radial club hand. *Journal of Hand Surgery* (American) **10**, 964–968.

Kay H. W. (1975) Clinical applications of the new international terminology for the classification of congenital limb deficiencies. *Inter-Clinic Information Bulletin* **14(3)**, 1–24.

Lamb D. W. (1977) Radial club hand. *Journal of Bone and Joint Surgery* **59A**, 1–13.

Littler J. W. (1953) The neurovascular pedicle method of digital transposition for reconstruction of the thumb. *Plastic and Reconstructive Surgery* **12(5)**, 303–319.

Snow J. W. & Littler J. W. (1967) Surgical treatment of cleft hand. Transactions of Fourth Congress, Society of Plastic Reconstructive Surgery. *Excerpt. Med. Found.* 888.

Starr D. E. (1945) Congenital absence of radius; method of surgical correction. *Journal of Bone and Joint Surgery* **27A**, 572–577.

Straub L. R. (1965) Congenital absence of the ulna. *American Journal of Surgery* **109**, 300–305.

Swanson A. B., Barsky A. J. & Entin M. A. (1968) Classification of limb malformations on the basis of embryological failures. *Surgical Clinics of North America* **48**, 1169–1179.

39

The Prosthetic Treatment of Congenital Upper Limb Deficiency

H.J.B. DAY

Introduction

Some cases of congenital upper limb deficiency need little physical help, some need prostheses, others may be suitable for reconstructive surgery, but all need and deserve careful assessment and long-term follow-up. The parents need substantial support from the moment of birth. They experience emotions of guilt and recrimination which may threaten their relationship when it needs to be closest. The support must provide positive answers rather than emotional platitudes. Early consultation is essential to answer their questions, both voiced and unspoken, about their child's future. Some parents want to cover up the abnormality with a prosthesis, perhaps as part of a process of denial, others are repelled by the thought of prosthetic replacement. So the relation between the type of deficiency and the advisability of a prosthesis and its nature and time of application requires sympathetic explanation. At this first consultation their central role in the team must be confirmed and the overall target agreed. This must be to help the child to see himself as having the smallest possible handicap both in childhood and throughout his adult life. To achieve this the programme must be flexible, and offer solutions which seem appropriate to the child's needs based on experience with other children who have similar deficiencies. However, in the long run only the child can decide whether to wear a prosthesis, and his decision will be taken in the light of his own experience, even though sometimes it will not be what his parents desired. Because this first consultation includes so much and is likely to be imperfectly remembered by the parents, it has been found invaluable to record it and to allow the parents to keep the cassette as an *aide-mémoire*.

Transverse deficiencies

In considering the prosthetic management it is convenient to reverse the direction of development and describe first the treatment of distal levels of loss. Patients with transverse deficiencies at levels *distal to the carpometacarpal joint* and also those with longitudinal deficiencies of metacarpals and phalanges should not be fitted with prostheses, but be encouraged to develop mobility and competence. Suitable opposition devices should be provided as and when difficulties arise, but there is no point in providing a 'solution' unless a problem exists. Usually the first requirement is for a simple device to hold a knife for eating. Other opposition devices may be needed later for use in sports and hobbies. At some stage, perhaps when starting or changing schools, embarrassment may be noted. This is another problem for which a solution must be found. A simple cosmetic glove with the deficient parts replaced by foam inserts usually cures the embarrassment, although in most cases the device is worn only occasionally because it hinders function. This does not matter providing the problem of embarrassment has been overcome. In those cases where there is an adequate metacarpal length, a socket carrying curved fingers can be 'clipped' on to the metacarpal region and opposition achieved between these fingers and the thumb, if present, or to an artificial thumb mounted on a cuff round the lower forearm. In this latter case opposition is achieved by palmar flexion.

Cases of *transverse total carpal deficiencies,* providing there is no significant forearm shortening, should also be left free initially to gain competence and dexterity. A cuff with a volar plate will allow the use of a knife for eating. At a later stage, because the child has pronation/supination ability, a socket which transmits this movement can be made. If it is to be fitted with a split hook and operated by a cord from a loop round the opposite shoulder, a reaction point will be provided by a separate socket brim near the elbow.

The *transverse forearm deficiency* is the most common of all congenital limb deficiencies, and the level of loss is usually at or about the junction of the upper and middle thirds of the forearm. At this level early prosthetic fitting is desirable, and a simple foam-filled prosthesis is fitted at four to six months. This enables the child to perform bimanual 'pat-a-cake' activities in the midline, improves sitting, and later standing, balance, and accustoms the child to the idea of wearing a prosthesis. It also usually pleases the parents and helps them in their acceptance of the deficiency. In the early stages a simple suspension system is needed, but once the child has become used to the prosthesis a self-suspending supracondylar socket can be employed. A wrist rotary/disconnect will be added at about 15–18 months. The soft, mouldable hand can then be interchanged with a split hook, and most children will achieve purposeful operation of this by 18–24 months. In recent years the Child Amputee Prosthetics Project (CAPP) terminal device (Fig. 39.1a) has become popular because it provides a more efficient grip and children seem to acquire control earlier than with a split hook. Many parents find its appearance less disturbing than that of a split hook, although others do not like the soft teeth which give the device a somewhat reptilian appearance. It is important to provide an ordinary cosmetic hand for social occasions, and vital for the child to be trained by a skilled occupational therapist. If the child uses a split hook or CAPP device competently most parents will accept it quickly. As interests widen, other interchangeable terminal devices may be needed. Mechanical hands in which the thumb opposes to the index and middle fingers as a chuck grip provide reasonable cosmesis, although the mechanical disadvantage of their geometry and the stiffness of the glove limit the grip strength.

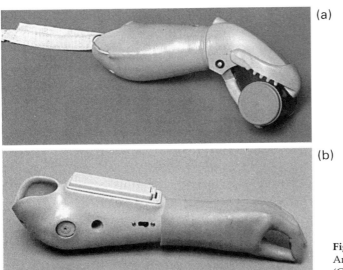

(a)

(b)

Fig. 39.1 (a) The Child Amputee Prosthetics Project (CAPP) terminal device. (b) Myoelectric prosthesis.

In the early 1970s Sorbye (1977, 1980) found an advantage in fitting young children with myoelectric hands, and as a result a small electric hand became available in 1978, and there are now a range of sizes (Fig. 39.1b). At that time the Department of Health and Social Security in the United Kingdom instituted a trial in which children between 3½ and 4½ years old with levels of loss in the middle third of the forearm were fitted with such hands. The trial (DHSS 1981, Mendez 1985) ran for three years and demonstrated that many children benefitted from such a prosthesis. Since 1981 the programme has been expanded, and children up to 17 years of age and with other levels of loss are now being fitted. If the prosthesis is fitted to all children whose level of loss is neither too proximal to require accessory suspension and control nor so distal that the completed prosthesis will be too long, about two-thirds appear to benefit. The remainder, who may acquire great competence with myoelectric devices, nevertheless may prefer to wear a conventional prosthesis or none at all. It is, however, wrong to fit it on a trial basis. The fact that the myoelectric prosthesis is seen by relatives, friends, and peers as highly desirable places great stress on the child if he does not like it. Therefore a proper assessment should be made as to whether benefit is likely, and it is thus desirable to concentrate assessment, fitting, and training in a few centres which can develop expertise based on a large experience. Since 1978, 233 children with forearm deficiencies have been formally assessed at Manchester, and 179 have been fitted.

Because the needs of children change with their development the assessment can only be valid at the time, and some who do not appear likely to benefit at one age may well require such a prosthesis a year or two later. The boy who is committed to a split hook at the age of 12 may well want the better cosmesis and freedom from harness at 14 or 15 years. The changing needs can also work in reverse and perhaps account for those who want to change from a myoelectric prosthesis after a few years. Of the 179 patients fitted in Manchester some 149 are still wearing their prostheses. A number of children with carpal deficiencies have been fitted with, and benefit from, myoelectric prostheses, particularly as they retain pronation/supination. However, frequently, particularly when the child is small, such fitting will make the arm too long. Electric hands can, of course, be controlled in other ways. Those with some longitudinal deficiencies such as ulna total, rays 2,3,4,5, total, with hypoplasia of the radius, have a short forearm with a single digit which can best control the hand by two microswitches mounted in the socket. Another version offers a positional servo control in conjunction with a harness in which a small transducer converts a light mechanical pull into a change in inductance. A similar inductor in the hand is varied by the motor which moves the fingers. An error circuit compares the two inductances and switches the hand accordingly so that with no pull the hand is closed, a full pull of 1 cm completely opens it, and a ½ cm pull causes the hand to stay in the half-way position. Thus the wearer has excellent control with positional awareness.

Transverse, arm total, down to forearm total deficiencies, i.e. those with a level of loss equivalent to between a shoulder and elbow disarticulation, are fitted first with a simple foam prosthesis whose endoskeletal structure is unjointed but preflexed at the elbow. The age of fitting may be a little later (6–9 months), as there is a conflict of interest in that the prosthesis is a help in sitting but a hindrance in lying. A little later an elbow joint which has a friction 'lock' can be added and voluntary elbow flexion from a shoulder cord can usually be obtained at 18–24 months. One may add a split hook as a 'passive' gripper until it can become activated by the incorporation of an elbow lock. The disadvantage of the conventional sequential control of elbow flexion–lock–terminal device is that it is robotic and few children can transfer as much power to the terminal device as they would like. However, most find little difficulty in obtaining elbow flexion by the operating cord, and this is fortunate, as although electric elbows are available few are small in size, all are heavy, and most provide little real usable power. Thus the hybrid system in which the body-powered elbow flexion is combined with an electric hand becomes attractive. If the level of loss is in the lower half of the humerus the hand can be controlled by electrodes placed over biceps and triceps (Fig. 39.2). Perhaps surprisingly, the children learn in a few minutes to flex the elbow by rounding the shoulders without giving any biceps signal, thus completely separating the movements. If the level of loss is higher, the positional servo hand can be used with the transmitting transducer worked either by 'hunching up' the shoulder or by blowing out the abdomen.

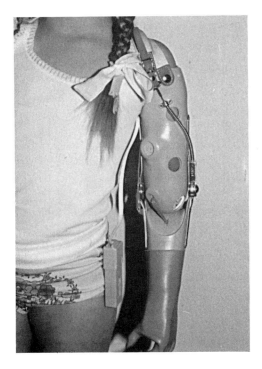

Fig. 39.2 Hybrid arm — body-powered elbow flexion combined with an electric hand.

Bilateral transverse, arm total deficiencies do not often present. In the past gas-powered prostheses of varying complexity have been used, but most of the children discarded them in favour of foot use. Indeed it is most important to encourage children with gross arm deficiencies to use their feet. The positional servo type of electric hand seems attractive in this case, but the inability to position the hands effectively because of the lack of suitable electric elbow and shoulder units at present limits the application.

Longitudinal deficiencies

Longitudinal deficiencies of the phocomelia type, in which the arm is very short, or indeed where the hand is attached direct to the shoulder, are best left without prostheses, providing that the hand has active movement, and that in the bilateral case one or both hands can reach the mouth. If a prosthesis is indicated it is usually desirable to allow the hand to protrude through an aperture in the socket so that the advantages of sensation and fine manipulation are retained. It may be possible for the hand to operate mechanical locks or gain control of an electric arm by means of switches. However the majority of these children become very competent with their natural hands and are best helped by dressing sticks and other aids to enlarge their reach.

Conclusion

No attempt has been made in this brief account to describe all the prosthetic options, but merely to indicate certain lines of treatment. No child will use a prosthesis unless he finds it advantageous, and we must ensure by frequent review that the prosthesis offered is matched to his changing needs.

References

Department of Health and Social Security (1981) Report on the trial of the Swedish myoelectric hand for young children. London: DHSS.

Mendez M. A. (1985) Evaluation of a myoelectric hand prosthesis for children with a below-elbow absence. *Prosthetics and Orthotics International* **9**, 137–140.

Sorbye R. (1977) Myoelectric controlled hand prostheses in children. *International Journal of Rehabilitation Research* **1**, 15–25.

Sorbye R. (1980) Myoelectric prosthetic fitting in young children. *Clinical Orthopaedics and Related Research* **148**, 34–40.

40

Total Management of the Limb-Deficient Child

E.G. MARQUARDT & H.U. BUFF

Introduction

Rehabilitation is usually split up into phases of medical, educational, social, and vocational rehabilitation or habilitation. This may result in a danger to the handicapped child: procedures which should be concurrent may be carried out successively, leading to false interpretation. As a result a hierarchy of command or priority may be imposed without justification and may be harmful to the child. In the Heidelberg special unit for limb-deficient children it has been demonstrated that both in-patient and out-patient medical treatment is far more successful if, from the beginning of the rehabilitation programme, the psychological and educational aspects of the child's problems as well as parental counselling, both individually and in groups, are included. It is important that the parents are involved from the very onset of the programme.

From 1959 until 1962 some 250–300 dysmelic children were treated each year. In 1970 there were 419 out-patient attendances of children with limb deficiencies attending for a first examination or follow-up and treatment; in 1973 this number was 603, and in 1983 1750 children attended. This does not signify an increase of limb deficiencies in general; instead the patients come from longer distances and different countries. The average length of stay of hospitalized dysmelic children was 42.4 days in 1970, 34.4 days in 1983, and 16.4 days in 1984. In keeping with these numbers the demands on the out-patient clinic have increased considerably. Children are only hospitalized (together with their mother or father until the age of three) in the event of an operation becoming necessary. At a later age the mother or father is present during the day while at night she or he stays within the clinic area or in a hotel nearby.

Experience with the enormous number of multiple limb-deficient children during the thalidomide episode has permitted the development of clear treatment concepts for different kinds of limb deficiencies and different age groups. Because of the great danger of the limb-deficient child developing emotional disturbances often followed by intellectual retardation, emphasis must be placed again on the urgent need for co-ordination between medicine, psychology and pedagogic therapy in the treatment programme for limb-deficient children.

Psychological and medical problems following the birth of a dysmelic child

The severe shock each mother sustains after giving birth to a limb-deficient child is a reality. The way in which the mother overcomes the acute shock and accepts the problem has a great influence of her child-rearing practices and the success of the habilitation programme. If she is well adjusted and understanding in her child-rearing practice, the child will be exposed to greater varieties and degrees of sensory stimuli during development and have a better opportunity to grow up psychologically normal. On the other hand, unaccommodating mothers impede normal development and often also the necessary treatment. Overprotection and excessive care as well as prolonged hospitalization and 'home hospitalism' are frequently the cause of emotional and intellectual disturbances, which are often more serious than the physical handicap itself.

Often the background for the mother's future attitude is determined in the maternity hospital. Even today the personnel of many maternity hospitals do not know how to treat or to converse with the mother of a newly born limb-deficient child. Frequently, the child is hidden for weeks or even months from the mother's view. Insecurity, tension and incorrect education of the mother and father only deepen the psychological shock and make the rehabilitation programme more difficult. The physician, the nurse, and often friends and relatives, may exhibit embarrassment and, in the guise of pity, express the wish that God may take back this poor child. This unfortunate attitude fosters the wish or thought of death and later evolves into an overprotective attitude towards the child. To prevent this development, the following is proposed:

The delivery physician should take the time for an objective and quiet conversation with the child's mother. He should enlighten her about the child's handicap in realistic ways: and if possible he should present the child to her personally and, at the same time, inform her about present treatment possibilities and practical assistance. The opportunity for the mother to take care of and to play with her child and show her affection is important. As soon as she realizes her child's abilities and that a positive solution is possible, it becomes much easier for her to adjust, to assume a positive attitude towards her child, and to adopt normal child-rearing practices. At this point it should be emphasized again how important is it that the physically handicapped infant should, if possible, remain with his mother instead of being referred to an institution for custodial care. If psychological and practical assistance is offered in time, and if the mother and father do their share in the total treatment programme of the child, and are provided with proper counselling and education, a therapeutic milieu which contributes significantly to psychotherapy will have been created.

Medical rehabilitation

The medical rehabilitation of the limb-deficient child includes the following:
1 Training of potential and residual abilities.
2 Correction of dislocations and abnormal posture.
3 Supplying prostheses, orthoses, orthoprostheses, and technical aids, as needed, including adapted clothing, seats and vehicles.
4 Surgical procedures required to improve and maintain residual and potential function, and — if indicated and possible — to improve appearance, mostly in combination with prostheses and orthoprostheses.

1 Training of residual abilities

An important example of the training of potential and residual abilities is the armless child with normal lower limbs. If the feet remain uncovered from the very beginning, the infant will use them for touching and grasping and will be able to experience and to comprehend the environment naturally. This grasping is a very important precondition for the use of the feet as hands in the best and most natural way. By bringing both feet together around an object, the child will achieve a three-dimensional grasp which will lead to three-dimensional thinking.

For all armless children the free mobility of the hip and knee joints and of the spine is most important. However, many limb-deformed children, especially those whose deformities are a result of thalidomide, have spinal problems, such as round back and scoliosis, as well as knee and hip problems that need special therapy. Corrective exercises, especially Vojta therapy, should be practised daily at home and under supervision of a physiotherapist to prevent, as far as possible, the fixed round back and progressive scoliosis. Parents should be taught these exercises, including swimming. The whole training programme must be built up systematically and regularly under constant supervision.

In the thalidomide population there will be found, in addition to the typical longitudinal deficiencies, especially of the radius and the thumb, a development disorder of the vertebral discs and vertebral bodies which has occurred in early embryonic life. In many children this produces fusion of the frontal parts of the vertebral bodies. The training programme has to relieve the pressure on the anterior edges of the vertebral bodies; nevertheless, one still sees in many of these people a serious kyphosis with anterior fusion and bridging of many vertebral bodies of the lumbar and thoracic spine.

2 Correction of dislocations and abnormal posture

Club hands should be orthopaedically corrected immediately after birth. Correction of the club hand performed by traction and corrective exercises should be carried out in many small steps. Early operative centralization of the ulna in bilateral club hands should mostly be avoided because of the severe functional losses which often occur. Details of the Heidelberg treatment concept may be found in the following publications: Marquardt (1969), Marquardt & Popplow (1971), Marquardt (1972), Marquardt (1980), Marquardt (1980/1981), Marquardt (1983), Martini (1980), Neff & Marquardt (1979).

Dislocation of the hip and scoliosis need to be considered and evaluated in relation to the total functional pattern, and especially with regard to the co-ordinated action of the lower and upper extremities and the mouth. Congenital dysplasia and dislocation of the hip is usually treated by Vojta therapy, triple diapers, Pavlik harnesses and splints, according to the severity of the disorder. This also applies in the case of arm malformations. However, if a complete hip dislocation is noted at birth in an armless child, function in the so-called teratologically dislocated hip must be maintained as much as possible because of the compensatory functional use of the feet as hands in later life. Reduction of such a dislocated hip will lead to early osteoarthritis and diminished use of the feet as hands, especially in the activities of daily living.

Another important example of the need to veto corrective surgery is found in progressive scoliosis. In otherwise normal children the spine is straightened and fusion performed at the age of 10–15 years. In the case of an armless or phocomelic child such an operation might destroy later independence. Early Vojta therapy and electrical stimulation, as well as swimming and normal physical training, should be the alternative approach in these children. If corrective surgery cannot be avoided, very careful judgement must be made as to how many segments and what degree of correction can be allowed. All measures have to be integrated into the concept of total management.

3 Prostheses

Prosthetic fitting and training of the child should be done in the presence of mother, father, or both. The parent(s) should be with the child in the physiotherapy department, in the occupational therapy department, in the prosthetic/orthotic workshop; in this way they see and experience all the steps of fitting, alignment, and training, and grow together with their child's physical and psychological problems. During their stay in the hospital they usually have more time for the child than at home. The child experiences the mother, father, or both in a situation similar in some ways to a vacation. Father, mother, and child learn together, but also mix with other children and their parents, and very often learn from them in a friendly atmosphere.

When the parents and child go home, all know about the prostheses and about their programme for the next period of time. They maintain contact with other parents, exchanging addresses, experiences, know-how and opinions, and give help to each other. On the other hand, a good result in fitting and training of a child with upper or lower prostheses cannot be expected if the child is hospitalized and homesick. In these circumstances the child will develop a close link in terms of cause and effect between the prostheses and his disability, and this destructive link will accompany the patient throughout life.

Practical remarks. In children with unilateral below-elbow (BE) or above-elbow (AE) stumps, fitting is started at the age of nine months with the mitten prosthesis. At the age of about 2½ years the first active grasping device is fitted, usually a hook or a CAPP grasper. Myoelectric-controlled prostheses are possible from the age of three or four years, but they are heavy and susceptible to breakdown. They need much maintenance, which interferes with the child's activities and education. For these reasons fitting of the first myoelectric prosthesis is delayed until the age of 10–12 years, and then only in selected patients. In 80% of patients the change from body control to myoelectric prosthesis is easy, provided that there are enough myoelectric potentials. About 10% need a short muscle training period. All, however, need special occupational therapy.

Parallel to the training of the body's own resources, pneumatic-powered prostheses were developed for the armless, and during the last few years a more sophisticated electrically powered prosthesis has been produced. Both have been rejected by more than 90% of congenital amelic persons. However, the electrically powered prosthesis has been found to be of value in trauma-derived abrachia.

During the first years of life infants with bilateral arm stumps will be supplied with simple cuffs or sleeves which can be equipped with spoons, forks, crayons, etc. At the age of 2½ years the fitting of a body-powered prosthesis is started, allowing bimanual activity. Myoelectric and/or electromechanically controlled functions are added later, dependent upon the child's needs and abilities.

Fitting the lower extremity malformations with prostheses and orthoses begins at the age of 11–12 months, dependent upon the child's psychological and motor development. In all severe bilateral cases, pelvic support is provided with a deep centre of gravity and stubbies, which provide a stable system. Depending on the kind of deformity, the state of the muscular system, and the degree of balance achieved, the pelvic support is shortened and functioning prostheses are provided with flexion and abduction hip joints and replacement of the stubbies by SACH feet. Artificial knee joints are added later, at first with a lock and finally with a swing phase unit. All of this is possible if the child has normal arms or sufficiently developed upper extremities to hold one or two canes.

The difficulties increase in the cases of bilateral upper and lower extremity phocomelia or amelia. In such severe cases the children are helped by fitting with ball-bearing, hip rotation joints or a parallelogram construction. However, for travelling long distances or on uneven ground these children must have adequately powered wheelchairs or cars.

In all of these cases good results are obtained when the parents are full members of the clinical team.

4 Surgical procedures

Numerous surgical procedures have been developed to improve and maintain residual and potential functions in dysmelic children. By using the techniques of hand surgery, including the operating microscope, in the case of both upper and lower limbs it is now possible to undertake surgery even in the first year of life. As in the case of prosthetic fitting, the presence of the mother (or father) is very important for the child. A baby or a young child is much quieter and needs less medication for pain and less sedation if the mother or the father is present and able to hold the child, to play with him and take care of him with the supervision of the nurse. Medications are the responsibility of the nurse. For more than 10 years there has been no increase in post-operative wound infections. Experience in co-operation with the parents in the ward and also in the out-patient clinic is now considerable and has been very rewarding. If difficulties occur the source of these difficulties must be identified. Sometimes the parents cannot fully understand the nature of strict clinical requirements. One must be prepared for such situations, and after a quiet explanation excellent co-operation is usually obtained (Marquardt 1983). If there is confidence in the parents' co-operation and abilities, the child is allowed home or to a nearby hotel for further out-patient care at a much earlier stage than some ten years ago.

Practical remarks. In longitudinal limb deficiencies the tibial defect is the most important example of a defect for which the rehabilitation programme requires surgery and prosthetic fitting in early infancy (Jones *et al.* 1978). In tibial defects the fibula bypasses the knee and the ankle joint. The feet cannot bear the weight of the body, and without surgery these children move about on their knees or buttocks, or they use a wheelchair. During the last 20 years the following treatment concept has been developed:

If the femoral condyles and the knee capsule are normal and the child is not older than one year, the Brown procedure (1965, 1971) is indicated. This procedure is intended to lead to the construction of a knee joint between the femoral condyles and the head of the fibula. At a second stage the distal end of the fibula is fused with the astragalus or calcaneus as recommended by Blauth and Hepp (1978). After the first year of life knee disarticulation is 'the treatment of choice' (Kruger 1981), provided that the femur is almost normal. In proximal focal femoral deficiency (PFFD) or hypoplastic femora, fusion between femur and fibula is preferred, as well as between fibula and astragalus or calcaneus (Marquardt 1983). The child will grow up and be well served with a succession of effective prostheses or orthoprostheses. In partial defects of the tibia the osteomized fibula is fused with the tibial rudiment and the distal fibula with the astragalus or calcaneus.

Conclusion

The principle to be followed in the early rehabilitation of limb-deficient children is the development and training of all body resources, especially all sources of sensory feedback, posture and balance, and three-dimensional grasp. The process of total rehabilitation begins in early infancy and integrates medicine, orthopaedic surgery, occupational therapy, physiotherapy, prosthetics and orthotics, education, psychology, social work and, if desired, spiritual help; through this process the child will become and remain part of the family constellation. Each limb-deficient child must be given an optimal chance for normal integration into society. It is fundamental to ensure that these patients manage their lives, not only in a functional sense, but also in relation to their jobs, their family life, their sex life, their free time and hobbies.

Children with severe limb deficiencies can learn how to drive specially equipped vehicles, electric wheelchairs, and, later, cars, all of which enable them to become mobile and independent, and to learn and perhaps to practise a profession. Armless children manage their daily life by using their feet as hands. In the case of children with bilateral aplasia of the tibia as well as in other severe malformations of the limbs, one can improve the quality of life by early effective operations. However, no matter what operations have been performed, whether they be knee disarticulations or Brown procedures, these children remain dependent on prostheses or orthoprostheses for the rest of their lives. If properly rehabilitated and fitted they can walk and are able to climb staircases and to go to a regular school. Of prime importance is that they can grow up in normal competition with others.

The ultimate goal of becoming independent of a wheelchair is often impossible in patients with total limb deficiencies. However, the decision whether the child goes to a special school or to a regular school depends more often on the social than the physical situation.

Limb-deficient children have to build their own scales of values and must learn to understand and accept without bitterness and self-loathing the reactions of so-called normal persons. One is often asked whether these severe malformations could not have been diagnosed earlier during pregnancy so that an abortion could have been performed. Sometimes students with limb deficiencies, perhaps due to thalidomide, are sitting in the same lecture theatre as the non-disabled and hear that such a disabled life should, in the opinion of their 'normal' colleagues, have been killed during pregnancy; but the non-disabled have always entertained such ideas. It is easy to demonstrate how seemingly hopeless severely disabled children have progressed and become law students, students of computer science, of political science, journalists, social workers, businessmen, commercial clerks, etc. It must be understood, however, what great difficulties may be encountered in finding a suitable training course. Equally, jobs for limb-deficient children with limited intellectual abilities can be extremely difficult to find. Those who are fortunate to have normal limbs should open their minds to learn and understand the disabled. A world without the enrichment of the personal aura and spirit of persons who manage their life with disabilities — each in his individual special way — would be a poor world. It should be realized that a man is not a man solely because of possessing arms and legs, but rather because of his mental abilities, his soul and spirit.

References

Blauth W. & Hepp W. R. (1978) Die angeborenen Fehlbildungen an den unteren Gliedmaben. In *Chirurgie der Gegenwart,* Band 5, pp. 1–50. Hewegungsorgane. Munich: Urban und Schwarzenberg.

Brown F. W. (1965) Construction of a knee joint in congenital total absence of the tibia (paraxial hemimelia tibia), a preliminary report. *Journal of Bone and Joint Surgery* **47A**, 695–704.

Brown F. W. (1971) The Brown operation for total hemimelia tibia. In *Selected Lower Limb Anomalies, Surgical and Prosthetic Management.* (ed. Aitken G. T.), pp. 20–28. Washington D.C.: National Academy of Sciences.

Jones D., Barnes J. & Lloyd-Roberts G. C. (1978) Congenital asplasia and dysplasia of the tibia with intact fibula. Classification and management. *Journal of Bone and Joint Surgery* **60B**, 31–39.

Kruger L. M. (1981) Lower limb deficiencies. In *Atlas of Limb Prosthetics: Surgical and Prosthetic Principles* (American Academy of Orthopaedic Surgeons), pp. 522–552. St. Louis: C. V. Mosby.

Marquardt E. G. (1969) The total treatment of the limb deficient child. Horowitz Lecture, 1968. In *Rehabilitation Monograph* 44, pp. 1–52. New York University Medical Center.

Marquardt E. G. (1972) Steigerung der Effektivatat von Oberarm prothesen nach Winkelosteotomie. In *Rehabilitation,* pp.244–248. Stuttgart.

Marquardt E. G. (1980) The multiple limb deficient child. In *Atlas of Limb Prosthetics: Surgical and Prosthetic Principles* (American Academy of Orthopaedic Surgeons), pp. 595–641. St. Louis: C.V. Mosby.

Marquardt E. G. (1980/1981) The operative treatment of congenital limb malformation. The Knud Jansen Lecture. *Prosthetics and Orthotics International.* Part I (1980), Vol. 4, 135–144; Part II (1981), Vol. 5, 2–6; Part III (1981), Vol. 5, 61–67.

Marquardt E. G. (1983) A holistic approach to rehabilitation for the limb deficient child. Thirty-first John Stanley Coulter Memorial Lecture. *Arch. Phys. Med. Rehabil.* **64(6)**, 237–242.

Marquardt E. G. & Popplow K. (1971) Das Dysmeliekind im Rahmen der Gesamtrehabilitation. In *Rehabilitation von Mehrfachbehinderten und Dysmeliekindern,* pp. 52–104. Frechen: Bartman Verlag.

Martini A. K. (1980) Klumphandkorrektur nach Wachstrumsabschlub. In *Handchirurgie* 12, pp. 229–233. VLE – Verlags GmbH: Brlangen.

Neff G. & Marquardt E. G. (1979) The radial clubhand. *Chir. plastica (Berl.)* **4**, 279–287.

SPECIAL PROCEDURES IN
AMPUTATION SURGERY

41

Plastic Surgery in Stump Reconstruction

N.I. KONDRASHIN & B.V. SHISHKIN

Successful rehabilitation of patients after limb amputation depends greatly on the state of the skin of the stump. Walking on a prosthesis often results in damage to blood and lymph circulation, traumatization of neural formations, and impairment of skin receptor functions. All these disorders cause the development of various pathological processes in the stump tissues and particularly in the skin.

Clinical experience has shown that defects and diseases of the stump occur all too frequently. The causes of their formation are quite different:

The extent and severity of the trauma accompanied by the degloving of the skin often over large areas.

The use of circular or guillotine methods of amputation.

Insufficient use of partially elevated skin-flaps at the skin closure of the primary operation.

Use of skin grafts or flaps with low functional characteristics.

Too fast growth of a bone stump in children.

Improper prosthetic design or fitting and prolonged use of a prosthesis.

Accordingly plastic surgery of stumps is necessary for a number of patients. Indications include the following:

Traumatic defects of the skin due to the primary amputation; chronic unhealed wounds; trophic ulcers of the stumps; and painful or ulcerated scars.

Localized areas of skin with signs of definitive atrophy and degeneration.

Scarring situated on functionally important sites of the stump where the skin is closely adherent to the underlying tissues.

Deficiency of skin in the case of planned lengthening of the stump or pathological stump bone growth in children.

Thick scarring causing stump deformation or formation of contractures at the nearest joint.

Scars disfiguring the exterior of the stump.

Not every type of plastic procedure is necessarily suitable for providing adequate skin cover. For example, the low functional characteristics of free split skin-flaps require that this type of plastic operation should be regarded solely for temporary cover of a post-operative wound, thus making it possible to carry out further skin plastic reconstruction of the stump later. Similarly, skin covering of stumps repaired by means of plastic operations based on the use of flaps like the temporary tubular nutritional pedicle cannot be considered functionally sound because the circulation and innervation of these flaps are not fully restored even after a considerable time. As a result, ulcers usually occur in the area of local pressure on the stump.

More recently plastic surgery with flaps based on a vascular and neurovascular pedicle as well as free skin grafts employing microsurgical techniques have become common practice. These methods are also applied in the plastic surgery of the amputation stump.

Extensive clinical experience has convinced the authors that from a functional point of view skin cover restored by a local plastic technique is the most suitable. From 1967 to 1977, 157 patients of the Clinical Department of the Central Research Institute of Prosthetics underwent 175 skin plastic operations, of which 167 were performed by local plastic techniques. Nevertheless, local plastic surgery possesses a necessarily limited potential to cover skin defects, which is why reamputation of the stump was performed because of a deficiency of available local skin in 71 cases operated on for removal of large defects.

New methods of skin plastic surgery for covering extensive skin defects of stumps have been developed at the Institute. These are the methods of massive cutaneous–subcutaneous flaps on a nutritional base, grafted from the neighbouring areas of the stump and from more proximal segments. The main principles of the method are as follows: preliminary preparation, designed to create great mobility and expansibility of skin areas subjected to the operation; the covering of defects, especially on functionally important sites of the stump; the rational use of the anatomical and physiological characteristics of skin on the operated stump area and the proximal segment; extensive mobilization of skin with subcutaneous cellular tissue, taking due account of local blood circulation and innervation; flap formation on a wide proximolateral base; and, finally, staged use of the method in total and subtotal lesions of the stump skin cover. The method has been employed mainly for the closure of defects on below-knee, above-knee, and hip disarticulation stumps. Overall, 182 operations on 153 patients of different age groups were performed on lower limb stumps as a result of trauma.

The skin plastic technique has made it possible to cover scar defects on large areas of the stumps. In the case of single use of the method, the area of the flap achieved on below-knee stumps was 150 cm^2 (Fig. 41.1); on above-knee stumps 200 cm^2 (Fig. 41.2) and on stumps after hip disarticulation 300 cm^2 and more (Fig. 41.3). The method was applied two or three times to patients with a total or subtotal skin lesion. All the results of skin plastic surgery both in the short and long term have been good.

The functional state of the grafted flaps has been considered quite satisfactory. After a period of tissue recovery, usually from four to six weeks, it was possible to proceed to early walking in a training prosthesis and thence to definitive prostheses. Follow-up of patients for up to seven years has shown that restoration

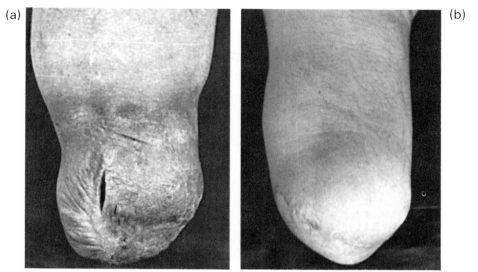

Fig. 41.1 The below-knee stump. (a) Before the operation. (b) After the operation.

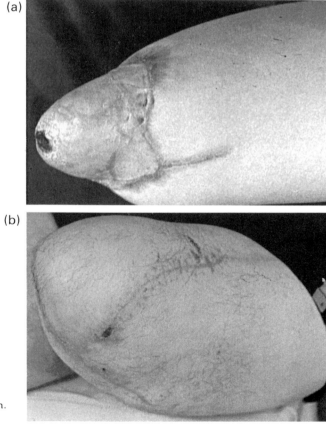

Fig. 41.2 The above-knee stump. (a) Before the operation. (b) After the operation.

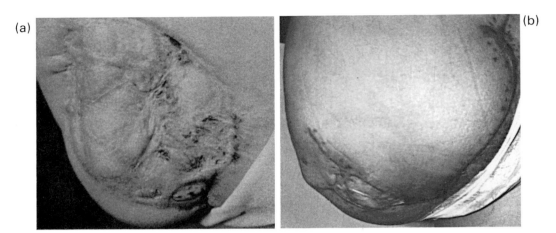

Fig. 41.3 The hip disarticulation stump. (a) Before the operation. (b) After the operation.

of skin cover of the stump has enabled patients to use the prostheses for the most part without restrictions. Many patients have returned to their work. The use of the described technique of plastic surgery has made it possible to avoid reducing the length of the stump bone. The number of reamputation procedures performed in the clinic has been reduced to one-third.

In conclusion it should be noted that the developed technique of skin plastic surgery for extremity stumps possesses incontestable advantages and can be recommended for wide application in clinical practice.

42

The Management of Short Stumps

A.N. KEIER, A.V. ROZHKOV & O.Y. SHATILOV

Introduction

Short stumps present certain difficulties in prosthetic fitting due to the anatomical characteristics and concomitant defects. The results of prosthetic fittings, especially in short humeral and femoral stumps, are often ineffective because of the poor fitting between such stumps and the prosthetic socket, with marked piston-like movements and hence poor control of the artificial limb.

The existing methods of lengthening short extremity stumps by means of free auto- or allotransplants (Tychonov 1949, Godunov & Keier 1969) require the existence or creation of redundant soft tissues at the stump end, but the results have not always been as good as they might be, due to atrophy of the transplant. In order to increase the length of the stump, to abolish contractures, rough, easily injured extensive scars, painful neuromas, and other defects, and to improve the effectiveness of prosthetic replacement a number of operative procedures have been developed. The development of a distraction method of stump lengthening has produced satisfactory results in 137 patients with short above-elbow and below-elbow stumps and short above-knee and below-knee stumps. The possibility of short stump lengthening in the absence of soft tissue redundancy at the stump end, and filling the bone defects in the process of lengthening, is a well-known characteristic of the distraction method using an external bone fixator. In these cases the stump can be lengthened by two or three times its original length.

Upper limb stump lengthening

Lengthening of humeral stumps in adults is carried out by means of a transverse or oblique osteotomy of the humerus and the application of the distraction device, which consists of a ring and an arc connected by three threaded rods. The stump can be lengthened by distraction of 1–1.5 mm per day, and thus by as much as 60–90 mm in two months. Lengthening in children is possible by disruption of the epiphyseal zone.

Lengthening of forearm stumps (Fig. 42.1) is performed by means of osteotomy

of the ulna alone or of both ulna and radius. The distraction device consisting of
two rings is applied. After osteotomy of the ulna only two pairs of transfixion nails
are passed through the bone. However, in children the process of distraction
sometimes results in lengthening of the radius also due to the influence on the
proximal growth zone of the radial bone through the periosteal membrane. The
stump is cylindrical after lengthening of the two bones of the forearm, but filling
the diastasis between the bone fragments takes 2–3 weeks more.

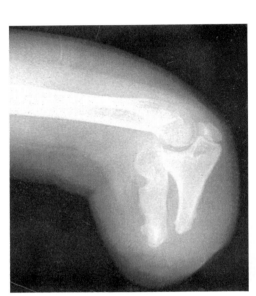 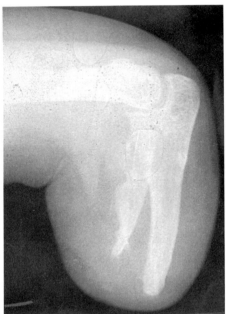

Fig. 42.1 Forearm stump before and after lengthening.

Lower limb stump lengthening

Lengthening of short femoral stumps is performed by means of an osteotomy and
distraction with the use of the device consisting of an arc and a ring (Fig. 42.2).
Traction of a growth zone makes lengthening possible in the case of congenital
short stumps with a distal growth zone. This technique produces a femoral stump
formation even if only a very small rudiment of femoral bone exists. Lengthening
of the shank stump is performed by disruption of the growth zone of the tibia
alone in children (Fig. 42.3). As a rule the growth zone continues to function. In
adults lengthening is performed by means of an r-shaped osteotomy of the tibia.
This type of osteotomy leaves the insertion of the patellar ligament intact on the
proximal fragment of the tibia and preserves the normal position of the patella. A
below-knee prosthesis has been designed which enables the patient to walk with
a moderate load on the stump end during the stump-lengthening process. The

(a) (b) (c)

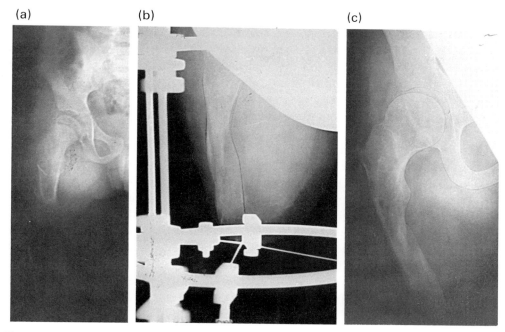

Fig. 42.2 Above-knee stump. (a) Before lengthening. (b) During lengthening with the distraction apparatus. (c) After lengthening.

(a) (b) (c)

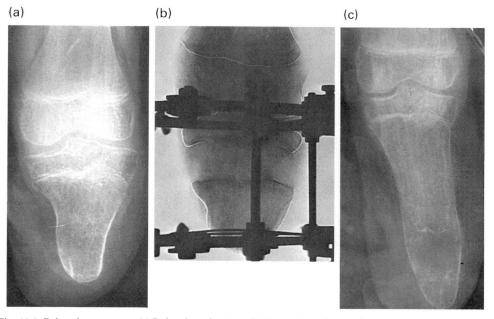

Fig. 42.3 Below-knee stump. (a) Before lengthening. (b) During lengthening by disruption of the growth zone. (c) Stump lengthened by 10 cm.

patient becomes more mobile throughout the treatment period, and this promotes stump muscle function, improves the blood supply to the stump, and encourages faster bone regeneration. A few patients have been subjected to lengthening of two stumps at the same time; this procedure has not affected the time of formation of bone regeneration (Fig. 42.4).

Surgical procedures

Short humeral stumps are often accompanied by scarred contractures and a conglomeration of painful neuromas in the axillary area which limit the use of a prosthesis. Such patients need special surgical treatment. The scars in the axilla are excised, and the conglomeration of painful neuromas is dissected out, together with the neurovascular bundle, and displaced from the prosthetic socket pressure zone and buried beneath pectoralis major. Then a tongue-shaped flap is cut from the scapular area and used to cover the defect in the axilla. In order to increase the functional length of the stump the tendon insertions of pectoralis major, latissimus dorsi, and subscapularis to the humeral stump are often dissected free as a preliminary procedure. By this means adduction contractures have been

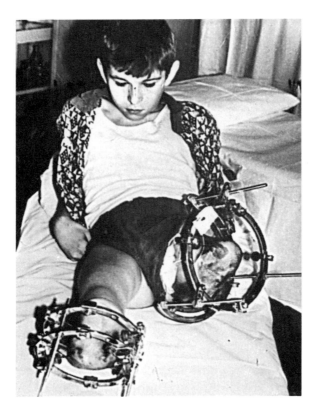

Fig. 42.4 Simultaneous lengthening of above- and below-knee stumps using the distraction apparatus (Ilizarov 1971).

eliminated, stumps have been lengthened by 3–4 cm, and recurrence of painful neuromas in the axilla has been prevented in 25 patients. Traditional methods of plastic surgery (a round pedicle, Indian, Italian, free grafts) are successfully used for covering wound defects on the stumps of different segments. Displacement of a thoracodorsal full-thickness flap including its neurovascular base is employed to cover significantly large defects of cutaneous integuments on the humeral stumps. Displacement of full-thickness grafts from remote parts of the body including the underlying muscle is also performed, in some cases using microsurgical techniques.

The incontestable advantages of weight-bearing Pirogoff stumps have encouraged the development of methods of displacement of a calcaneal tuberosity to the proximal parts of the shank or hip, by microsurgery, in cases of traumatic amputation. As a result of grafting the calcaneal tuberosity the stump is lengthened and becomes weight-bearing.

After the above-mentioned reconstructive operations patients were fitted with, and have successfully used, active above-elbow prostheses, forearm prostheses, external-control prostheses and below-knee prostheses with total-contact sockets of PTB with cuff suspension, PTS, or KBM design.

References

Godunov S. F. & Keier A. N. (1969) Free bone plasty for lengthening of short arm stumps. *Acta Chirurgica Plasticae (Praha)* **11**, 163–174.

Ilizarov G. A. (1971) Osnovnye printsipy chreskostonogo kompressionnogo i distraktsionnogo osteosinteza. *Ortop. Travmatol. Protez* **32**, 7–15.

Tychonov V. M. (1949) Short thigh stump in children, its lengthening and preparation for prosthesis. *Tr. Tsentr. Nauchnoissledov. Inst. Protez. Moskova* **72**, 258.

PROSTHETIC TECHNOLOGY

43

Computer-aided Design and Computer-aided Manufacturing in Prosthetics and Orthotics

B.L. KLASSON

Introduction

Computer-aided design (CAD) and computer-aided manufacturing (CAM) are now being introduced in prosthetics, orthotics, and orthopaedic footwear. What we have seen so far is either experimental or perhaps only plans for projects, but there are reasons to believe that this new development will be very fast and change not only patient service, but also the professional roles. We are facing what is sometimes called the third industrial revolution. The first one was the substitution of manpower by external power, like steam in manufacturing, the second one was the introduction of automation, and the third one is a general utilization of the microcomputer. It is important to understand what CAD and CAM are and what they can offer us, but it is equally or more important to realize the more general implications of this new technology and of the third industrial revolution.

What is CAD?

Design is a creative, intellectual process, based on such things as the specification of the aim, knowledge of physics, manufacturing, components, materials, calculation of strength, etc., experience from other designs, talent, intuition, skill, and hard work. Design is artwork based on science.

The design process covers many activities, some of which are:

Generation of ideas.
Creation of geometrical shapes.
Calculations.
Experiments.
Simulation.
Development of manufacturing data.

The design approach may be:

Iterative.
Direct.
Choice from alternatives.

In the iterative approach a preliminary solution is developed through intuition or experience. Then the solution is analysed with reference to the demands that were specified for the product. If the specification is not satisfied, the solution is modified, and remodified if necessary, until it is acceptable, or until the designer is convinced that no solution is possible. In the direct approach, an analysis of the problem is used for the direct development of an acceptable solution. If choice from alternatives is used, many alternatives, all of them satisfying the specification, may be generated. After analysing all the alternatives, the designer selects and finalizes the best one. These approaches all fall into the following general design process:

Specification.

Selection of design strategy.

Solution of the design problem.

Checking of the design.

Preparation for manufacture of the design.

During the 20th century manufacturing may be said to have increased in efficiency by 1000%, but design by only 20%. The reason is that it has been possible to increase the efficiency of manufacturing dramatically by means of machines, which has not been the case for design. The most important progress in design was the introduction, about two decades ago, of the computer as an aid for fast calculation. The calculation volume in a design can be very large. The next step, now being developed and applied, is the introduction of descriptions of geometrical configurations such that they can be stored in computer memories, along with interactive graphic terminals, where the configurations can be displayed, or imaged, and modified by the designer. This is computer-aided design or CAD.

CAD is only at the beginning of its development, but it is already very powerful, especially if combined, or interfaced, with calculation of strength (FEM — finite element method) and simulation of the designed object in operation. Such comprehensive applications are, however, very demanding as far as computer power is concerned. Contemporary CAD systems may not be very convenient for a unique design, but as a 'library' of knowledge is accumulated the economic efficiency increases. It may not be practical for the design of a 'mark I', but it is much more efficient in modifying mark I to produce 'mark II', 'mark III', etc. The philosophy is that if the best abilities of man are combined with the best abilities of the computer the result will be better than if man made it alone. The computer can amplify the designer's memory, support his analytical and logical ability, and take over repetitive routines. The designer will then supply creativity and experience to the design process, control it, and organize the information about it. The following (economic) reasons for the use of CAD are frequently mentioned:

Avoid duplication of work.

Simplify studying three-dimensional geometries avoiding physical models.

Simplify input of data for analyses and display of results.

Simplify documentation of the product.

Store experience and information from previous designs.

What is CAM?

CAM is computer-aided manufacture. Unfortunately there is no general agreement as to how much is included in CAM. In the U.S.A., CAM covers the preparations for manufacture as well as the manufacture itself. In Sweden CAM covers the preparations only. In this presentation the U.S. concept of CAM is applied.

One of the economic reasons for using CAD is that time-consuming steps, other than the design in the process of production, can be integrated into the system. The most obvious operation is then the connection to numerically controlled production machines. Interfacing CAM to CAD is obvious and rational, but CAM can be used, and has been used for a long time, without CAD.

CAM has been applied for a much longer time than CAD, and it is less critical than CAD as far as the introduction of computer-aided socket design is concerned. In this context it is sufficient to understand CAM's potential in being connected to CAD for automatic manufacturing.

Interaction between man and computer

The first reason why CAD and CAM have been possible is, of course, the development of the microcomputer by Intel in 1970. The basis for the interaction between man and computer is visualized in Table 43.1 (Besant 1983). This comparison between man and computer is, however, only true for a short time. The fourth generation of computers will be much faster, maybe 1000 times, than today's computers, resulting in higher capacity. The computer will then further approach man's intellectual brilliance as it can work so much faster. When, however, the fifth generation of computers (Feigenbaum & McCorduch 1984) is available in the 1990s, it will be time to revise completely Besant's comparison. Several authors (Balkhausen 1978, Evans 1979) forecast that there will be very little need for technicians doing manual work and controlling machines in the industries of 1990. Expert systems with artificial intelligence and computer-based knowledge and computer-aided manufacturing will remove man from most of his remaining top positions in the comparison.

Applications in prosthetics, orthotics, and orthopaedic footwear service

Although it is agreed that the services can now be performed to a very high standard, it is also agreed that at least three serious problems remain, viz. reproducibility, capacity, and costs.

The lack of reproducibility derives from the fact that both measurement and modification techniques are not reproducible. They are the result of an individual's interpretations, judgement, and skills. This leads to some unfortunate consequences:

Table 43.1 Characteristics of man and computer. Reproduced with permission, from Besant (1983).

	Man	Computer
1 Method of logic and reasoning	Intuitive by experience, imagination, and judgement	Systematic and stylized
2 Level of intelligence	Learns rapidly but sequential. Unreliable intelligence	Little learning capability but reliable level of intelligence
3 Method of information input	Large amounts of input at one time by sight or hearing	Sequential stylized input
4 Method of information output	Slow sequential output by speech or manual actions	Rapid stylized sequential output by the equivalent of manual actions
5 Organization of information	Informal and intuitive	Formal and detailed
6 Effort involved in organizing information	Small	Large
7 Storage of detailed information	Small capacity, highly time-dependent	Large capacity, time-independent
8 Tolerance for repetitious and mundane work	Poor	Excellent
9 Ability to extract significant information	Good	Poor
10 Production of errors	Frequent	Rare
11 Tolerance for erroneous information	Good intuitive correction of errors	Highly intolerant
12 Method of error detection	Intuitive	Systematic
13 Method of editing information	Easy and instantaneous	Difficult and involved
14 Analysis capabilities	Good intuitive analysis, poor numerical analysis ability	No intuitive analysis, good numerical analysis ability

1 The fitting procedure is sometimes, if there are many failures, a prolonged, painful, frustrating, depressing, expensive, and maybe physically destructive, experience for the patient.

2 Probably too many patients are left with badly fitting devices.

3 The fitting programme is more expensive than is necessary.

Furthermore, the lack of reproducibility is also a serious bottleneck in research and development. No prosthesis is better than the fit (the interface between the stump and the prosthesis), irrespective of the sophistication of the rest of the prosthesis. Often when a new prosthetic component is subject to evaluation, it is not possible to isolate the quality of the new component from the quality of the fit.

The inadequacy of contemporary service capacity has been reported repeatedly through the years. One of the most recent (Jacobs & Murdoch 1985) concludes: 'Recognizing the size of the problems of prosthetics and orthotics services in the developing countries the traditional approaches from the industrial world have failed in solving them.'

The cost of prosthetics, orthotics, and orthopaedic footwear supplies may not be high when compared to the other components of care in a rehabilitation programme, but in some areas of the world the costs of prostheses of contemporary standard are prohibitive. Even in economically favoured countries the cost is now seen as a problem.

CAD and CAM will improve reproducibility and capacity and will cut down the costs. In addition they will support research and development to improve the fitting principles and methods. Consequently integration of the appliances with the human body will be much better.

The principles of CASD

The first step in current CAD/CAM projects in prosthetics is to find a way to arrive at an optimal socket shape from information about the stump. This is computer-aided socket design (CASD). The second step is to find a rational way to manufacture the socket. The third step is to find a way to modify the socket, if needed, after checking it on the stump. The problems in orthotics and fitting orthopaedic footwear are rather similar to those in prosthetics.

James Foort started to get interested in CASD as early as the beginning of the 1960s. His idea was that a limited amount of significant measurement on a stump is sufficient to define the shape of an adequate socket after the data have been processed to fit to a model. The model, which is a program in the computer, performs modifications in a way similar to the prosthetist's deformation of the stump when making a cast. The model actually represents experience from thousands of fittings. It is a common misunderstanding that the model is the final shape. The model is the transformation from the measured profile to the socket shape.

In Foort's current system the measurements used for the PTB prosthesis are the conventional anteroposterior and mediolateral measurements at the knee, plus an anteroposterior measurement each inch or each quarter-inch down the stump. When these measurements are fed into the CAD computer, the shape is generated and presented on the monitor screen. It is possible to look at selected cross-sections, modify the shape, and see the new result. When the prosthetist is satisfied by the result presented on the monitor, the first CAD step is finished and the information can be used in the CAM step for automatic manufacture of the socket.

Such a system is already a reality through joint efforts between Vancouver and London, as described in Chapters 44 & 45. It is fast. The CAD processing takes about ten minutes, numerically controlled carving of a mould another ten minutes, and making the socket in a Rapidform machine a further 30 minutes. The entire process, therefore, takes about 40 minutes to one hour. There is no need for a big, central computer in this system: an IBM personal computer or similar is adequate. The fact that it is adequate points out one limitation of the system. This limitation is not a criticism of the entire project. The joint project between the Medical Engineering Research Unit of the University of British Columbia, Vancouver, and the Bioengineering Centre of University College, London, is a total project interfacing measuring, design, and manufacture. All individual steps have to be simplified as much as possible initially. When the whole process is under control, the details can be refined. The potential of the project is much more interesting than the fit of the sockets coming out of the Rapidform machine at the present time. An evaluation of this project, based upon patient trials now, would probably be an evaluation of the socket concept and not of the value of CAD/CAM. It would miss the point if not very carefully performed. The classical PTB concept has already been modified or replaced in many places.

Socket design possibilities

The James Foort concept uses limited profile information from the stump to generate the total shape of the socket. On the other hand, it is agreed that good surface fit is important. One example is when the medial flare of the tibia is used for weight-bearing. Consequently, there is a need for a measurement technique that can feed surface information to the computer, and the computer must be powerful enough to process this information. Furthermore, there is clearly a need to control the volume of the socket, at least if it is not open-ended. Many doctors and prosthetists are of the opinion that the stump tolerates very little change in its original volume; thus any modification of the shape has to be compensated for somewhere else in the socket. There is also, therefore, a need for a measurement technique that can feed volume information to the computer and for a computer powerful enough to handle it. This leads one to the conclusion that measurement techniques constitute the most interesting area for research and development. The computer requirements, concerning hardware as well as software, are very much defined by the character of the input data. The three important questions are:

1 What is a good fit?

2 What information is necessary to achieve a good fit?

3 Which processing of the information is necessary to arrive at a good fit?

How is this solved in current practice? It is interesting to note that there are at least two commonly used approaches to this problem:

1 'A plaster cast is taken to obtain a replica of the shape to be fitted as a first step. As a second step the prosthetist modifies the replica further by adding and

subtracting plaster to generate a different shape which he knows from experience will provide optimal comfort.' (Fernie *et al.* 1985).

2 'A plaster cast is taken in such a way that the pressure and force distribution in the final socket are created in the cast by application of forces during the casting. Minor, if any, modifications are performed on the plaster positive as a second step.' (Holmgren, personal communication).

It is the author's view that the use of the second approach was the key to Holmgren's internationally recognized success as a fitter, and the reason is that it is a straight application of physics (*see later*). The first approach is not. It is rather an iteration, with obvious drawbacks:

1 More 'trial and error', and consequently higher costs.
2 A tendency and perhaps an acceptance of a less than good final result.

In more general terms there are three basic principles available when measuring the stump:

1 The stump is not deformed when measuring and only the surface is measured.
2 The stump is not deformed when measuring and both the surface and the interior are measured (X-ray, etc.).
3 The stump is deformed during measuring.

The trend right now is that scientists try to find ways of avoiding the third principle, successfully applied by prosthetists all over the world, in favour of the first and second ones. This is possible if:

1 Statistical documentation shows that the modification from the shape of the 'free' stump to the shape of a good fit follows mathematically definable laws or rules.
2 The data available from measurement and other available means are adequate for the purpose. This has led to a focusing of interest on:

    Further development of James Foort's concept, utilizing photographs or videodigital interpretation of silhouettes (in the sagittal plane).

    Surface scanning by means of light (laser, moiré shadow, etc.).

    CAT (computer-aided tomography) scanning. CAT offers the possibility of actually studying the bone/soft tissue distribution in the stump and using this information to determine the ideal modification of the shape.

It is, however, possible to combine CAD with a measurement technique that not only deforms the stump but also, actually during the course of measurement, physically creates the shape of the ultimate fit, allowing for patient reaction. One justification for this statement is the fact that automatic, computerized palpation devices are now being developed for diagnosing cancerous mammae. It is the author's view that interest will soon be refocused on the third principle. The reason stems from the question, 'What is a good fit?'. A good fit is primarily defined not by a particular shape of socket, but by the accommodation of the forces or pressures between the stump and the socket, to provide for comfortable and harmless weight-bearing, stabilization, and suspension. All forces are transmitted from the socket to the skeleton of the patient via soft tissues. Generally speaking, soft tissues transmit forces in two ways, hydrostatically and elastically. The 'elastic' force transmission appears to be the most critical one as far as fit is concerned. The force chooses the 'stiffest' way through the soft tissues. A uniform force or pressure distribution can be achieved even through a thin layer of soft tissues between a bone surface in the stump and the socket, but a local mismatching will change the pressure distribution, which may result in pain or damage.

The late Gunnar Holmgren, one of the world's foremost prosthetists, known for his combined analytical capacity and manual skill, used to say that he wanted to create or simulate the working conditions for the stump when casting (and make a minimum of modifications to the cast afterwards). He applied pressures and checked the result, and the shape resulted from the application of pressure. He shared the opinion of many prosthetists that modifying a socket is not a matter of adding or shaving away a few millimetres here or there; it is, rather, a matter of modifying the pressure distribution when making the cast.

It is the writer's opinion that the real breakthrough in CASD will take place when the system can simulate the socket on the stump, i.e. when we have an active computer-aided stump measurement technique. We will have to wait very long for this. This concept has for a long time been included in at least one development project. In the meanwhile, the work on the more 'iterative' principles is continuing, and should not be underestimated. Computer-aided equipment is very good at iterations (trial and error). The faster the system is, the better the result.

The strength and potential of CAD–CAM

The following points identify the strengths of CAD–CAM; reasonable insight and an open mind may well permit the identification of others.

1 Although the results may be primitive, it is already possible to design and manufacture a prosthetic socket using a CAD/CAM system.

2 All aspects of socket fit which have been discussed can be included if the measurement technique allows for surface and volume control, including the application of load at selected areas. This is possible with CAD using contemporary technology (although a lot of development may be required).

3 CAD/CAM is reproducible.

4 All modifications of a socket shape are quantitatively controlled and simply documented.

5 CAD and CAM are backed up by enormously strong industries with good profit, huge research and development resources, and good salesmen.

6 Computer technology is an important subject in schools and universities.

7 Computer technology is so strong in itself that it may be easily sold to less informed politicians and other 'decision makers'.

8 CAD–CAM interfaced with computer-aided production planning offers cheap mass production of items where each unit is unique or 'tailor-made' (e.g. Cabbage Patch doll).

The last point is extremely significant as far as orthopaedic footwear is concerned.

It is frequently stated that the service of the tailor and the shoemaker, making individual shoes, will soon be back on a wide scale. But they will be computerized (CAD–CAM). We are likely to see this within a few years. It is obvious that such a manufacturing system will easily be able to handle most of the problems related to the manufacturing of shoes for deformed feet.

CAD and CAM are only two examples of what the microcomputer can be used for. Others are:

CAPP   computer-aided process planning
CAP   computer-aided planning
CAQ   computer-aided quality assurance
CAE   computer-aided engineering
CAT   computer-aided tomography
CIM   computer-integrated manufacturing

and, of course: computerized setting, word-processing, book-keeping, literature retrieval, medical diagnostics, autopilots, time measurements, musical synthesizers, alarm systems, etc., etc. This is only the beginning of the third industrial revolution, and there is much more to come!

All these uses of the microcomputer have at least one thing in common: they replace previous methods and occupations. *No professional role is safe from change!* It is not only that new technology replaces routine work in production and administration (Klasson 1985), but computerization of medical and legal procedures will change also the roles of doctors and lawyers, to mention just two intellectual professions (Evans 1979). It may be difficult to accept the totality of the third industrial revolution, and it is perhaps even more difficult to accept the speed of its implementation, except for those who have already been affected by it. There are numerous examples of how professions have become obsolete and people have lost their jobs in this process, and there is an obvious need for eye-opening amongst a lot of people who refuse to see what is happening. There is enough history available to get an idea about what we are in for. This is not the place for a case review, but the writer would strongly recommend reading Evans (1979), Balkhausen (1978) and Feigenbaum and McCorduch (1984). Evans and Balkhausen may not represent the latest experiences and opinions, but on the other hand it is interesting to see how true their forecasts have proved to be over just a few years. There is a need for all professions to apply a strategy for the future (Klasson 1985), including the professions in our clinical teams. The most important component of such a strategy is that *the education systems must prepare the young people for the future, and not for the past!*

What is then the future in prosthetics and orthotics? The following personal opinions of the author may at least initiate a discussion:

1 Conventional technology has only to a limited extent been utilized in P/O service.

2 The most advanced application of technology is not necessarily the same as application of the most advanced technology.

3 Advanced technology, like CAD and CAM, will improve the patient service.

4 Advanced technology in P/O is not the same as advanced rehabilitation. 'Who is the best prosthetist, the one that is able to make the best possible prosthesis, or the one who is able to convince the patient that he has got the best possible prosthesis?' (Klasson 1985).

5 Other important components are the psychological and the social ones. It turns out that all the members of the clinical team spend a significant, maybe dominant, part of their efforts on communication with the patient and his family. The communication is a therapeutic effort.

6 There has been an unfortunate tendency for the clinical P/O team to emphasize the medical, surgical, and technical aspects, with high scientific quality, in their meetings and public events, but to exert only small, summary efforts on the other aspects.

7 There is a need now to change this. If not, our fascinating, stimulating, and fruitful work may by mistake be replaced by computerized diagnosis, computerized robot surgery, CAD–CAM fitting, computerized training machines and procedures, and computerized check-out.

8 The solution is not to try and avoid advanced technology. Such an approach is doomed to fail.

9 Time is now so fast that you do not see the future until it has passed.

References

Balkhausen D. (1978) *Die Dritte Industrielle Revolution. Mikroelektronik unser Leben Verandert.* Dusseldorf: Econ-Verlag.

Besant C. B. (1983) *Computer-aided Design and Manufacture,* 2nd Edition, pp.16–17. Chichester: Ellis Horwood.

Evans C. (1979) *The Mighty Micro: the Impact of the Computer.* London: Gollancz.

Feigenbaum E. A. & McCorduch P. (1984) *The Fifth Generation Artificial Intelligence and Japan's Computer Challenge to the World.* London: Michael Joseph.

Fernie G. R., Griggs G., Bartler S. & Lunai K. (1985) Shape sensing for computer aided below-knee prosthetic design. *Prosthetics and Orthotics International* **9**, 12–16.

Jacobs N. A. & Murdoch G. (eds) (1985) Report of ISPO workshop on prosthetics and orthotics in the developing world with respect to training and education and clinical services. Moshi, Tanzania. Copenhagen: ISPO, 94.

Klasson B. (1985) Computer aided design, computer aided manufacture and other computer aids in prosthetics and orthotics. *Prosthetics and Orthotics International* **9**, 3–11.

44

Shape Management: Systems Concepts and the Impact of Information Technology

M. LORD & R.M. DAVIES

Introduction

The present will be seen by historians as another industrial revolution, when new technologies emerged which transformed the operation of industry and commerce. Information technology and advances in materials are both highly significant factors in this changing face of the industrial society. These changes may be equated in broad terms to two key issues in lower limb prothetics — shape management and structural integrity. This chapter and that which follows explore the opportunities which emerge when the new technologies are firmly grasped and applied in a total system to the solution of problems in shape and structure.

Shape management of non-geometric doubly curved surfaces is applicable to lower limb prostheses in the areas of socket design, cosmesis design, and alignment. The last application may not be obvious at first, but the relative location of two non-geometric shapes (foot and socket) must be based on considerations of their shapes. Structural integrity is an issue in most of the components of the limb except soft coverings. It can be incorporated into the design of the shaped components, as in a Rapidform socket (Davies & Russell 1979) or an exoskeletal limb, or provided for separately.

While a primary application of information technology will be to generate customized shapes, for example in computer-aided socket design, and a primary application of new materials will be for structural reasons, e.g. strength-to-weight ratio, it would be wrong to attempt merely to equate information technology with shape management, and advances in materials with structural integrity. Without realization of the interaction between all four components many exciting opportunities for systems improvements could remain unexploited. For example, forming processes for the new materials allow the routine manufacture of shapes hitherto impossible; information technology facilitates the analysis and design of structural components previously inconceivable. The interplay between shape management and structural factors cannot be ignored.

This chapter concentrates on the possibilities arising primarily out of the use of information technology, using shape management as an example. In the next chapter the potential of new materials and forming processes is presented. Neither chapter gives a state-of-the-art review of the technologies, which is available extensively elsewhere and referenced in the text. Rather the emphasis is placed on the development of an awareness of what can be achieved by employing a total system concept, and putting together the component parts in a new yet logical way.

The example of CASD/CAM

An early demonstration of information technology used in the production of lower limb prostheses is to be seen in computer-aided socket design/computer-aided manufacture (CASD/CAM). The essential processes involved are shape data acquisition, shape data manipulation in digital form, and physical realization of the socket thus designed. The component parts of the first implementation of a CASD/CAM system are described in a special issue of *Prosthetics and Orthotics International* (Vol. 9, April 1985). A laser shape sensor (Fernie *et al.* 1985) can be used as an alternative to the normal caliper measurement input to an IBM-based CASD program (Saunders *et al.* 1985). The socket design is fed out onto a computer numerically controlled (CNC) carver (Saunders *et al.* 1985, Lawrence *et al.* 1985) and a socket produced over the positive on an automatic vacuum-forming machine (Davies *et al.* 1985). The system designs and produces below-knee sockets of the patellar tendon-bearing type.

Research and debate will no doubt continue on the possible technical implementations of each of the stages of this process in isolation. Body shape measurement techniques using various mechanical, optical, and ranging techniques have been widely developed (Rouse 1984, Harris [in press]). Digital manipulation of non-geometric surfaces is a special application within the general area of surface contouring (Duncan & Mair 1983). CNC machine technology is widely available in industry. It may ultimately be possible to go directly from the data file to the socket without generation of an interim positive. However, taken in isolation, it may be impossible to define the specifications for any of the stages. Usually the technologist working within the specialized area has made implicit if not articulated assumptions about the rest of the system, which may or may not be valid. The most exciting aspect of this work is the operational systems that are enabled by the technology. Merely to employ the new technology piecemeal in place of the old within the same operational framework would be to suppress latent potentiality. An entirely new approach is possible as a direct result of the technical innovation, and this can be engineered to the great benefit of the patient.

Operational logistics — who and what goes to whom?

Consider the CASD/CAM implementation described above. As Saunders shows, the entire socket fitting process can take as little as one and a half hours if successful at the first try — a time which will surely be reduced as the technology improves.

This fact alone has tremendous implications for service operation. With a similar approach to the generation of the other components for the limb, the prospect of the 'one-day delivery' as routine practice comes ever closer. However the 'instant' socket does assume the juxtaposition of the patient, prosthetist, computer, CNC carver, and socket generator in time and space. Is this a realistic goal? From the one extreme of a centralized facility that caters for wide areas on the basis of a short residential stay, through to the other extreme of a travelling workshop touring the neighbourhood doing domiciliary limb fitting, one can envisage many ways to combine all the ingredients. Even these extremes may be optimal given new technologies and social considerations. For example, in Jaipur (Childs 1985) the development of an appropriate limb which can be fitted in a matter of hours has provided a constant stream of self-referred patients from a wide area. No possibility should be dismissed without consideration of the total system.

However, information technology also offers the facility of rapid communication over distances, and would permit the divorce of, say, the measurement and socket design process from the socket manufacture, without the delays incurred in shipping plaster casts back to the central fabrication plant. Virtually a 'return of post' service on sockets could be offered in response to data transmitted by telephone. When CASD programs are sufficiently well developed that iterative fittings are the exception, this may offer a realistic approach for large operations. A small dedicated company geared to producing only CASD/CAM sockets could offer the type of facility provided by the photographic developing concessions.

There is an interesting balance between the various factors of shape measurement, sophistication of the computer program, and availability of the socket fabrication system. In a naive guess one can propose the premise that the better the shape measurement and the computer generation of the primitive socket, the less is the need for subsequent on-screen modifications and iterative fittings. The Saunders CASD program relies on very simple caliper measurements, and although the generation of the primitive socket has evolved to reasonable sophistication it is anticipated that the prosthetist will make routine use of the extensive facilities provided for on-screen modifications. The more the modification is left to the judgement of the individual prosthetist, the greater is the likelihood that iterative fitting may be necessary. In that case, the need for on-site socket fabrication is heightened. At the other extreme, another approach to CASD is being developed at the Bioengineering Centre, London, based on obtaining a complete shape definition of the stump followed by automatic computer rectification. By more sophisticated shape-sensing it is hoped to trade off the need for extensive on-screen sculpting, and to hit a high first-time success rate from automatic rectification. The development teams for both of these approaches are working in close collaboration; it is anticipated that from experience with the extreme systems, a mid-way optimum will eventually be reached.

The economics of the exercise will be dependent on geographic factors, mobility of the patient population, cost of the suite of equipment, and manpower costs.

The balance of these factors is changing, not least due to the rapidly advancing technology. It is in the nature of information technology that the second generation of computer-aided socket fitting systems will doubtless have a reduced cost and smaller physical size than that currently described.

Changing role of the prosthetist in the system

The impact of CASD/CAM on the prosthetist is often seen only in relation to the switch from manual to computer rectification. This is of course an important aspect, as Klasson (1985) describes. The prosthetist of the future will need to be more of an engineer/scientist than at present to operate with such equipment. However, there are other systems implications. In the U.K. and elsewhere, it is common that the prosthetist who sees the patient does not himself oversee the complete manufacture of the socket and mounting. Often the hardware passes out of the control of the prosthetist at the stage when a cast has been taken and marked out, with a few written comments on alignment. Unfortunately, there will be several points along the road to limb production where individual judgement will be made on the shape management factors, leading to an ambiguous interpretation. The prosthetist is out of control in a sense, and the patient is often aware of the intervention of the 'factor' between himself and his prosthetist. CASD/CAM introduces the possibility for the prosthetist to prescribe completely the socket and alignment at the design stage, so that the same socket and alignment can be produced if necessary many times over. This puts the responsibility back on to the prosthetist, where it should be. It also gives him a firm base from which to refine his decisions in a systematic and scientific way, and also to describe accurately to others those decisions for teaching (Fernie *et al.* 1984) or other purposes.

Cosmesis and data banking

As mentioned in the introduction, shape management is an integral concept in the generation of cosmesis. The ideal external shape of a lower limb prosthesis for the unilateral amputee is the mirror image of the existing limb, giving some licence for subjective improvements on nature if desired. However this shape is often not achievable because the structural components of the limb go outside the desired mirrored shape. With information fed into the computer on the shape of the natural limb, and the alignment and dimensions of the structural components of the prosthesis, a blend should be achievable to yield a best-compromise cosmetic shape. The physical realization of the outer shape as defined in a computer to produce an acceptable cosmesis has not yet been explored. In the systems sense it would be more profitable to think in terms of a single process which can realize an article with the desired internal and external shape, possessed of the necessary structural integrity, to yield, for example, a complete below-knee prosthesis down to the ankle or below.

In generating CASD/CAM sockets, digital data become available for the socket shape and perhaps also the stump shape. These data can be stored in very compact form for subsequent use. Such a data bank will allow subsequent transmission to any location for an exact repeat or modification to the existing socket, in many instances eliminating the need to call the patient in for recasting or socket copying. Also, a wealth of data will become available for scientific studies. As examples, the long-term effects on stump shape by the use of a particular socket shape, or the fluctuation of shape from the primary amputee to the established user, might be established.

Conclusion

A few of the operational systems enabled by the introduction of information technology into shape management have been discussed. The direction of the technological developments must be seen in the context of the entirely new systems opportunities now feasible, and not as a replacement item by item of component parts of the existing system. Although the first impact of information technology in lower limb prosthetics is on shape management, it is not restricted to this area.

Acknowledgements

The work of the Bioengineering Centre is primarily funded by the Department of Health and Social Security.

References

Childs S. (1985) The Jaipur limb — an Indian success story. *Therapy Weekly* **11(38)**, 6.

Davies R. M. & Russell D. (1979) Vacuum formed thermoplastic sockets for prostheses. In *Disability* (eds Kenedi R. M., Paul J. P. & Hughes J.), pp.385–90. London: MacMillan.

Davies R. M., Lawrence R. B., Routledge P. E. & Knox W. (1985) The Rapidform process for automated thermoplastic socket production. *Prosthetics and Orthotics International* **9**, 27–30.

Duncan J. P. & Mair S. G. (1983) *Sculptured Surfaces in Engineering and Medicine*. Cambridge: Cambridge University Press.

Fernie G. R., Halsall A. P. & Ruder K. (1984) Shape sensing as an educational aid for student prosthetists. *Prosthetics and Orthotics International* **8**, 87–90.

Fernie G. R., Griggs G., Bartlett S. & Lunau K. (1985) Shape sensing for computer aided below-knee prosthetic socket design. *Prosthetics and Orthotics International* **9**, 12–16.

Harris J. D. (in press) *Proceedings of 3rd International Symposium on Surface Topography and Spinal Deformity, Oxford, September, 1984*. Gustav Fischer Verlag.

Klasson B. (1985) Computer aided design, computer aided manufacture and other computer aids in prosthetics and orthotics. *Prosthetics and Orthotics International* **9**, 3–11.

Lawrence R. B., Knox W. & Crawford H. V. (1985) Prosthetic shape replication using a computer controlled carving technique. *Prosthetics and Orthotics International* **9**, 23–26.

Rouse D. J. (1984) *Modern Orthopaedic Footwear Practice*. Report of a workshop to define clinical criteria for a Computer-Aided Design and Manufacturing System. Research Triangle Institute, North Carolina. Sponsored by the National Institute of Handicapped Research, Washington, Contract No. 300-83-0236, 4.16-4.18.

Saunders C. G., Foort J., Bannon M., Lean D. & Panych L. (1985) Computer aided design of prosthetic sockets for below-knee amputees. *Prosthetic and Orthotics International* **9**, 17–22.

45

Materials and Processing Systems

R.M. DAVIES & M. LORD

Introduction

The possible applications of modern engineering methods extend far beyond the use of computers and graphic systems to define prosthetic sockets. Additional future applications may include the means of production of complete prostheses at all levels and subsequently the extension of the concepts to orthoses, body support systems, and orthopaedic footwear. In terms of systems and specifications, the results of the information and materials revolutions seem likely to lead to reductions in delivery times, costs, and weights of appliances, in addition to increases in reliability, strength, and field life. The processes can be conducted at clinical facilities by plug-in, self-contained machines. And these in turn will be compact, automated, and foolproof. Alignment definition will be specified and replicated as well as shape definition — the latter encompassing cosmesis as well as socket shape.

The patient must be the ultimate judge of the value of the work. He must be able to answer 'yes' to the question 'Is there significant improvement in fit, comfort, function or delivery time?'. Thus the new technology is employed with constant reference to patient feedback.

The philosophy adopted to date has been to reduce the dependence on the artisan, and instead to distil his expertise into specially developed automated sytems. This has meant the introduction of microprocessor controls and computer-aided design (CAD) techniques into prosthetics. It is part of the rationale to use computer techniques to determine the prosthetic requirements of the patients and then computer-controlled automated machines to fabricate the prosthesis (Lawrence & Davies 1981). Any later advances in the state of the prosthetic art would simply mean an update in software.

The processes being replaced in prosthetics have their roots in artisan methods. The harness maker, the aircraft metal worker, the cabinet maker, and the armourer has each left his mark. Workers in the field were often wearers of devices themselves. These people were innovators by nature, often basing the modifications on their original art and craft or on the needs they wished to satisfy as wearers.

Since 1945, research organizations have played a major role in the development of improvements. They have engaged in the formulation of new information, the systemization of artisan practices, the development of tools, devices, and techniques, and the introduction of new materials. The formulation of new information must continue, but the technologies which have emerged during the past few years make further refinement of artisan methods inappropriate. Instead, the technological advances in computer-based information manipulation, along with new materials, are being exploited to break out of many longstanding constraints. These will make a real impact on standards of treatment, delivery times, and reliability.

Materials

Thermoplastics are removing a number of old design limitations imposed by working with more traditional materials (Foort et al. 1984). The apparently unlimited design freedom made available is already being exploited in industry for everything from bicycles to car body parts and engines. Indeed a plastic-engined racing car has appeared and competed on the track at Daytona Beach. The engine is quiet because of the plastic's acoustic insulating properties, produces 238 kW (320 hp), and weighs only 68 kg.

Designers have not been slow to exploit other properties of thermoplastics. There is no corrosion; colour can be throughout instead of surface only; field life is at least doubled; but, most important of all, thermoplastics can be moulded and therefore shaped. In many fields of engineering, these properties have heralded the dawn of a new era in design and manufacture. They can also radically alter and upgrade the bioengineer's contributions, not least in prosthetics.

In socket work it is necessary to cover the desired range of socket sizes whilst restricting the draw ratio. Starting off with something that approximates to the finished shape implies a double deformation technique; first by injection moulding (to mass-produce thermoplastic preforms cheaply) and then by vacuum-forming to the definitive shape. Materials hitherto were oriented towards one or other of the methods of deformation, whereas this application calls for a material suitable for both methods. In addition, it has to possess first-rate post-formed mechanical properties. The materials shortlist shrinks to two or three likely materials, of which one of the co-polymers of polypropylene is preferred.

There are up to 14 variables that can be adjusted during the injection moulding process. Preforms that look the same as each other are obtainable from various permutations. Laboratory investigations, however, reveal that they are not the same, and an instrumentation exercise must be carried out on the moulding machine in order to define the optimal settings for moulding preforms. Although the moulding conditions are controlled in this way, and all raw material is released against a British Standard specification, this specification is very broad and unacceptable variations can sometimes occur. Consequently, it has been found necessary to check samples from batches using a technique of biaxial deformation, carried out at a particular strain rate.

Rapidform

Several years ago the Rapidform technique for automatically fabricating thermoplastic sockets was developed and brought into service (Davies & Russell 1979). These sockets were the first thermoplastic sockets in clinical service, and they proved to be highly successful. They were accurately formed, hygienic, extremely tough, slightly resilient, and very reliable. In fact there have been no mechanical failures of any socket, and some have been regularly used by patients for over six years. They are rapidly fabricated, and they are cheap. The Rapidform machines form consistently high-quality sockets without the need of a skilled operator. The U.K. government's Central Office of Information (COI) made a film of the process about four years ago. It is entitled 'Fit a Limb' and was part of the *Living Tomorrow* series. The U.K. Department of Health and Social Security provided Rapidform machines for their limb centres, and private purchases were also made by some major limb manufacturing firms.

Rapidform is central to the high-technology methods for prosthetic supply. It was the first of the modules to be developed, and with ten machines in use in artificial limb and applicance centres and in private firms has manufactured over 16 500 sockets up to July, 1985. These sockets are on average one-third of the weight of their conventional counterparts and can be used in modular or conventional leg prescriptions and at above- or below-knee levels of amputation. They are comfortable, sturdy, lightweight, and inexpensive. Fig. 45.1 shows the most recent version of the Rapidform and also a collection of typical sockets formed by the machine.

(a)   (b)

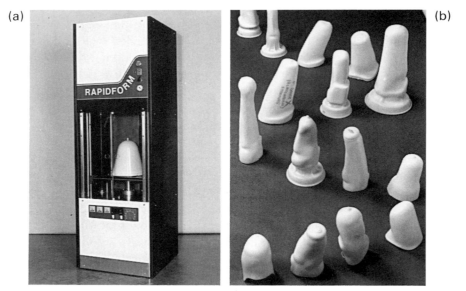

Fig. 45.1 (a) The Rapidform machine for AK and BK socket forming. (b) Typical Rapidform thermoplastic sockets including AK, BK and Syme levels.

In the context of the overall modernization of the field however, Rapidform is one module in the supply process — automatically forming over a plaster positive or over a carved wax model which in turn has been computer-shaped; then interfacing with a plastic tapered column prosthesis structure. The time-span of the operation (20 min) is compatible with that of the other modules of the automated system. The socket can be fabricated without operator attention while the operator carries out another action of a comparable time-cycle. For example, new shape data could be prepared and completed sockets trimmed so that a continuous production stream is maintained.

Thermoplastic shanks

The successful development of the Rapidform socket fabrication system was followed by a semi-automated system for rapidly and cheaply fabricating a below-knee system called tapered column prostheses. This technique fabricates thermoplastic shin sections by rotationally casting the required section in a specially controlled machine (Coombes *et al.* 1985a). The tapered columns are extremely light and strong. They interface via plastic alignment couplings (Coombes *et al.* 1985b) at either end to the socket and the foot. These sections are fabricated quickly and cheaply. A typical below-knee prosthetic system comprising a Rapidform socket, tapered column and alignment couplings, and a SACH foot weighs just under one kilogram. It has an exceedingly good fatigue life. An above-knee system is being finalized. An option exists for supplying tapered columns by injection moulding. Two options are also being explored for providing complete alignment capability, and the early field experience is promising.

Rotational moulding, in addition to having a time-cycle compatible with the other modules with which it would be working in parallel (not series), provides an opportunity for 'tuning' the prosthesis to the patient's requirements by varying the wall thickness. Thus a frail patient can be supplied with a lightweight limb, and a robust user can have a very sturdy limb — and these from the same system, with fabrication on the spot for fitting and delivery on the same visit. Laboratory testing has taken them well past the internationally agreed structural standards (ISPO 1978). Fig. 45.2a shows a cutaway view of a tapered column BK prosthesis. The socket is vacuum-moulded, the shank is rotationally moulded, and the jacked alignment units are injection-moulded.

This technique also holds the promise of producing an exoskeletal structure of cosmetic form for the fabrication of ultralight prostheses (Fig. 45.2b). With the other modules in place, it advances in significance. Thus, because CAD has the potential for dealing with alignment and cosmesis, including the shapes of the socket and foot of the prosthesis, the outer contours can be completely defined and the requisite mould equally defined.

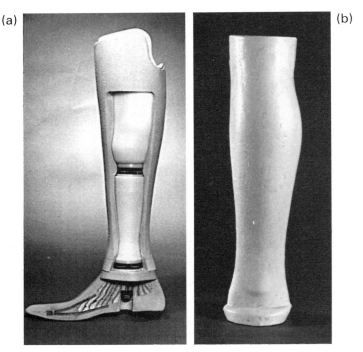

Fig. 45.2 (a) A tapered column BK prostheses with the cosmesis cut away to show the vacuum-moulded socket, the rotationally moulded shank, and the injection-moulded jacked alignment units. (b) A thermoplastic, rotationally moulded, exoskeletal shank.

Computer numerically controlled (CNC) carving

The fabrication of the socket requires a positive mould that represents the rectified shape of the stump. A CNC machine uses co-ordinate data from CAD to cut and shape a wax blank. This carved wax is the model of the rectified stump shape over which the thermoplastic socket will be Rapidformed.

Computer numerically controlled carving is well established in industry, and a number of systems are available. Prosthetics applications, however, do not call for the stiffness and precision of industrial machines, and a purpose-built carver such as that being developed by the Bioengineering Centre offers certain advantages. It is capable of a deep cut (up to 75 mm) since it is milling only wax or foam, not metal. Thus a shorter carving time is achieved. Its operation is as follows. A wax blank is mounted in the chuck of its rotary table. The table rotates the blank as the cutting tool moves along the length of the blank while moving up or down. All motions are directed by a microprocessor controller, which receives its data on where the tool tip must be from the computer which is used to design the required shape.

It is intended that fixtures and special wax blanks will be used so that minimal carving will be required to obtain a given shape. Work could be scheduled so that carved blanks could be used again on smaller sized objects. Sufficiently inexpensive, the dedicated carver could be adjacent to the client so that, with all essential elements within reach, trial prostheses could be delivered within the composite timespan of module operations.

Conclusions

The CAD shape definition system typically takes ten minutes to define the required shape (using a few key measurements taken from the patient). The CNC machine then takes about ten minutes to produce the former representing the stump shape. This is used in Rapidform to fabricate a socket in 20 minutes. In parallel with this socket preparation, the shin section (tapered column) is rotationally moulded.

From the above, it can be seen that a patient can be measured and fitted with a prosthesis within a very short time, even with trimming and adjusting. Because of the low cost and high speed of the process, it becomes preferable to manufacture and issue a new prosthesis than to undertake repairs.

Developments in the two areas of information and materials technology have permitted these current advances. The graphical and computer-based methods of acquiring and manipulating shape data replace plaster work. Thus sockets and cosmetic shapes can be specified, stored, and subsequently recalled and/or modified. These methods permit the compact permanent storage of thousands of patients' shapes for quick recall. Thus a duplicate prosthesis can be fabricated immediately from no more than an identity number. A data bank is also compiled in this way, allowing the extraction of statistical information which has never been obtainable in the past.

Modern thermoplastic materials, the second technology permitting the current advances, have the great advantage over conventional structural materials (wood, metal, and even carbon fibre) of microprocessor-controlled formability. It is this property which marries so happily with the information technology. However, these materials have a number of other attractive features including lightness, high strength, low cost, and corrosion resistance.

New and much more flexible choices are made available in organizing supply systems. These range over completely local (even portable) fabrication to central fabrication, but with many possible variations in between, which make use of modems and telephone data transmission systems.

The benefits to patients have been stressed, but the impact on the manufacturing industries will also be profound. Extrapolating from other fields, it is possible to see the initial reservation giving way as the power of computer-based design and manufacture is revealed. In addition, small companies become relatively more viable as the 'economies of scale' of the earlier methods are reversed. The features of these systems which give general advantage are increased quality, reliability, and productivity. But the special features which will transform medical equipment supply are flexibility, ease of customization, and enhanced product development options.

Acknowledgements

The work of the Bioengineering Centre is primarily funded by the U.K. Department of Health and Social Security.

References

Coombes A. G. A., Lawrence R. B. & Davies R. M. (1985a) Rotational moulding in the production of prostheses. *Prosthetics and Orthotics International* **9**, 31–36.
Coombes A. G. A., Knox W. & Davies R. M. (1985b) Thermoplastic alignment couplings for prostheses. *Prosthetics and Orthotics International* **9**, 37–45.
Davies R. M. & Russell D. (1979) Vacuum formed thermoplastic sockets for prostheses. In *Disability* (eds Kenedi R. M., Paul J. P. & Hughes J.), pp.385–90. London: MacMillan.
Foort J., Lawrence R. B. & Davies R. M. (1984) Construction methods and materials for external prostheses — present and future. *International Rehabilitation Medicine* **6**, 72–78.
International Society for Prosthetics and Orthotics (1978) *Standards for lower limb prostheses; report of a conference.* IPSO, Philadelphia Pa.: ISPO.
Lawrence R. B. & Davies R. M. (1981) Thermoplastics for prosthetic applications. *Journal of Biomedical Engineering* **3**, 289–293.

46

Alignment and Gait Optimization in Lower Limb Amputees

M. SALEH

Introduction

In current prosthetic practice the final prescription is derived by combining the prosthetist's manual skill and experience in gait assessment with current component technology. In the words of Eberhart *et al.* (1954) 'the pattern of walking exhibited by an individual represents his solution to the problem of how to get from one place to another with minimum effort, adequate stability, and acceptable appearance'. For the amputee, it is doubtful whether these criteria can be assessed adequately using subjective methods alone. This chapter explores the potential role of gait analysis techniques in the precise matching of the prosthesis to the user. This fine tuning of prosthetic prescription may increase the number of successful fittings, improve the amputee's overall performance, and enable younger amputees to engage in more physical pursuits both at work and leisure; it may also reduce long-term sequelae such as back pain. It has been termed *gait optimization.*

Gait analysis systems, whether simple or complex, are designed to measure the temporal and spatial characteristics (kinematics) and force characteristics (kinetics) of gait. Two kinematic parameters are of particular interest: the time–distance measurements, for example step length, velocity, and single support time; and the joint angles. The former may be measured very simply with minimal equipment (Robinson & Smidt 1981), the latter with goniometers (Jansen & Orbaek 1980), photographic techniques (Sutherland & Hagy 1972), television cameras (Jarrett 1976), and optoelectronic devices (Mitchelson 1977). Kinetic measurement of the ground reaction forces may be made with mechanical or piezoelectric force plates describing six main components of the ground reaction force, i.e. vertical force, anteroposterior and mediolateral shear forces, torque about the vertical axis, and the 'x' and 'y' co-ordinates of the centre of pressure. Automated gait analysis systems (Jarrett 1980, Taylor *et al.* 1982) record kinematic and kinetic data in real time and are capable of calculating external joint moments (the product of the ground reaction force and the perpendicular distance from the line of action of that force to the centre of the joint concerned). These moments must be counteracted by equal and opposite internal moments provided by tension in ligaments and muscle contraction.

Gait optimization will be considered under three main headings — the amputee, the prosthesis, and the assessment methods (Fig. 46.1).

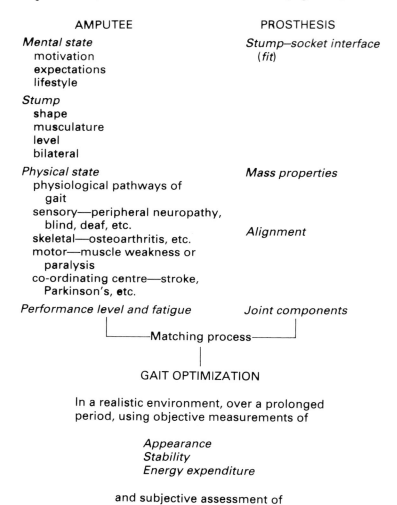

Fig. 46.1 Amputee and prosthetic interactions in gait optimization.

The amputee

In Dundee, 87% of lower limb amputations are performed for peripheral vascular disease, 80% of the patients are over 60 years of age (Dundee Limb Fitting Centre

1981), and 75% have multiple physical impairments (Troup 1976). Many of these physical impairments directly influence the 'physiological pathways of gait' (Fig. 46.1) and may critically influence the amputee's potential for rehabilitation, in contrast to the young amputee, who is often seen to walk well with a poorly adjusted prosthesis. Other physical constraints affecting the success of a prosthetic fitting include proximal amputation levels, bilateral amputees, and the adequacy of the stump to accept and control a prosthesis. The amputee's motivation, expectations, and lifestyle must be considered, and his fatigue and exercise tolerance impose further restrictions on the fitting process.

The prosthesis

There are four main areas of interest in optimization — the stump–socket interface or *fit,* mass properties, alignment, and joint components.

The stump–socket interface

The amputee's stump has a unique configuration, and to achieve total contact the socket must be matched precisely to it, albeit modified to effect efficient force transference and comfort; this exercise should be repeatable with built-in contingencies for slight changes which occur in the stump with time. Computer-aided design (CAD) and computer-aided manufacture (CAM) are now being developed for sensing stump shapes and the design and manufacture of sockets. The stump is easily deformed, and Klasson (1985) has emphasized the importance of being able to simulate the effect of the socket on the stump, and this must be considered both statically and dynamically during force transmission in the gait cycle. It is possible to measure interface pressures by inserting transducers into the socket liner (Pearson *et al.* 1973). In Pearson's study, however, only four small transducers were used, providing information over a small area of the interface only. A much more satisfactory arrangement would be a matrix array of transducers, providing a pressure profile of the whole of the interface during gait. The provision of an ideal socket for an amputee has far-reaching implications, not least with regard to optimization in the rest of the fitting and alignment process.

The mass properties of the prosthesis

Traditionally, the weight and balance point or mass centre of the prosthesis was a direct consequence of the materials selected for its manufacture rather than ballistic requirements. There is considerable interest in so-called ultra-lightweight limbs at present, and with that an unsubstantiated belief that lowering the prosthetic mass would lead to a reduction in the amputee's metabolic energy expenditure (Convery *et al.* 1984).

The propulsive effort of locomotion is provided by forces generated at push-off and the kinetic energy of the swinging limb. The magnitude of these push–pull forces may be calculated using Newton's first law of motion, $F = m \times a$. Thus, lowering the overall mass of the prosthesis would lead to a reduction in the muscular effort required for effective push-off, but it would also reduce the kinetic energy generated in the swinging limb. The position of the centre of mass of the prosthesis, by affecting its inertial properties, will also alter its projectile characteristics. The situation is analogous to moving the weight of the pendulum of a grandfather clock. If the weight is moved down, the inertial properties increase, and as the motor mechanism is the same the clock will slow down.

Perhaps one of the most valuable contributions that can be made using low-mass prostheses is the determination of the optimum mass characteristics of the prosthesis using an iterative approach. This method was elegantly demonstrated by Simon (1981) when he studied the gait of a 35-year-old above-knee amputee using a lightweight prosthesis weighted in both the thigh and shank. The amputee did not like the unweighted limb, or weighting of the thigh or shank three inches above the ankle. The preferred situation was weighting of the shank 11 inches proximal to the ankle, which corresponds closely to the position of the mass centre in the natural situation. Altering the mass characteristics of the limb did not change the gait kinematics apart from the cycle time, but significant changes were noted in the external joint moments at both hip joints. He concluded that the young amputee was controlling gait kinematics at the expense of increased muscular activity at proximal levels.

In a study of 25 consecutive below-knee fittings, using a Berkeley jig, at the Dundee Limb Fitting Centre, the prosthesis fitted with an alignment device was shown on average to be 30% heavier than the delivery limb, and a change in the mass centre of over 1 cm was noted in 18 cases (Saleh *et al.* 1983). Gait analysis was performed on five amputees, each using their own completed prosthesis and a specially fabricated optimally aligned prosthesis fitted with an alignment device. Significant differences in gait were noted by the amputees but not by the prosthetist; these differences were clearly demonstrated using the measurement system. In order to exclude the possibility of slight differences in socket fit and heel bumper density, three further amputees were assessed at dynamic alignment and three weeks later on completion of the limb. The previous results were confirmed, but on this occasion the amputees were not aware of any difference. Fig. 46.2 shows a typical example of a knee angle diagram and Fig. 46.3 a hip moment diagram, comparing dynamic alignment and delivery prostheses. It seems likely that younger, fitter amputees will prefer heavier limbs than their geriatric counterparts.

Prosthetic alignment

In current prosthetic practice, the optimum alignment for an amputee is achieved during the dynamic alignment process by subjective assessment. This comprises visual observations of gait deviations by the prosthetist and the amputee's

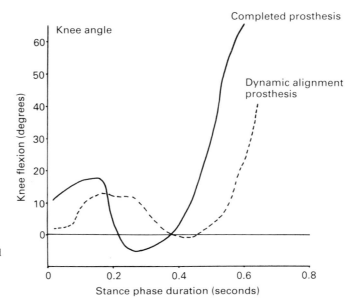

Fig. 46.2 Knee angle plotted against stance phase for a below-knee amputee.

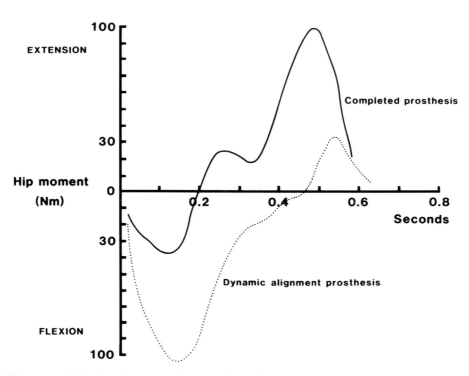

Fig. 46.3 Hip moment plotted against stance phase for a below-knee amputee.

comments regarding his comfort, stability, and performance. In a study by the author (Saleh 1981), deliberate anteroposterior misalignments were made in five below-knee amputees, and their gait was assessed both by visual observation and by an automated gait analysis system. Subjective methods of assessment were found to be inadequate on three counts. Firstly, the geriatric amputee's comments were often found to be unhelpful. Secondly, visual observation conducted by an experienced clinical team was found to be an unreliable clinical skill. Finally, the amputee's responses to misalignments were not always apparent in the appearance of gait as predicted by Radcliffe (Radcliffe & Foort 1961); however, changes could be seen in time–distance, force, and moment data consistent with instability and complex compensatory responses (Saleh 1984). When visual observation was compared to biomechanical analysis and quantitative measurements (Saleh & Murdoch 1985) the observers recorded 22.2% of the predicted gait deviations and were unable to comment on 15.5% of all the required observations. Step length and step time were noted to be the most difficult parameters to assess visually, followed by ankle–foot observations in stance phase and finally ankle–foot function in swing phase and knee function observations. In contrast, the quantitative measurement system was found to be very sensitive in picking up gait deviations. Fig. 46.4 shows a stick figure diagram of a below-knee amputee deliberately misaligned anteriorly.

In a parallel but more extensive series of studies by Zahedi *et al.* (1983a) on above- and below-knee amputees, subjective methods produced a range of alignments acceptable to the amputee. However, the amputee's gait changed significantly (Zahedi *et al.* 1983b). Zahedi confirmed the need for measurements of the proximal segments and the contralateral limb, and also noted complex neuromuscular compensatory responses (Zahedi *et al.* 1985), he concluded that it was possible to select biomechanically the most suitable alignment from the range of otherwise acceptable alignments for any one patient.

The range of alignments achieved merely reflects the inadequacy of subjective methods of assessment, and the amputee's tolerance to this range is likely to depend on his age and fitness. Gait analysis is advocated, but an elegant idea worthy of mention is the use of motorized alignment devices which are controlled by telemetry, designed by Hobson in Winnipeg (1972).

Joint components

Joint components are generally selected from the wide range available according to the limb centre's practice and budget, the prosthetist's experience, and those types preferred or available, especially with respect to modular systems. It would seem self-evident that the joint selected will influence the amputee's performance, not only because of its mass characteristics but also its particular design characteristics. Goh *et al.* (1984) compared the characteristics of two ankle–foot mechanisms in common use today, the SACH and uniaxial feet. These two feet

Fig. 46.4 Stick figure diagram of the stance phase of gait as affected by an anteriorly misaligned prosthesis. Markers outline the hip, knee, ankle and forefoot. Note the early occurrence of foot-flat at 13.5% and heel-off at 61% of stance phase compared to 18% and 70% respectively with the same prosthesis optimally aligned. Reproduced with kind permission of the British Editorial Society of Bone and Joint Surgery (Saleh & Murdoch 1985).

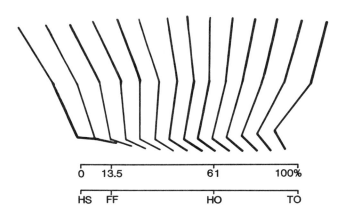

are quite different in design, and in general the amputee preferred the foot that he was accustomed to. Little change was noted in the kinematic parameters of gait, or in fact in proximal or contralateral limb joint moments, but significant changes were noted in the vertical force pattern reflecting differences in stance phase loading (Fig. 46.5). It would seem likely that gait analysis may have a role to play in the development of these components and the identification of those best suited to particular amputee groups.

In summary, gait analysis has a major role to play in the selection of the mass characteristics and alignment of prostheses for individual amputees and in the research and development of sockets and joint components for particular amputee groups.

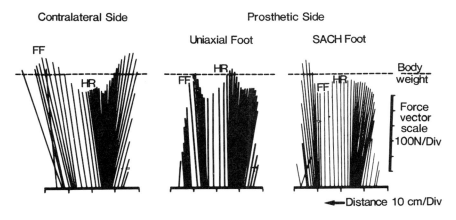

Fig. 46.5 Typical force vector diagrams of a below-knee amputee. Reproduced with kind permission of the Editorial Board of *Prosthetics and Orthotics International* (Goh *et al.* 1984).

Gait assessment

Atha Thomas (1944) stated 'in the proper fitting and alignment of the amputation prosthesis, knowledge of the structure and function of the normal joints of the lower extremity as well as of the relation of the joint axes to each other is essential. Also of value is an understanding of the mechanics of normal locomotion and its relation to the pathomechanics of the gait with a prosthesis'. There seems no doubt that more sensitive kinematic and kinetic measurements will aid gait optimization.

Using automated gait analysis systems, a large body of data is created. These data must be reduced to pick out sensitive parameters, and these parameters must be displayed in a way that is easy to understand and analyse. The lack of normative data and knowledge regarding the effects of alignment and mass changes on particular kinetic and kinematic parameters are limiting factors in the present ability to use gait analysis for optimization. The use of symmetry indices as described by Hannah (1983) is not, in the author's opinion, a satisfactory way of optimizing gait, since the amputee is asymmetrical and deficits on the prosthetic side are to some extent compensated for by reactions occurring in the contralateral limb. For maximum information generation, spatial measurements of the whole of the body and contralateral limb must be made and multiple steps recorded over differing terrains. Finally, four main groups of quantitative measurement parameters will be considered.

1 *Time–distance measurements.* These parameters are considered by most workers to be the basic descriptors of gait and would seem to be consistent in successive recordings of the same individual (Murray *et al.* 1964). They are considered necessary for the proper interpretation of other more complex parameters (Lamoreux 1971, Grieve 1968, Andriacchi *et al.* 1977). They are sensitive descriptors of gait changes (Andriacchi *et al.* 1977) and Perry *et al.* (1979) consider the velocity and single support time to reflect the amputee's mobility and support characteristics respectively. In the author's study, the stance phase duration was found to be a useful indicator of acclimatization and fatigue (Saleh 1981).

2 *Joint angles* may display against time (Eberhart *et al.* 1954) or as angle–angle diagrams (Grieve 1968). There seems to be no doubt that these are very sensitive parameters of change in both mass characteristics and alignment. They have another advantage in being easy to interpret when plotted graphically (Fig. 46.2).

3 *Ground reaction forces* provide valuable information regarding weight transfer, stability during stance phase, and push-off force. They are sensitive to alignment changes and joint component characteristics.

4 *External joint moments.* Solomonidis (1980) demonstrated the value of anteroposterior hip moments in the assessment of above-knee modular systems,

and other workers demonstrated the value of external joint moments as indicators of neurophysiological control (Simon 1980, Saleh 1981). The external joint moments at the ankle and knee, and to a lesser extent at the hip, have also been shown to be sensitive indicators of misalignments (Saleh & Bostock 1985).

In conclusion, subjective methods of assessment are inadequate for gait optimization. Gait measurement would appear to be valuable in selecting the prosthetic alignment and mass characteristics for each individual amputee and in the research and development of sockets and joint components. It is necessary for centres or institutions interested in both prosthetics and gait analysis to collaborate in the collection of baseline data regarding the effects of mass and alignment on measured gait parameters. In the future, but perhaps a long way off yet, is the possibility of feeding the amputee's unique description into a computer, where a general formula based on the requirements for socket fit, optimum mass, alignment, and preferred joint components is considered, and a definitive prosthesis automatically manufactured.

References

Andriacchi T. P., Ogle J. A. & Galante J. O. (1977) Walking speed as a basis for normal and abnormal gait measurement. *Journal of Biomechanics* **10(4)**, 261–268.

Convery P., Jones D., Hughes J. & Whitefield G. (1984) Potential problems of manufacture and fitting of polypropylene ultralightweight below-knee prostheses. *Prosthetics and Orthotics International* **8**, 21–28.

Dundee Limb Fitting Centre (1981) Records of all the in-patient admissions to the Dundee Limb Fitting Centre, 1965–1980. Tayside Health Board, Department of Occupational Medicine, Ninewells Hospital, Dundee.

Eberhart H. D., Inman V. T. & Bresler B. (1954) The principal elements in human locomotion. In *Human Limbs and their Substitutes* (eds Klopsteg P. E. & Wilson P. D.), pp. 437–471. New York: McGraw-Hill.

Goh J. C. H., Solomonidis S. E., Spence W. D. & Paul J. P. (1984) Biomechanical evaluation of SACH and uniaxial feet. *Prosthetics and Orthotics International* **8**, 147–154.

Grieve D. W. (1968) Gait patterns and the speed of walking. *Biomedical Engineering* **3(3)**, 119–122.

Hannah R. E. (1983) The effect of prosthetic alignment changes on below-knee amputee gait. International Society for Prosthetics and Orthotics, IV World Congress, Imperial College, London, Book of Abstracts 84.

Hobson D. (1972) A powered aid for aligning the lower limb modular prosthesis. *Bulletin of Prosthetic Research* **10(18)**, 159–163.

Jansen E. & Orbaek H. (1980) Reproducibility of gait measurement using the Lamoreux goniometer. *Prosthetics and Orthotics International* **4**, 159–161.

Jarrett M. O. (1976) A television/computer system for human locomotion analysis. PhD Thesis. Glasgow: University of Strathclyde.

Jarrett M. O. (1980) A clinical system for three dimensional gait analysis. Biological Engineering Society, 20th Anniversary International Conference Proceedings, London, 24–27.

Klasson B. (1985) Computer aided design, computer aided manufacture and other computer aids in prosthetics and orthotics. *Prosthetics and Orthotics International* **9**, 3–11.

Lamoreux L. W. (1971) Kinematic measurements in the study of human walking. *Bulletin of Prosthetic Research* **10(15)**, 3–84.

Mitchelson D. L. (1977) CODA: a new instrument for three dimensional recording of human movement and body contour in orthopaedic engineering. In *Orthopaedic Engineering: proceedings of the orthopaedic engineering conference held in Oxford, September 1977* (eds Harris J. D. & Copeland

K.), pp. 128–138. Oxford Orthopaedic Engineering Centre and Biological Engineering Society.

Murray M. P., Drought A. B. & Kory R. C. (1964) Walking patterns of normal. men. *Journal of Bone and Joint Surgery* **46A**, 335–360.

Pearson J. R., Holmgren C., March L. & Oberg K. (1973) Pressures in critical regions of the below-knee patellar-tendon-bearing prosthesis. *Bulletin of Prosthetic Research* **10–19**, 52–76.

Perry J., Bontgrager E. & Antonelli D. (1979) Footswitch definition of basic gait characteristics. In *Disability: proceedings of a seminar on rehabilitation of the disabled in relation to clinical and biomechanical aspects, costs and effectiveness* (eds Kenedi, R. M., Paul J. P. & Hughes J.), pp. 131–135. University of Strathclyde, Glasgow. London: MacMillan.

Radcliffe C. W. & Foort J. (1961) *The patellar-tendon-bearing below-knee prosthesis.* Revised Edition. Berkeley: Biomechanics Laboratory, University of California.

Robinson J. L. & Smidt G. L. (1981) Quantitative gait evaluation in the clinic. *Physical Therapy* **61(3)**, 351–353.

Saleh M. (1981) A study of the effects of prosthesis alignment changes on the gait of below-knee amputees. MSc Thesis. Dundee: University of Dundee.

Saleh M. (1984) The use of gait analysis in below-knee prosthetic alignment. International Society for Prosthetics and Orthotics, United Kingdom Scientific Meeting, Manchester. Abstract ISPO Newsletter, 27–29.

Saleh M. & Bostock S. (1985) The use of external joint moments as an indicator of prosthetic misalignment. International Society for Prosthetics and Orthotics, United Kingdom Scientific Meeting, Warwick.

Saleh M. & Murdoch G. (1985) In defence of gait analysis: observation and measurement in gait assessment. *Journal of Bone and Joint Surgery* **67B**, 237–241.

Saleh M., Jarrett M. O. & Spiers R. W. (1983) The effects of mass properties of prostheses on the gait of below-knee amputees with special reference to dynamic alignment. International Society for Prosthetics and Orthotics, IV World Congress, Imperial College, London, Book of Abstracts, 82.

Simon S. R. (1981) On mass properties of an above-knee prosthesis. Workshop on the clinical application of gait analysis, Bonar Hall, University of Dundee. 30th March–1st April.

Solomonidis S. E. (1980) Modular artificial limbs. *Second report on a Continuing Programme of Clinical and Laboratory Evaluation. Above-Knee Systems.* London: HMSO.

Sutherland D. H. & Hagy J. L. (1972) Measurement of gait movements from motion picture film. *Journal of Bone and Joint Surgery* **54A**, 787–797.

Taylor K. D., Mottier F. M., Simmons D. W., Cohen W., Pavlak R., Cornell D. P. & Hankins G. B. (1982) An automated motion measurement system for clinical gait analysis. *Journal of Biomechanics* **15(7)**, 505–516.

Thomas A. (1944) Anatomical and physiological considerations in the alignment and fitting of amputation prostheses for the lower extremity. *Journal of Bone and Joint Surgery* **26A**, 645–659.

Troup I. M. (1976) The assessment of amputation level and management of stump environment in peripheral vascular disease. Thesis submitted for the Diploma of Rehabilitation, Dundee, May 1976.

Zahedi M. S., Spence W. D., Solomonidis S. E. & Paul J. P. (1983a) The range of optimum alignment in lower limb prostheses. International Society for Prosthetics and Orthotics, IV World Congress, Imperial College, London, Book of Abstracts 85.

Zahedi M. S., Spence W. D., Solomonidis S. E. & Paul J. P. (1983b) The effect of variations in limb alignment on amputee gait: a quantitative study. International Society for Prosthetics and Orthotics, IV World Congress, Imperial College, London, Book of Abstracts 86.

Zahedi M. S., Spence W. D., Solomonidis S. E. & Paul J. P. (1985) The need for quantification of the alignment process. International Society for Prosthetics and Orthotics, United Kingdom Scientific Meeting, Warwick.

47

The Influence of Alignment on Prosthetic Gait

M.S. ZAHEDI, W.D. SPENCE & S.E. SOLOMONIDIS

Introduction

Human motion can be described as the harmonious and co-ordinated movement of the limb segments relative to each other. The lower limbs are mainly responsible for locomotor activity and can be considered as levers with articulations at various levels. The relative positions of the joints, coupled with the muscular interplay, achieve the displacement of the body from one place to another with, it is thought, minimum expenditure of energy. Loss of segments and joints through amputation disrupts this natural mechanism and results in loss of function. As part of the rehabilitation process a prosthesis is provided, which attempts to replace lost parts and function.

Although a prosthesis replaces the amputated parts, the sound limb compensates for the shortcomings of the system. Whilst some compensation is acceptable and perhaps not apparent to an observer, excessive compensation is noticeable in terms of an abnormal gait pattern and increased energy expenditure by the patient. Increased quality of prosthetic replacement will reduce the degree of compensation required. Considering one aspect of the 'quality' of the prosthesis, viz. the positioning of the joints and the angulation of the segments, 'the alignment', it can be demonstrated that this can influence the performance of the amputee during locomotion.

Recent advances in the field of study of human locomotion have resulted in a better understanding of the underlying biomechanical principles of human movement. There are now better facilities for the measurement of the kinetics and kinematics of the body. Using such measuring systems it is possible to demonstrate that the ambulation process is an interrelation between the ground reaction force and the orientation of the joints and segments.

Studies on alignment (Zahedi *et al.* 1986) carried out at the University of Strathclyde have shown that there is a range of acceptable alignments for any one amputee. One would therefore expect that these acceptable alignments would have an influence on the gait. It is the purpose of this presentation to quantify the effect of various alignments on the amputee's gait.

Methodology

Ten below-knee and ten above-knee amputees, mean age 61, s.d. ±11.9, and mean activity level 23.3, s.d. ±11.5 (Day 1981) participated in the study. One prosthetist was responsible for casting and fitting all patients with Otto Bock modular prostheses. Total-contact, quadrilateral suction sockets and patellar tendon-bearing sockets were fitted to the above-knee and below-knee patients respectively. Five prosthetists were involved in aligning the prostheses and in verification of the acceptability of the prostheses. More than 300 alignments were performed, and all alignment configurations measured. The alignment of the prosthesis was defined as the relative geometrical position of the socket to the knee (for above-knee cases) and to the foot. Individual component reference points were defined and related to a known axis system based on the bolt hole at the top of the SACH foot. Alignment parameters were then defined relative to this origin (Zahedi *et al.* 1986). Several custom-built devices were used to obtain accurate measurements of the component reference points and subsequent calculations provided alignment parameters in terms of tilts and shifts (accuracy: tilts±1° and shifts±1 mm).

Objective evaluation of the patient's gait, in addition to the prosthetist's subjective assessment, was performed using several kinetic and kinematic measuring systems. Temporal–distance parameters were measured using footprints. Markers were placed on the major joint centres of the upper and lower limbs, the pelvis, and the sternum for whole-body kinematic analysis using 3D cinephotography running at 50 frames/second. The Strathclyde TV/computer/force platform system was used for measurement of kinetic data of both lower limbs. Prosthetic loading data were obtained by means of a six-component strain-gauged pylon transducer incorporated into the shank of the prosthesis; an electrogoniometer measured knee flexion. The data collected from the above devices, in conjunction with the alignment measurements, allowed calculation of the forces and moments in three dimensions at the ankle, knee, and hip joints in the specified reference axes systems shown (Fig. 47.1) during stance phase.

In the adopted sign convention, forces are positive when they act from a distal to proximal direction along the positive direction of the relevant axis, e.g. F_X is positive when acting along the positive direction of the *x* axis (Fig. 47.1). Moments are positive when they are due to external forces acting on the body which tend to cause clockwise rotation, the system being viewed along the positive direction of the relevant axis. A list of abbreviations and other notation used is given at the end of the chapter.

The data from the cine system were digitized; the remaining kinetic and the kinematic data were sampled through a 32-channel 16-bit analogue to digital converter of a PDP11/34 mini-computer. All data were sampled at 50 Hz, except those from the pylon transducer, which were sampled at 200 Hz. Software was developed for signal processing (e.g. sorting, filtering, and averaging) to compute the results and present them in tabular or graphical form.

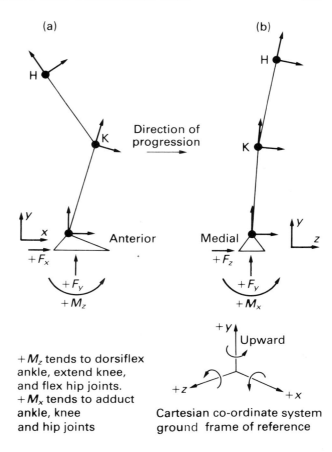

Fig. 47.1 Sign conventions and frames of reference used in the calculation of load actions at the hip, knee and ankle. (a) AP view, (b) ML view, from rear — right leg

$+M_z$ tends to dorsiflex ankle, extend knee, and flex hip joints. $+M_x$ tends to adduct ankle, knee and hip joints

Cartesian co-ordinate system ground frame of reference

Results and discussion

One of the main findings of this study was that an amputee may be satisfied by more than one alignment (Zahedi *et al.* 1986). Fig. 47.2 illustrates a typical example of alignment configurations which resulted from one patient on one prosthesis dynamically aligned by one prosthetist on 19 occasions. It is clear that a number of so-called 'optimum' alignment configurations are obtained. In other words there is a range of acceptable alignment which is satisfactory to both patients and prosthetists. However, it is evident that a true optimum alignment configuration which has the characteristics of optimum function and comfort is a unique configuration, and the position that the patient accepts is not necessarily the true optimum alignment. It is further evident that the prosthetists under the present method of fitting are unable to achieve this optimum position at will. The range of alignments is not of the same magnitude in the AP and ML view for any one patient, and it also changes when other prosthetists align the same patient. However, it should be pointed out that only specific configurations of limb geometry

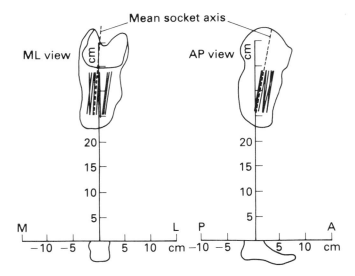

Fig. 47.2 Socket position and orientation for 19 acceptable alignments by one prosthetist on one patient.

within these ranges are acceptable.

The influence of various alignment configurations on the amputee's gait pattern can be quantified by measuring a number of kinematic and kinetic parameters. Perhaps rather unexpectedly it was found that acquisition of kinematic data alone could not detect small variations in gait patterns. Moreover, the instrumentation available does not permit the quantification of the variability in a series of successive steps. On the other hand, the kinetic parameters can detect small differences in gait and provide quantification of step-to-step variation on the prosthetic side. However, the kinetic data do not provide information on, for instance, the displacements of the body segments or on the temporal–distance parameters. These parameters are sometimes necessary in order to provide a complete understanding of amputee locomotion.

In this chapter, examples of amputee locomotion analysis based on kinetic information are discussed.

Kinetic parameters

Consideration of the results for prosthetic loading obtained from the pylon transducer showed that in all cases there were significant step-to-step variations. These variations were different from one channel to another. Also, as expected, they were different from one subject to another. The individual steps for each channel were superimposed to show the 'repeatability envelope', which describes the magnitude of the step-to-step variation. This variation was expected, and has also been reported by Winter (1984) for the normal subject. He found significant step-to-step variations in the load actions at the joints, and that this variation changed at the various levels of the limb.

The loss of a limb results in greater step-to-step variations. In fact, in most of the amputees tested there was a trend for a larger magnitude of repeatability envelope for the above-knee amputee than the below-knee amputee. As with normal subjects, the magnitude of the repeatability envelope depends on the individual. It was also found that if three equally acceptable but geometrically different alignments on the same subject with the same prosthesis are considered, the magnitude of the repeatability envelope varies from one alignment to another (Fig. 47.3). The ML bending moment showed largest differences in the repeatability envelopes due to alignment variations in the majority of the subjects. Furthermore, there are differences in the magnitude and pattern of the force and moment traces that are attributable to various alignments. For the purpose of comparison, it is necessary to employ a means of averaging these signals. However, due to fluctuations in the stance phase time, a simple averaging technique could not be employed without distorting the data. A Fourier analysis technique (Zahedi 1985) was therefore adopted, which time-normalized the signals before averaging was carried out. Using this technique, it was thus possible to discuss the biomechanical effect of different alignments. Examples of comparative representative signals are shown in Fig. 47.4.

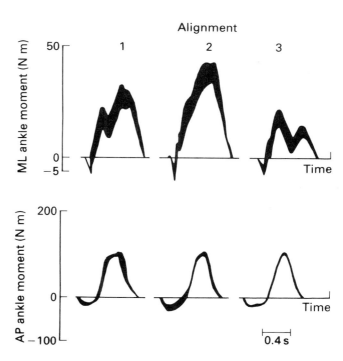

Fig. 47.3 Repeatability envelopes for AP and ML ankle moments for three acceptable alignments on one patient.

Effect of misalignment

Figs. 47.5 and 47.6 show loading patterns for two conditions on one prosthesis:

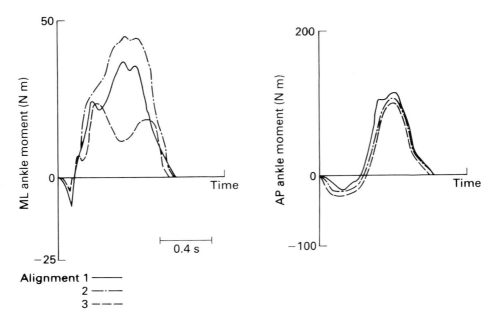

Fig. 47.4 Comparison of normalized and averaged traces of ankle moments for three acceptable alignments on one patient.

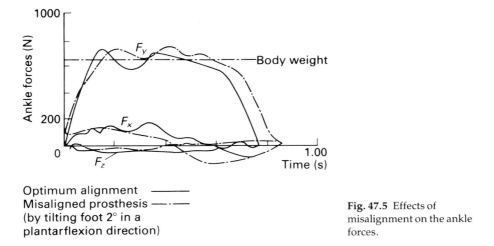

Fig. 47.5 Effects of misalignment on the ankle forces.

(a) An acceptably aligned prosthesis (so-called 'optimum'); and

(b) Same prosthesis but deliberately misaligned to increase the AP tilt of the foot in a plantarflexion direction by 2°.

Examination of the load actions at the ankle joint shows that the prosthesis with the misaligned foot has resulted in a reduced duration of the positive AP shear force (F_X) (Fig. 47.5), indicative of a shorter heel contact to foot-flat phase. The magnitude of the plantarflexion moment about the ankle (Fig. 47.6) is reduced, which confirms the less dorsiflexed position of the foot during early stance phase. During late stance there is an increase in moment tending to cause dorsiflexion, illustrating a larger resistance to roll-over.

From the trace of the knee extension moment, it is seen that the misalignment has resulted in a reduction of the extension moment. This is somewhat contrary to that expected. It is believed that, as there is no change in AP hip moment pattern, this difference is caused by a change in the knee joint centre in relation to the ground reaction force vector line. Due to the later reversal of the AP shear force from positive to negative (Fig. 47.5) in the acceptable alignment as compared to the misalignment, the geometry of the limb is reckoned to have a dorsiflexed foot and the body must therefore be well forward of the limb during the late stance. The increase of the foot AP tilt by 2° (in a plantarflexion direction) does not necessarily result in a plantarflexed foot. However, it would increase the posterior inclination of the limb, and the body in turn would be positioned further back. Consequently the distance between the knee joint centre and the load line during the roll-over would be reduced in comparison with the corresponding acceptable alignment. This would result in the reduction of the knee extension moment. Furthermore, this small change in AP tilt of the foot, which would have been thought insignificant, has resulted in a change in the ML shear force (F_Z) and thus influences the ML stability.

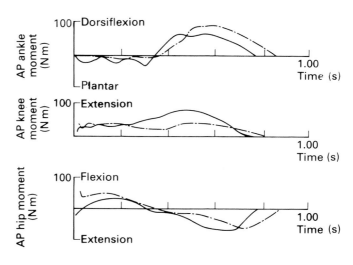

Fig. 47.6 Effect of misalignment on the AP ankle, knee and hip moments.

Optimum alignment ———
Misaligned prosthesis—·—
(by tilting foot 2° in a plantarflexion direction)

Thus, it can be seen that although it is possible to extract a substantial amount of information from the kinetics of the prosthetic side, in order to obtain verification of some of the above statements reference had to be made to additional data relating the position of the body segments to the ground reaction resultant force and to the measurement of the alignment configurations. It may be concluded that at present, for a complete biomechanical evaluation, the availability of both kinematic and kinetic information is essential.

It should be pointed out, however, that although a 2° change in the AP tilt of the foot appears to be insignificant there have been many occasions during this study when such small alterations to the so-called 'optimum' alignment resulted in a prosthesis that was totally unacceptable to the amputee.

Comparison of two acceptable alignments

Two alignment configurations, produced on the same prosthesis, and which were both acceptable to the patient and prosthetist, are shown in Fig. 47.7. The alignments were measured and the hip–ischium line was taken as the datum for superimposition, assuming that these are two points on the patient's anatomy with a fixed relationship to each other. The anteroposterior view (Fig. 47.7a) indicates that 'alignment 1' is inherently unstable, the foot is slightly more dorsiflexed and

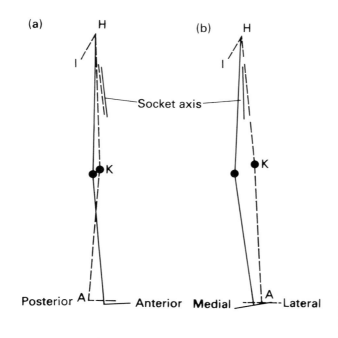

Fig. 47.7 Comparison of the geometrical configuration for two acceptable alignments for an above-knee amputee. (a) AP view. (b) ML view, from the rear.

further behind, and socket AP tilt is reduced compared with 'alignment 2'. The position of the knee joint in 'alignment 2' relative to the hip–ankle line would tend to indicate that this is a stable setting, much more so than 'alignment 1'. Considering the mediolateral view (Fig. 47.7b), 'alignment 2' appears to result in a narrower walking base and has a larger ML tilt (adduction angle) of the socket.

Considering the prosthetic loading results (Figs. 47.8 & 47.9) differences in the loading pattern are seen which can be attributed to the different alignment configurations. The graph of the AP shear force (F_x) for 'alignment 1' displays a longer duration of positive shear than that for 'alignment 2', and is of greater magnitude. This indicates a relative delay in obtaining the foot-flat position. This is due to the greater dorsiflexion of the foot and lower stability of the knee in 'alignment 1'. This results in a plantarflexion moment at the ankle greater in magnitude and duration. Due to the inherent instability of 'alignment 1' the rate

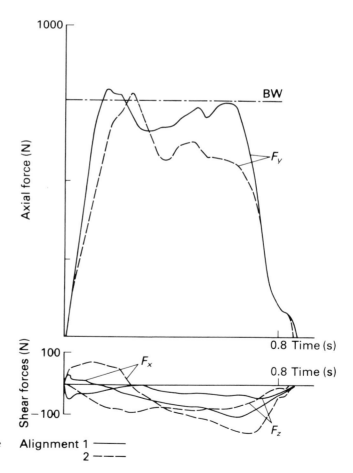

Fig. 47.8 Comparison of ankle forces for alignments 1 and 2.

Alignment 1 ——
2 – – – –

of loading of the prosthesis is slower and the hip extension moment is greater, reflecting the amputee's willingness to load an unstable prosthesis.

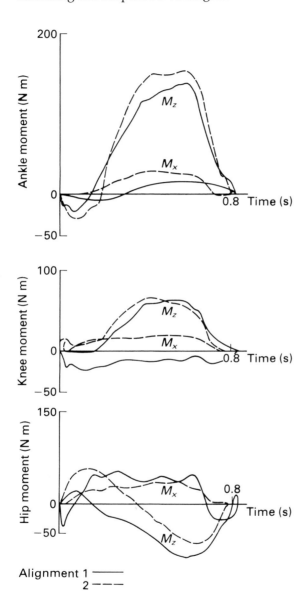

Alignment 1 ——
          2 – – –

Fig. 47.9 Comparison of AP and ML ankle, knee, and hip moments for alignments 1 and 2.

As can be seen in the diagram of knee moment (Fig. 47.9), both alignments display extension moments: one by means of geometry and one by amputee action, as is verified by the increase in hip extension moment for 'alignment 1'. In late stance, the foot of 'alignment 1' being further behind has resulted in an increase of the dorsiflexion moment due to the body to ankle geometrical relationship. Further, the amputee offloads the prosthetic side sooner, which indicates a shorter step (prosthetic to sound) must be taking place as the amputee loses support from an effectively shorter keel (due to the foot being behind) and dorsiflexed foot. Finally, in the AP view the hip flexion moment required to break the knee in late stance is smaller in the case of the inherently unstable set-up.

Fig. 47.7b shows the alignments in the ML view and there are obvious differences in the bending moments (Figs. 47.8 & 47.9). On 'alignment 2' the amputee at heel contact is less stable due to the foot position and its attitude relative to 'alignment 1'. Thus an effort is made to bring the load line within the support area. This is seen by an adductor action during early and late stance (Fig. 47.9, M_X curve). During the remaining part of the stance phase, stability is mainly achieved by abductor action as expected. In the case of 'alignment 1' the limb provides a stable walking base and allows the amputee to use the abductors in an expected manner throughout the stance phase. This is further reflected by the differences in direction and magnitude of the ML shear force (F_Z) (Fig. 47.8). At the knee and ankle levels differences in ML bending moment are merely a reflection of the resultant load line relative to the geometry of the limb. Whilst both these alignments were considered to be acceptable at the time of dynamic alignment, after consideration of the above analysis it is perhaps possible to suggest that a better alignment would consist of 'alignment 1' with the foot brought forward. This would have the effect of prolonging the single-limb support and the subsequent increase in step length. However, this proposed alignment has to be verified by the amputee. Overall, however, it is suggested that 'alignment 1' is better than 'alignment 2'.

Conclusions

For an amputee walking on a certain prosthesis, a step-to-step variation in the gait parameters exists. This variation can be quantified and described by an envelope. The overall signal pattern and the size of these envelopes are directly influenced by the alignment configuration. In other words, the alignment of a prosthesis has a direct effect on the amputee's gait pattern. A technique for comparing representative signals has been developed. Although small differences in gait pattern can only be detected by considering kinetic parameters, for complete understanding of amputee locomotion both kinetic and kinematic data are necessary. Using biomechanical analysis, it is possible to select the most suitable alignment from a number of acceptable alignments. Currently, this is a time-consuming process due to the method of data reduction and handling. However, it is foreseen that a clinical method, based on the development of appropriate instrumentation and analysis for optimizing alignment, will become a reality.

Abbreviations and notations

AP   Anterioposterior
ML   Mediolateral
I   Ischium
A   Ankle
K   Knee
H   Hip
F_x AP shear force
F_y Axial force
F_z ML shear force
M_x ML moment (abduction/adduction)
M_y Axial torque (inward/outward)
M_z AP moment (flexion/extension)

References

Day H. J. B. (1981) The assessment and description of amputee activity. *Prosthetics and Orthotics International* **5**, 23–28.

Winter D. A. (1984) Kinematic and kinetic patterns in human gait: variability and compensating effects. *Human Movement Sciences* **3(1/2)**, 51–76.

Zahedi M. S. (1985) Study of alignment in lower limb prostheses. PhD Thesis under preparation. Glasgow: University of Strathclyde.

Zahedi M. S., Spence W. D., Solomonidis S. E. & Paul J. P. (1986) Alignment of lower limb prostheses. *Journal of Rehabilitation Research and Development* **23(2)**, 2–19.

48

Cosmesis: Thoughts and Prejudices

R.M. KENEDI

Rehabilitation as a process has two main facets: restoration of function to the maximum possible and re-establishment of the 'body image' in a form acceptable to the individual and to society. The importance of body image has always been recognized. (One is reminded of the conversation between George Bernard Shaw and a very pretty young woman sitting next to him during a dinner party. The very personable young lady proposed to Shaw that they should 'join' in producing an offspring, since it would have her looks and Shaw's brains. Not unreasonably Shaw countered this by pointing out the other and perhaps undesirable possibility of the baby having *his* looks and *her* brains!)

Everyone has at least three different 'body images'. Firstly there is the 'on-face' image of oneself, a very familiar static image that one sees in the mirror. This may range from unappetizing to impressive, depending on the time of day and the activities of the night before. Its primary characteristic is, however, its static nature. The second image is that which other people have of oneself. This is essentially a dynamic image. Here an important point arises. In a crowd, for example, one is more aware of deviations from the normal dynamic appearance than of abnormality *per se*. Thus, for example, if somebody walks with a limp this is noticeable because it deviates from the normal body movement on an 'even keel'. However, if someone could, for example, be provided with a form of completely abnormal locomotive facility (say wheels instead of feet) which would nevertheless permit such 'even keel' body movement with minimal deviation from the normal 'dynamic' image, the gross abnormality of wheels instead of feet would probably escape the notice of the ordinary passer-by. The third image is perhaps the most important — this is one's own inner image of oneself, and is generally a composite of features and characteristics that one would like to be. Thus in most instances it bears little resemblance to either the static or the dynamic image. This inner image, however, has one very specific characteristic: it requires the integrity of the intact physical body. Any impairment, be it a pimple on the face or the loss of a limb, can embarrass and destroy this inner image. One of the major needs of rehabilitation is to assist the impaired to rebuild this inner image so as to regain their confidence in accepting, and in being accepted by, society.

A major part of the rehabilitation process consists of the rebuilding of these 'body images'. The first obvious requirement is efficacy of the aesthetics of the prosthesis/orthosis itself. To quote one obvious shortcoming — while the 'body' of the artificial limb has perhaps improved with advances in materials science, the cosmesis of the joints of the prosthesis is still at the stage where the individual wearer has to evolve his or her own cosmesis compensation. Thus a young above-knee amputee will perhaps wear a knee bandage when in shorts as a socially acceptable way of disguising his glaringly non-natural prosthetic knee. Another such compensatory approach might be capitalization on the 'dynamic' nature of the public image. This, because of the public's casual perception under the usual dynamic conditions, would permit the provision of devices with superficial, although acceptable, cosmesis but with functionally supranormal performance. This, in turn, would possibly commend such devices to the impaired, as the better than normal performance could conceivably compensate for the shortcomings of the cosmesis. Carrying this a stage further brings about the possibility that in the near future the impaired will be provided with a wardrobe of devices of varying degrees of functionality and cosmesis, and the device appropriate to the occasion (functional and/or cosmetic) will be selected.

Yet another factor influencing the level of cosmesis necessary is the receptiveness of the public at large to body configuration other than normal. Public attitudes at present can vary from, at one extreme, contemptuous enmity arising basically from fear, to socially integrative acceptance at the other extreme. One relatively new and promising influence is the increasing popularity with children of all ages of today's science fiction heroes. Creatures more grotesque than the worst deformed are readily accepted as human and humanized companions. E.T., Chew Bacca and even perhaps Darth Vadar still come in the fairly standard configuration of eyes, ears, limbs, etc. but possess also wholly non-human yet apparently not only acceptable but likeable characteristics. The advent of these, coupled with the increasing variety of robots endowed with human appreciative emotions (R2D2 and C3PO of *Star Wars* are good examples), will hopefully condition generations to come to be much readier than the present to accept a wider variation in human norms than heretofore.

In summary, the effectiveness of cosmesis in rehabilitation is influenced by many factors originating from within and outwith the impaired. The degree of success achieved in rebuilding the static, dynamic and inner images may contribute to or detract from the cosmetic success. In this context it is important to remember that rehabilitative solutions often considered inadequate by the professional clinic team handling the patient may nevertheless satisfy the patient. This particularly obtains with elderly patients who are reactivated rather than rehabilitated for independent living. The professional idea of what the patient should look like does not always coincide with the patient's concept as to what he or she wants to be like. Broadly the right combination of function and cosmesis is one which enables the impaired to compensate for his/her 'difference' from the normal and at best to convert that difference into an asset.

49

The Role of the Consumer

P. DIXON

If I think back 25 years, no one would have been asked to present any comments on this subject, as it was not recognized; indeed it did not exist! The consumer was the object which lay between the surgeon's created stump and the manufacturer's prosthesis. Often he got in the way. Having worked for those years not only to get the consumer recognized as a person, but also to establish his right to be involved, I am delighted to have been asked to write about his role as if it has really become recognized.

There are two levels of activity that have to be catered for in this role; firstly the consumer as an individual, and secondly the consumer as a representative of the general problems of all the amputee consumers. It is obvious that the consumer must stand on his own feet as soon as possible, both physically and metaphorically. It should be accepted as normal that he joins in the discussions of the clinic team, to question and to contribute. By and large, amputees are normal intelligent people, who find themselves in a frightening situation. Frightening, because they are often not told the facts, good or bad, that they have to face. This does not need to be the situation. The consumer has the right to be involved so that his fears from ignorance are reduced in these conversations, in ordinary language, and not larded with the jargon of the so-called professionals.

It is easier for the extrovert consumer, of whom the late Sir Douglas Bader was more than life size, to look after his own interests, but, having done so, he should do as Douglas Bader did and help the more reticent to look after themselves.

It is important that the consumer has available to him a simple complaints procedure such as provided in the National Health Service. The British Limbless Ex-Servicemen's Association (BLESMA) started one in each artificial limb and appliance centre with the blessing of the Department of Health and Social Security. But someone in power did not like it, and it was soon found that the complaints cards were not replaced in the holder. If that scheme were reintroduced, and added to it the right of each patient to seek help from his community health council to act as the 'patient's friend' we could deal with the very real complaints that exist.

The equally important but much more complex activity of representation is one that I have promoted for some 30 or more years. BLESMA has had 55 years' experience of protecting the interests of the disabled, and we are concerned that it should continue to be done properly even after BLESMA has declined substantially in numbers.

It is no use telling a minister or senior civil servant that you think something is wrong. They will merely reply that they know it is not! You have to be able to present a case as if it were to a court of law. The facts must be indisputable, the reasoning logical, and the solution economically possible. Unless you can do this you might just as well spit into the wind.

So the consumer must be prepared to become knowledgeable in all matters of the Limb Service. This is no easy task. He must keep up with the ever-changing technology, the changing needs, and, as ever, the changing people in and out of the Service. Each time the staff in charge change, he has to revert once again to a new approach. All this has to be done if he hopes even to begin to deflect the enormous state machine in a new direction.

The consumer will have to read, listen, and learn about such things as amputation surgery, which will lead back to understanding the reasons for amputation and the urgency of correct diagnosis; the role of physiotherapy in the pre- and post-operative phases of treatment; post-amputation recovery and the ideal conditions for primary fitting. He will wish to ask questions and obtain answers. What prosthesis should be fitted and why? How soon can a definitive limb be fitted? What is the rehabilitation plan and who should manage it? What occupation is recommended for the amputee and what is needed in terms of therapy and vocational counselling? What about the rehabilitation of the family as it applies to home and work? How is the amputee to get to work and what barriers have to be overcome? Who is doing research in all these areas? What is already known? What is the optimum solution in each case?

All this knowledge has to be absorbed and checked constantly. To ensure its availability it requires a competent well-managed organization that has people who can liaise with others to acquire information from anywhere in the world. There have to be resources to employ high-calibre people, resources to finance studies, research, training and so on. The organization must be able to mobilize the vast body of voluntary effort, both members and friends, from whom it will gather facts and experiences and for whom the whole business of representation must be beneficial.

If the British Amputee Sports Association, the National Association for the Limbless Disabled, or Opportunities for the Disabled are to achieve their objectives in representation then they have a lot of work to do in the next decade, during which time BLESMA will continue to decline in members and maybe also in ability. I hope that from these groups a competent body will arise, because without an independent outlook, based on personal and current experience, the amputee will not be so well provided for as he is today.

In the structure for the Limb Service recommended by the McColl Working Party Report (1986) we expect to see the consumer well represented, not by some prima donna, but by a hard-nosed grass roots professional consumer. This representation must operate at the highest level, and equally the involvement of the amputee must penetrate the Service at all levels and include counselling and an individual complaints management.

Reference

Review of artificial limb and applicance centre services: the report of an independent working party under the chairmanship of Professor Ian McColl (2 vols.) (1986). London: DHSS.

50

Cultural Considerations and Appropriate Technology in Orthopaedics for Developing Countries

W. KAPHINGST & S. HEIM

Introduction

To talk about a 'developing country' suggests that such an entity exists and is well defined. Certainly it would be presumptuous to assume that a report restricted to a relatively small population necessarily covered all the thousands of tribes and millions of people worldwide. Even considering the African continent alone, it seems presumptuous to put forward a generalization which is truly valid. Varieties in the development of different peoples do not permit of a uniform opinion, but in these countries the extended family is still to be seen as the basic element for almost the whole sphere of living together, whereas the industrial society has created many changes in the traditional way of life. The family still takes charge of many problems and is still to be seen as a kind of traditional 'social insurance'. Family members may be aged or ill, they may be students or handicapped, but whatever the circumstances their family will try to solve any problems that may arise in a mutual way. Any member may hope for assistance from other family members, but equally he must be prepared to substitute for his family fellows. Agriculture is the main source of income in African families, and they are living near subsistence level most of the time; thus each hand is essential for common work. Each of the children, the elders, and even the disabled, is employed according to his capacity.

Clearly it is necessary to provide orthopaedic appliances appropriate to the need for a handicapped member of the family as soon as possible. The work of the disabled has to be done by someone else for as long as orthopaedic care is unavailable; the family, moreover, is burdened with such care as is necessary for the disabled member.

Cultural considerations

The demand for orthopaedic appliances is more urgent and necessary in many cases than is presumed from the point of view of the industrial nations. It may be more important than it is in an industrial country with all its social security measures.

The influence of the cultural background requires explanation in addition to more or less obvious socioeconomic aspects of orthopaedic technical care. For example, a religious Indian needs all his limbs in order to gain access to eternity. He requires to visit the places of sanctity barefoot, and thus it is most important that his feet are retained or substituted in all their natural parts (toes, etc.) in order to be accepted. Furthermore, a prosthesis must be so designed to permit traditional praying seated in a cross-legged position, producing a real challenge to the prosthetist!

Many of those customs or rules required by religious belief are not found in African countries, but similar situations do arise. Members of the Chagga tribe, living in the Kilimanjaro region, must be 'complete' when buried. After an amputation of a leg as a result of an accident the severed member will be buried. This partial grave is situated on the same spot where the rest of the corpse will be buried; the ceremonies are identical.

The belief that diseases and accidents as well as their consequences are sent by God, or meant as a punishment for blunders within the family, is widespread in African tribes. Fast delivery of orthopaedic care releases the amputee from many questions in the village and from the contempt of his neighbours. It is therefore important that aesthetic criteria are considered along with those in respect of restoration of function. Orthopaedic restoration may be most important for the future living conditions of inhabitants of countries following the Charia laws. A hand or a foot is amputated as a punishment for theft in countries subscribing to these laws. Accordingly restoration is of paramount importance for someone who has lost an appendage as a result of injury. A demand for an aesthetic prosthesis is justified for these patients, quite apart from those demands required for proper functioning of the appliance. Shape and colour should simulate the remaining limb in order to be accepted by the family, neighbours, friends and fellow men. Despite all those arguments it is considered that in Africa the socioeconomic aspect of orthopaedic care is of greater importance than the psychosocial aspect. If it were not so prostheses would be fabricated which offered cosmesis but no real function. All the efforts made in recent years in adapting technologies to local needs demonstrate that function is required and receives priority.

Appropriate technology

The catch phrase for the second part of this contribution is 'appropriate technology'; this phrase is much used by the international agencies and is often misunderstood. That is why appropriate technology should be considered in some detail. Are standardized, well-tested and sturdy technologies, such as those offered in Europe, really not fit for developing countries? There is no simple 'yes' or 'no' to that question. The technology of the industrial nations is in part of proven worth, in part too sophisticated, and often too expensive. Sometimes however, especially with regard to long-term use, it is even cheaper than so-called appropriate technology. It is frequently superior compared to local products but, it has to be said, sometimes totally inadequate.

What does the term 'appropriate technology' mean? Is it truly within the field of orthopaedic technology? Does it always mean a peg leg made from bamboo connected to a hand-woven socket made from sisal or bastfibre? Does a caliper always mean one made from roundsteel without joints — far from it! For clarification two definitions are offered. One is centred on the patient and the other on the appliance.

1 Appropriate technology in prosthetics/orthotics is produced under difficult conditions, is a functional adaptation of orthopaedic appliances, but nevertheless is always aiming at a qualified result to the benefit of the patient.

2 Appropriate technology concerns appliances made under the individually restricted possibilities of a certain country or region. They are made using locally available material, tools, and machinery. However, under all circumstances they should be produced following faithfully internationally recognized standards of function and fit. Furthermore these appliances should demonstrate adaptation to circumstances of climate, ease of repair, durability, low cost, and to the living standards and working conditions of the patient. The overlapping of 'simplified technology' with higher developed technology may be justified.

It seems evident that the priority is to adapt the appliance to the patient's needs. A fisherman stepping into water needs a different kind of prosthesis to a farmer growing maize on the slopes of mountains. Someone running a fashion boutique in the city needs a quite different appliance to a herdsman in the savannah.

The following criteria are considered to be important in describing an appliance as 'appropriate':

1 Low cost.
2 Local availability of materials.
3 Manual fabrication.
4 Climatic adaptation.
5 Durability.
6 Simplification of repair.
7 Simplification of processing technology.
8 Reproducibility by local personnel.
9 Technically functional.
10 Encompasses proper biomechanical fit.
11 Light in weight.
12 Meets the psychosocial demands of the patient.

Further discussion of these criteria is required. In one sense they appear to be mutually exclusive, but the situation becomes meaningful when individual priorities and compromises are sought, specific for a certain patient. The criteria mentioned above are therefore explored further.

1 Production costs are dependent on the price for components and on the manpower costs, i.e. ultimately on the input of time. Components may be cheaper

abroad or in the home country. As soon as they are ordered from abroad, by reason of moderate prices, criterion no. 2 cannot be fulfilled. If they are ordered in the home country, being cheaper, they may prove to be less durable and they will prove to be more expensive than foreign products in the end. However, components and subparts should be ordered in the home country whenever possible and practical, if only for reasons of independent development.

2 A guarantee is needed of permanent availability of semi-finished products. As soon as an orthopaedic appliance is modified in such a manner that it can be produced using local materials, a number of problems frequently emerge. Equally it does not help if a certain subpart is available only at certain times. If this is permitted to happen there is built in a constantly changing technical modification leading to restrictions in quantity and quality of production.

3 Orthopaedic appliances shall be manually producible in the developing country by use of simple tools. This demand is both appropriate and at first sight justified. However, the exclusion of accepted and rational procedures using machine tools will block an improvement in both quantity and quality of products as well as possible future development. 'Hand-carved' orthopaedic appliances will reach the required standards only so long as each co-worker becomes a real professional artist. In the real world this does not happen.

4 The appliance as a whole must be adapted to the climatic conditions in order to offer sufficient comfort to the patient. Only those taking a 'bath' in their own body sweat for several hours per day really know the justification for this criterion. Non-biomechanical parts of a prosthesis are also affected in terms of changes of volume and function by changes of climate. Wooden bearings for axles, for example, will shrink and swell, dependent on changes in atmospheric humidity, and they will lose their functional capability within a short time. Additionally, it should be pointed out that wooden prostheses are eaten by woodworms in East Africa. This is a climatic problem of a kind, since the woodworm procreates readily under those local conditions. An appropriate, non-toxic agent has not yet been found to combat the woodworm. A local wood protection is the use of diesel oil, but a prosthesis soaked with diesel oil and offering at the same time good service to the patient is not easily envisaged.

5 The 'throw-away' attitude of European and American production should not be transferred to the developing world. It is not possible in those countries to change modules or to prepare a new acquisition within a short time. Each appliance must be as durable as possible, especially in its wearing parts. So-called maintenance-free exchange parts are not feasible in developing countries, and accordingly components must be maintainable and repairable.

6 Simplification of repair must be pushed forward so that as many components as possible can be substituted by standardized local parts and so far that a low-level craftsman in a rural area will be able to undertake the repair. This is, of course, only possible with respect to mechanical parts and not for biomechanical parts, which must be repaired by a professional in order to avoid serious harm to the

patient.

7 Orthopaedic workshops must be equipped in an appropriate way. This means that an irreducible minimum of hand and machine tools is available. In ideal terms it is possible to pose three alternatives with an identical final result, e.g. producible by means of:

   (a) Solely manual (hand tools) methods.
   (b) Semi-mechanical (basic machine tools) procedures.
   (c) Small serial production (as far as components are concerned).

It is, in fact, a challenge to the practitioner, knowing the conditions in the developing world, to develop alternatives like these. This task can only be solved in the long term.

8 The whole technology of manufacture must be reproducible by the professionals in the country in question. It is senseless to import technical know-how which is incapable of independent, long-term, and autonomous reproduction. A good deal of this goal is attainable by the criterion mentioned under no. 7, but only where there are qualified personnel with the appropriate training and education. The organization of that training and education must be central to all efforts towards adapting to local circumstances.

9 The ideology of 'appropriate technology' must never lead to a loss of technical function to the point where it is held to be no more than an upgrading of substandard solutions accompanied by an unquestioning admiration. The professional must disassociate himself from such 'ideologists' and 'know-alls' in a sensitive but nevertheless distinct way, and convince them by arguments and evidence.

10 Technical function may be attainable even by non-professionals, so long as they are concerned solely with the application of their technical knowledge: the judgement of biomechanical function, however, must exclusively reside with the professional. Professionals have to be trained for as long as they are not available. It may be that sectional specialization may be admissable in the short term, but it is a questionable philosophy with respect to long-term rehabilitation and political aspirations. An orthopaedic appliance must not be of substandard quality in its biomechanical parts even when seen as an example of so-called 'appropriate technology'.

11 Making orthopaedic appliances as lightweight as possible usually requires a compromise with regard to criteria no. 2 and no. 5. Unfortunately compromises are to be found again and again. This is not a problem specific to the Third World, but a problem of orthopaedic technology in general. However, the weight problem is highlighted in a more dramatic way than in Europe or in North America, since there are no lightweight materials and no lightweight technologies available in the developing world.

12 Last but not least the patient hopes that his orthopaedic appliance will permit his reintegration with his work scene but also with other aspects of his private life and the community. A prosthesis is not only a tool, but is a substitute for a part of his body as well. Accordingly orthopaedic appliances should be produced with

an acceptable appearance whenever possible. The demands of the patient in this regard should be taken into consideration so long as they are not opposed to more important criteria.

The demand for an 'appropriate technology' includes, as demonstrated by the arguments mentioned before, a whole catalogue of measures partly opposing each other. It is important to achieve an international co-ordination in this field and to convince everyone interested in co-operation. Over the years it may be possible to submit results meeting the needs of the target groups, i.e. results which can be called 'appropriate' indeed.

PROSTHETIC STANDARDS

51

Standards in Physical Testing for Lower Limb Prostheses

J.J. SHORTER

Introduction

Structural testing of components and assemblies is an important and integral part of the design and development of prostheses for the lower extremity. Testing in a laboratory should not be considered to be a way in which the engineer satisfies his ego or just a method in which the purchasing authority can be satisfied. It should be a procedure whereby all members of the clinic team, perhaps most importantly the clinician, can be confident that the prosthesis is safe for the patient to use. Arguably, if the development of limb systems is stagnant, as it has been for periods in the past, there is little to be gained by testing, as information towards variations on a design can be acquired empirically. However, current development is rapid and accelerating, and with the arrival of new high-technology materials such as carbon fibre-reinforced plastic (CFRP) the need for thorough laboratory testing is increased.

It is important to remember that systems are being designed with the strength to weight ratio very much in mind, and therefore, almost by definition, margins of safety have to be no greater than necessary in order to achieve lightweight but structurally sound prostheses. Before actual test methods and load levels are considered, the different phases of testing employed during the development of a new system should be described. The following sequence of events shows clearly that acceptance testing is but one part of the overall test and evaluation programme.

Testing as a design tool. Stress analysis of complex structures by practical means rather than calculation using test equipment, e.g. stress pattern analysis by measurement of thermal emission (SPATE).

Materials testing. For example, testing of hybrid composites to obtain design data. Bond testing.

Testing or prototype equipment. Development testing to refine design of components.

Type approvals testing to standards set by purchasing authority. Work is progressing towards the establishment of both United Kingdom national and International Standards Organization standards for physical testing.

Field trials to supplement laboratory testing. Small-scale trial with regular feedback on technical as well as clinical aspects.

Environmental testing. Including accelerated wear tests, corrosion effects, etc.

Quality assurance testing. In-company testing of randomly selected production components and assemblies.

Test methods

The tests employed in the United Kingdom since about 1970 (coincidental with the introduction of the modular concept of limb construction) until the present time are of two basic forms: *static* tests represent peak loads encountered in service, and *cyclic* tests use a lower load level but represent commonly repeated loads on the limb during normal use with duration of test set to approximately five years' usage.

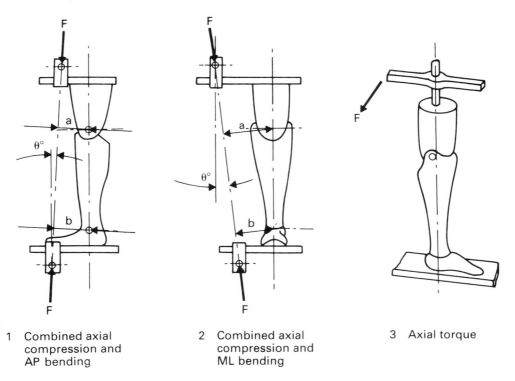

1   Combined axial
    compression and
    AP bending

2   Combined axial
    compression and
    ML bending

3   Axial torque

Fig. 51.1 Test method according to 'Philadelphia' recommendations.

The tests are arranged as shown in Fig. 51.1, so as to permit testing to be carried out using standard laboratory test machines with special end fixings to position the specimen in the geometrical configuration necessary to generate the required bending moments. This test philosophy enables not only the complete limb but also individual segments, such as the knee or ankle mechanisms, to be tested. This system has proved to be simple and effective, and there has generally been good correlation with field experience gathered through a formalized defect reporting system, giving us confidence in the design. The author's experience and resulting confidence is almost exclusively with this test method.

Following the activities of international working groups, and latterly within the framework of the International Standards Organization Technical Committee 168 (ISO TC 168), new test methods have been proposed. An example of these is given in Fig. 51.2 where, in the interests of increased realism, the geometry used has been modified to combine the axial compression, anterior/posterior (AP) and medial/lateral (ML) bending with one single applied load. The application of these defined loads also generated an axial torque. Again the testing can be carried out using standard test equipment with a single activator.

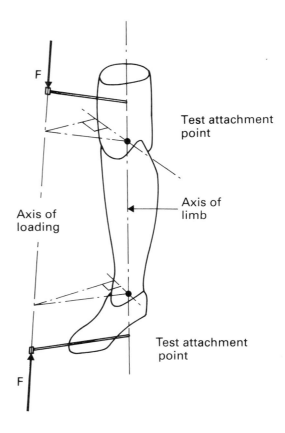

Fig. 51.2 Combined testing with single load application.

Load levels

Load measurement data have been collated from a number of laboratories including Berlin, Roehampton, and Strathclyde (ISPO Interlab). An example is the data presented by Mr D. Murray from the Biomechanical Research and Development Unit (BRADU) laboratory consisting of loads recorded using a strain-gauged shin tube on patients set a variety of tasks within the laboratory. Loads were measured during 1283 runs by 88 different patients involved in activities such as slow, normal, and fast run, and level walking, and included data relating to up and down ramp, up and down stairs, sidehill walking, and jumping down two steps. The measurement from slow, normal and fast level walking activities were sufficiently consistent to be taken as the basis for selecting cyclic load levels, whilst peak loads during other events were considered in relation to static load levels. From analysis of this data bank at the international meeting on physical testing at Philadelphia (Standards for Lower Limb Prostheses 1978), load levels were recommended (*see* Table 51.1) based on analysis of this information normalized for a 100 kg patient, and broadly speaking these have been used as the basis of testing in the U.K.

Table 51.1 Test loading values according to 'Philadelphia' recommendations.

	Axial load (N)	Axial torque (Nm)	Knee bending moments		Ankle bending moments	
			A/P (Nm)	M/L (Nm)	A/P (Nm)	M/L (Nm)
Static test	2500	35	230	150	250	70
Cyclic test	1350	20	120	80	140	±50

In the case of static testing, the load is applied over a period of 30 seconds and held at the level specified for 20 seconds and removed over 30 seconds. After the load has been removed, the specimen should not have suffered any permanent deformation. Loading is reapplied at the same rate and again the specimen should not have suffered any permanent deformation. Loading is reapplied at the same rate and this time the specimen is taken to failure, and the load level and mechanics of failure are noted. If a brittle failure occurs then a factor of safety of 2 over the specified load is applied; a ductile failure incurs a factor of safety of 1.5 for acceptance purposes.

Cyclic testing comprises 2×10^6 applications of the specified load at a frequency of 1 Hz. Patients would normally achieve approximately 5×10^6 steps in five years, therefore testing at 1 Hz would give a test of three months' duration. However, to accelerate the testing, loads are increased by a factor of 1.3 to complete the test at 2×10^6 instead of 5×10^6 cycles. Failure of components at lower endurance in the laboratory compare well with similar failures in service, confirming that 2×10^6 cycles gives five years' use on the heavy active amputee.

In the case of the combined-loading philosophy known as single-vector loading, it was considered unrealistic to add full values for Philadelphia-recommended axial compression plus AP bending, plus ML bending, as these peak loads did not occur simultaneously during the walking cycle. Therefore the peak load experienced during AP bending is used with AP and ML bending moments in proportion according to the Philadelphia recommendation (Table 51.2). Some torque is also generated, but as this does not reach the specified figure it might be necessary to employ a separate test to cover this aspect.

Table 51.2 Load levels proposes by U.K. delegation to ISO/TC168/WG3 for combined loading.

	Axial load (N)	Axial torque (Nm)	Knee bending moments		Ankle bending moments	
			A/P (Nm)	M/L (Nm)	A/P (Nm)	M/L (Nm)
Static test	2500	35	190	−125	240	−65
Cyclic test	1350	20	100	−65	130	−50

A/P bending moments causing tension on the posterior aspect of the limb are considered positive.

M/L bending moments causing tension on the medial aspect of the limb are considered positive.

There is a case for factoring the recommended loads to reduce the levels according to either the patient's weight, age, or activity rating, or indeed a combination of all these factors. However, caution should be exercised, as experience has shown that some lightweight amputees have generated extremely high loadings, far beyond that which could reasonably have been expected.

Supplementary testing

So far the main structural test schedule has been considered, but other supplementary tests are necessary in order to ensure that the limb will not be irreparably damaged during less regular but nevertheless normal use by the patient. One test which is extremely searching in respect of the structure is to load the limb at maximum knee flexion to represent a patient kneeling or crouching (Fig. 51.3). The line of application of load can be seen to be offset by a considerable distance and high moments will occur at the knee.

Durability testing of articulating joints in the lower limb by repeated flexion under load is carried out in some test houses as a method of assessing wear rates, but there is so far no agreement to have these included in the proposed international standards. In practical terms it is often difficult to reproduce on test equipment wear patterns that are truly representative of problems experienced in service.

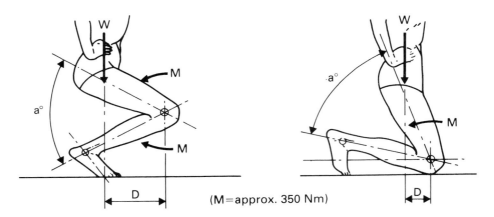

(M=approx. 350 Nm)

Fig. 51.3 Supplementary test for full extension of the knee.

Quite rightly, the ISO Working Group (Working Group 3, TC 168) has concentrated its initial efforts on tests designed to eliminate potential defects which could endanger the safety of the patient. Once this objective has been achieved the failure of components due to premature degradation or unacceptable wear can be considered. To a large degree, unreliable designs, which represent poor value for money in terms of longevity, will in any case be eliminated by market forces.

This short chapter has attempted to give the bare bones of a tremendous amount of work that has been undertaken over many years, and this has inevitably meant that much detail has been omitted. In conclusion there is a clear requirement to establish a realistic international standard for structural testing, and it is hoped that with new data becoming available the ISO working group will provide the solution. This should not inhibit innovation with the materials and techniques that are currently available. On the contrary, publication of these standards must provide the responsible engineer with reliable information on which to base his designs.

Reference

Standards for Lower Limb Prostheses (1978) Report of a conference held in Philadelphia, 1977. International Society for Prosthetics and Orthotics.

52

Nomenclature and Terminology

D.N. CONDIE

Introduction

Working Group 1 of the ISO Technical Committee 168 is concerned with nomenclature and terminology in prosthetics and orthotics.

The word 'nomenclature' is commonly used to describe a collection of names, and none would dispute the desirability of creating such a vocabulary of prosthetic/orthotic terms with corresponding definitions. In deciding upon the format of such a listing it is possible to consider the normal use of these terms and to organize the nomenclature accordingly. *Nomenclature* which is systematically organized in this way may be described as forming a *terminology*.

When the Working Group was formed in 1980 at St Andrews, it was agreed that the approach which would be adopted in tackling the task would be to consider the scope of a complete terminology in general terms initially, and then to proceed to identify and define the particular nomenclature necessary for each aspect in a systematic manner (Table 52.1). This approach had led to the development of three draft international standards (DIS), and work is continuing on the extension of the scope of the terminology.

Table 52.1 Proposed structure of prosthetic/orthotic terminology.

Scope			
Patient	Device/system		Personnel and procedures
Amputee congenital acquired	Prostheses Orthoses	General functional components	Prosthetic orthotic
Other			
Anatomical			
Activity level			

399

Draft international standards

Description of limb deficiencies present at birth

One of the first tasks of the Working Group has related to the collaboration with Working Group 2 on Medical Aspects of Terminology, under the Chairmanship of George Murdoch, to develop a draft standard based on the system of classification developed by the late Hector Kay of the Committee on Prosthetic Research and Development (CPRD) in the U.S.A. (Working Group ISPO 1974). This work is described in the section on congenital limb deficiency.

Prosthetics and orthotics vocabulary part 1: general terms

This part of the international standard establishes the vocabulary used to describe *prostheses and orthoses,* the *anatomy of those parts of the body most commonly fitted with prostheses,* and the *personnel* and *procedures involved in the practice of* prosthetics and orthotics.

Terms used to describe prostheses and orthoses

Basic terms defined in this section of the draft include:
   Prostheses–prosthetic devices. An externally applied device used to replace wholly or in part an absent or deficient limb segment. It includes any such device having a part within the human body for structural or functional purposes.
   Prosthetics. The science and art involved in treating patients by the use of prostheses.
   Upper limb prosthesis. A prosthesis used to replace the whole or part of the upper limb.
   Lower limb prosthesis. A prosthesis used to replace the whole or part of the lower limb.

Personnel and procedures

Important definitions proposed in this section of the draft include:
   Prosthetist. A person who having completed an approved course of education and training is sanctioned by an appropriate national authority to design, measure, and fit prostheses.
   Prosthetic technician. A person who having completed an approved course of training is sanctioned by an appropriate national authority to fabricate prostheses under the direction of a prosthetist.
   It is considered that these definitions, although not generally reflecting actual international practices, provide a clear indication of the preferred direction of further development with respect to education, training, and registration of prosthetic

personnel.
   Prosthetic/orthotic procedures defined include:
   Prosthetic/orthotic assessment.
   Prosthetic/orthotic casting and measurement.
   Cast modification.
   Tracing modification.
   Alignment.
   Bench assembly and alignment.
   Static alignment.
   Dynamic alignment.
   Finishing.
   Check-out.

Prosthetics and orthotics vocabulary part 2: terms relating to prostheses and wearers of prostheses

The first element of this draft standard specifies and defines the vocabulary to be used to describe the level of amputation in acquired amputations (Table 52.2). The major innovations adopted in this section on the strong insistence of the Canadian Standards Association relate to the replacement of the traditional below- and above-knee and elbow terminology with terms transtibial, transfemoral, transradial and transhumeral. The Working Group also preferred to adopt a standard approach to the description of amputations at a joint by preferring 'ankle disarticulation' to the more commonly encountered 'Syme' terminology.

Table 52.2 Terms used to describe the level of amputation in acquired amputation.

Level of amputation (acquired amputation)	
Lower limb	Upper limb
Partial foot amputation	Partial hand amputation
Ankle disarticulation	Wrist disarticulation
Transtibial (below-knee) amputation	Transradial (below-elbow) amputation
Knee disarticulation	Elbow disarticulation
Transfemoral (above-knee) amputation	Transhumeral (above-elbow) amputation
Hip disarticulation	Shoulder disarticulation
Hemipelvectomy	Forequarter amputation

   The development of further terminology to describe the structure and components used in a prosthesis has received considerable attention, although no specific proposals are yet available.
   The method adopted for this task has been to agree upon five basic categories

of components based on the principal function of the component.

Interface (components), e.g. socket, suspension.

Functional (components), e.g. terminal devices, joints.

Alignment (components).

Connective (components).

Cosmetic (components).

Work is now actively proceeding on the development of a system of terms and definitions which may be used to describe precisely the properties of particular components in each of these categories.

Conclusions

The purpose in developing a standard terminology for prosthetics and orthotics is to improve communication. Such a terminology, if adopted by designers, manufacturing companies, and clinical personnel when describing their products and reporting clinical experiences, would considerably reduce the confusion and doubt which often exists when attempting to interpret such literature.

Reference

Working Group, International Society for Prosthetics and Orthotics (1974) A proposed international terminology for the classification of congenital limb deficiencies (prepared by Hector W. Kay). *Orthotics and Prosthetics* **28(2)**, 33–48.

53

Lower Limb Amputation Stump Descriptions

M. WALL

Many different systems of stump classification have been developed (Persson & Liedberg 1983) but none has achieved universal acceptance. The reasons for this are many. The members of the clinic team in different countries working with different patients and different technical possibilities develop their own descriptors to meet their individual needs. An international system requires to be developed for one main reason, viz. it will be possible to compare one publication against another, one patient against another. The different care groups who might use a standardized form of stump description will include surgeons of different disciplines, other doctors, especially in rehabilitation and general practice, physical therapists and prosthetists and perhaps others. General acceptance of such a system would also be of interest to epidemiologists and government health officials. The system proposed must meet the needs of the different members of the clinic team and enable the description of the stump to be recorded in a way that can be easily incorporated in reports. It should be capable of inclusion in forms designed by the individual institution and also be computer compatible.

The main elements in any description will include:

1 Measurements.
2 Stump shape.
3 The condition of the skin of the stump.
4 The condition of the circulation of the stump.
5 The condition of the soft tissues of the stump.
6 Pain.
7 Proximal joint function to include range of movement and muscle power.
8 Certain features of the contralateral leg.

Soft tissue *measurements* are chosen because they are non-invasive, require no special equipment, can be made by any member of the clinic team and provide a proper relationship between longitudinal and circumferential dimensions. The number of measurements used must be no more than is necessary to give an adequate description of the stump and its shape.

Basic reference levels include the circumference at the crotch and at the medial joint line of the knee, even though the latter may be difficult to identify in obese subjects. The distal reference level is at the end of the stump with the subject standing, and the stump hanging vertically and unconstrained. Two circumferential measurements of amputation stumps are required:

(a) The circumference of the base, i.e. at the crotch in the above-knee or at the tibial plateau in the below-knee, case and

(b) At the 'fall-away' point, i.e. the point at which the slope of the stump shape steepens or curves in towards the end. A length measurement from this 'fall-away' point to the stump end helps in the appreciation of the stump shape.

Other circumferential measurements are needed in the disarticulation amputations and these will be described in those sections.

In both hemipelvectomy and hip disarticulation no measurements are possible, but the presence or absence of pelvic or femoral remnants must be noted.

Descriptions of the *shape* are restricted to conical, bulbous and cylindrical. Bulbous is self-evident, and the words 'cylindrical' and 'conical', provided they are not interpreted too literally, are equally descriptive. Prominence of the bone end should be included in the description, and in the particular case of the below-knee amputation it is important to record whether the fibula is prominent or not, i.e. extending beyond the distal end of the tibia. Equally, the state of the distal end of the tibia requires some mention should it not be smoothly contoured.

In descriptions of the *skin* of the stump one is concerned simply with the situation in general, namely the incision, sensitivity and scarring. Clearly many different descriptors could be used in providing a picture of the skin but it is sufficient to note whether the skin barrier is intact or not. There is no requirement to describe the incision in any detail but simply to record whether it is healed and mobile or otherwise.

Many factors concerning the *circulation* might well be recorded but it is enough to state simply whether the skin is normal or cyanotic, whether it is warm to the examining hand or not, and whether oedema is present. Excessive oedema is seen to be that which would force the patient to take off the prosthesis during the day or such that one would hesitate to fit the patient. The presence or absence of pulses is of interest but is not significant.

The *soft tissues* of the stump are described only in terms of the amount and the consistency.

Pain as an entity is always difficult to describe and is largely incapable of measurement. It is also important to make the differentation between spontaneous pain and tenderness. Presence of any palpable neuroma, pain after exercise, and presence or absence of phantom pain and similarly of pain in the proximal joint are noted.

Proximal *joint function* in terms of range of movement and power is noted.

In order that the description of the stump can be related to the patient as a whole, the *contralateral limb* needs some minimal dimensional description, i.e. the length from the crotch to the ground and the length from the medial tibial joint line to the ground. In addition, a simple statement as to whether the limb is normal or not is required.

In defining *levels of amputation* it is suggested that supracondylar and transcondylar amputations are above knee joint level and should be treated as such in the description. It is interesting to note that a foot ablation at ankle or Syme level performed in infancy may become in adult life a below-knee amputation and a new set of descriptions may have to be used on reaching skeletal maturity. The same applies in the case of a knee disarticulation performed in infancy and becoming in adult life an above-knee amputation, the distal end of the femur very often being hardly bulbous at all. Depending on the surgery intended and its performance, the level of the patella in the knee disarticulation amputation may vary. It is difficult, however, to describe its position with any exactitude. It is considered that the circumferential measurement of the femoral condyle is sufficient. The following are examples of how descriptions of amputations can be organized at different levels. In addition copies of forms used in the University of Uppsala to record findings are appended.

Hemipelvectomy

Measurement
Hemipelvic remnant   Absent/present

Skin of the stump
Incision   Healed/unhealed
                                  Mobile/adherent
General   Skin intact/ulcerated
                                  Sensation normal/sensation impaired
                                  No additional scarring/additional scarring

Circulation
Oedema   Non/minimal/excessive

Soft tissues of the stump
Amount   Adequate/inadequate/excessive
Consistency   Normal/flabby/indurated

Pain
Spontaneous pain   No/yes
Tenderness to palpation   No/yes — generalized/yes — localized
Palpable neuroma   No/yes
Pain after exercise   No/yes
Phantom pain   No/yes

Contralateral leg
Normal   Yes/no

Hip disarticulation

'Hip disarticulation' for the purposes of this paper includes disarticulation at the acetabular–femoral joint and also transfemoral section above the upper reference level as described for the above-knee level.

Measurement
Upper femoral remnant   Absent/present — not prominent
                                         Present and prominent

Skin of the stump
Incision   Healed/unhealed
                                         Mobile/adherent

General   Skin intact/ulcerated
                                         Sensation normal/sensation impaired
                                         No additional scarring/additional scarring

Circulation
Oedema   None/minimal/excessive

Soft tissues of the stump
Amount   Adequate/inadequate/excessive

Consistency   Normal/flabby/indurated

Pain
Spontaneous pain   No/yes

Tenderness to palpation   No/yes — generalized/yes — localized

Palpable neuroma   No/yes

Pain after excercise   No/yes

Phantom pain   No/yes

Contralateral leg
Normal   Yes/no

Above-knee amputation

Measurement

The upper reference level for length measurement should be the crotch, defined as the highest point of the limb at which it is possible to obtain a circumferential measurement parallel to the ground with the patient vertical. The lower point of reference for length measurement should be the end of the unconstrained stump hanging vertically at a plane horizontal to the ground. In the case of a flexion deformity, the upper reference level for length would be that at which a circumferential measurement is possible at right angles to the centre line of the stump, and the lower point of reference would be the plane of the end of the stump at right angles to the centre line of the stump. The length of the rounded or tapered portion of the stump should be measured from the 'fall-away' point (at which the radius of the stump began) and the plane at the end of the stump, with the patient standing.

The following measures should be recorded:
1 Length from crotch to end of stump.
2 Circumference at the crotch.
3 Circumference at the 'fall-away' point.
4 Length from 'fall-away' point to end of stump.
5 Length from crotch to the ground.
6 Length from crotch to the medial joint line of the contralateral limb unless the contralateral limb is also the site of an amputation, in which case specify:

    Above-knee
    Knee disarticulation
    Below-knee
    Syme amputation
    Partial foot

and omit measurements 5 and 6.

Stump shape
Cylindrical
Conical   With or without prominent end of femur
Bulbous

Skin of the stump
Incision   Healed/unhealed
                          Mobile/adherent

General   Skin intact/ulcerated
                          Sensation normal/sensation impaired
                          No additional scarring/additional scarring

Circulation
Colour of skin   Normal/cyanotic

Temperature   Warm/cold (to the examining hand)

Oedema   None/minimal/excessive

Soft tissues of the stump

Amount	Adequate/inadequate/excessive
Consistency	Normal/flabby/indurated

Pain

Spontaneous pain	No/yes
Tenderness to palpation	No/yes — generalized/yes — localized
Palpable neuroma	No/yes
Pain after exercise	No/yes
Phantom pain	No/yes
Pain in proximal joint	No/yes

Joint function
Hip

range of movement	Flexion/extension	
	Abduction/adduction	
power	Significant reduction yes/no	

Contralateral leg

Normal	Yes/no

Knee disarticulation amputation

Measurement

The upper reference level for length measurement should be the crotch, defined as the highest point of the limb at which it is possible to obtain a circumferential measurement parallel to the ground with the patient vertical. The lower point of reference for length measurement should be the end of the unconstrained stump hanging vertically at a plane horizontal to the ground. In the case of a flexion deformity, the upper reference level for length would be that at which a circumferential measurement is possible at right angles to the centre line of the stump, and the lower point of reference would be the plane of the end of the stump at right angles to the centre line of the stump.

The following measurements should be recorded:
1 Length from crotch to end of stump.
2 Circumference at the crotch.
3 Minimum circumference of stump.
4 Circumference of femoral condyles.

5 Length from crotch to the ground.
6 Length from crotch to medial joint line of contralateral limb unless the contralateral limb is also the site of an amputation in which case specify:
    Above-knee
    Knee disarticulation
    Below-knee
    Syme amputation
    Partial foot.

Stump shape
Cylindrical
Bulbous

Skin of the stump

Incision	Healed/unhealed
	Mobile/adherent
General	Skin intact/ulcerated
	Sensation normal/sensation impaired
	No additional scarring/additional scarring

Circulation

Colour of skin	Normal/cyanotic
Temperature	Warm/cold (to the examining hand)
Oedema	None/minimal/excessive

Soft tissues of the stump

Amount	Adequate/inadequate/excessive
Consistency	Normal/flabby/indurated

Pain

Spontaneous pain	No/yes
Tenderness to palpation	No/yes — generalized/yes — localized
Palpable neuroma	No/yes
Pain after exercise	No/yes
Phantom pain	No/yes
Pain in proximal joint	No/yes

Joint function
Hip
   range of movement   Flexion/extension
                          Abduction/adduction

   power   Sigificant reduction yes/no

Contralateral leg
Normal   Yes/no

Below-knee amputation

Measurements

The upper reference level for length measurement should be the crotch defined as the highest point of the limb at which it is possible to obtain a circumferential measurement parallel to the ground with the patient vertical. The next reference level for length should be the medial joint line of the knee. The lower point of reference for length measurement should be the lowest part of the stump, at a plane horizontal to the ground at the end of the stump. In the case of a flexion deformity, the upper reference level for length would be that at which a circumferential measurement is possible at right angles to the centre line of the stump, and the lower point of reference would be the plane of the end of the stump at right angles to the centre line of the stump. The length of the rounded or tapered portion of the stump should be measured from the 'fall-away' point (at which the radius of the stump began) and the plane at the end of the stump, with the patient standing.

    The following measurements to be recorded:
1 Distance from medial joint line to end of stump.
2 Circumference at medial joint line.
3 Circumference at 'fall-away' point.
4 Length from 'fall-away' point to end of stump.
5 Record if cut end of fibula is above, level with, or below the end of the tibia.
6 Length from crotch to ground.
7 Length of contralateral limb from medial joint line to ground unless the contralateral limb is also the site of an amputation, in which case specify:
    Above-knee
    Knee disarticulation
    Below-knee
    Syme amputation
    Partial foot
and omit measurements 6 and 7.

Stump shape
Cylindrical
Conical
Bulbous

With or without prominent end of tibia
With or without prominent end of fibula

Skin of the stump

Incision

Healed/unhealed
Mobile/adherent

General

Skin intact/ulcerated
Sensation normal/sensation impaired
No additional scarring/additional scarring

Circulation

Colour of skin

Normal/cyanotic

Temperature

Warm/cold (to the examining hand)

Oedema

None/minimal/excessive

Soft tissues of the stump

Amount

Adequate/inadequate/excessive

Consistency

Normal/flabby/indurated

Pain

Spontaneous pain

No/yes

Tenderness to palpation

No/yes — generalized/yes — localized

Palpable neuroma

No/yes

Pain after exercise

No/yes

Phantom pain

No/yes

Pain in proximal joint

No/yes

Joint function

Hip
  significant reduction of range
  significant reduction of power

No/yes
No/yes

Knee
  range of motion
  power
  stable/unstable

Flexion/extension ☐☐
Significant reduction yes/no

Contralateral leg
Normal

Yes/no

Syme amputation

Measurements

The upper reference level for length should be the medial joint line. The lower point of reference for length measurement should be the lowest part of the stump, at a plane horizontal to the ground at the end of the stump. In the case of a flexion deformity, the upper reference level for length would be that at which a circumferential measurement is possible at right angles to the centre line of the stump, and the lower point of reference would be the plane of the end of the stump at right angles to the centre line of the stump.

The following measurements should be recorded:

1 Length from medial joint line to end of stump.
2 Circumference at medial joint line.
3 Minimum circumference of stump.
4 Circumference at 'fall-away' point.
5 Length from crotch to the ground.
6 Length from crotch to the medial joint line of the contralateral limb unless the contralateral limb is also the site of an amputation, in which case specify:

    Above-knee
    Knee disarticulation
    Below-knee
    Syme amputation
    Partial foot

and omit measurements 5 and 6.

Stump shape
Cylindrical
Bulbous   With or without prominent bone

Skin of the stump
Incision   Healed/unhealed
                           Mobile/adherent

General   Skin intact/ulcerated
                           Sensation normal/sensation impaired
                           No additional scarring/additional scarring

Circulation
Colour of skin   Normal/cyanotic

Temperature   Warm/cold (to the examining hand)

Oedema   None/minimal/excessive

Soft tissues of the stump

Amount	Adequate/inadequate/excessive
Consistency	Normal/flabby/indurated

Pain

Spontaneous pain	No/yes
Tenderness to palpation	No/yes — generalized/yes — localized
Palpable neuroma	No/yes
Pain after exercise	No/yes
Phantom pain	No/yes
Pain in proximal joint	No/yes

Joint function

Hip

significant reduction of range	No/yes
significant reduction of power	No/yes

Knee

range of motion	Flexion/extension ☐☐
power	Significant reduction Yes/no
stable/unstable	

Contralateral leg

Normal	Yes/no

Partial foot amputations

Measurements

1 The level of amputation should be defined at whichever of the following is appropriate:

Talonavicular

Tarsometatarsal

Transmetatarsal

with 1, 2, 3, 4, 5 as suffices relating to metatarsals divided.

Metatarsophalangeal

with 1, 2, 3, 4, 5 as suffices relating to toes removed.

2 The length should be recorded as the perpendicular distance between the anterior aspect of the tibia and the level of the end of the stump when the ankle is held in neutral position or as near to that position as possible.

Stump shape
Excessive bony prominence

Skin of the stump
Incision   Healed/unhealed
                                      Mobile/adherent

General   Skin intact/ulcerated
                                      Sensation normal/sensation impaired
                                      No additional scarring/additional scarring

Circulation
Colour of skin   Normal/cyanotic

Temperature   Warm/cold (to the examining hand)

Oedema   None/minimal/excessive

Soft tissues of the stump
Amount   Adequate/inadequate/excessive

Consistency   Normal/flabby/indurated

Pain
Spontaneous pain   No/yes

Tenderness to palpation   No/yes — generalized/yes — localized

Palpable neuroma   No/yes

Pain after exercise   No/yes

Phantom pain   No/yes

Pain in proximal joint   No/yes

Joint function
Hip
  significant reduction of range   No/yes
  significant reduction of power   No/yes

Knee
  range of motion   Flexion/extension   □ □
  power   Significant reduction Yes/no
  Stable/unstable

Ankle
  Range of movement   Flexion/extension □□
  Power   Significant reduction
  Stable/unstable

Contralateral leg
Normal   Yes/no

Reference

Persson B. M. & Liedberg E. (1983) A clinical standard of stump measurement and classification in lower limb amputees. *Prosthetics and Orthotics International* 7, 17–24.

ANKLE DISARTICULATION
AND TRANSTIBIAL AMPUTEE

Date of examination .... Examiner ....

Name

Overall situation

AMPUTATION Diabetes   1   Trauma 3
DIAGNOSIS   Other vascular   Tumour 4
            disease   2   Other   5

Not fitted before   1   Date of previous
Renewal   2   renewal   ....

Reason for present ....
consultation   ....

Described side   Right 1
Bilateral amputees: Use two forms   Left 2

ACTIVITY LEVEL: Average for age   1
               Exceptionally active   2
               Exceptionally low activity   3

JOINT FUNCTION KNEE Stable   1   HIP
   Normal   1   Instability 2   Normal 1
   Not normal 2   Not normal 2
Limited movements   Other conditions   Specify:.........
Record deficit only   None   1
                        Descr. below 2

SHAPE   Cylindrical 1
                        Conical   2
Comments ....   Bulbous   3

Flexion

Extension

SKIN SITUATION   Normal 1   INCISION   OK 1
   IN GENERAL   Sores 2   Not healed   2
                             Fold or adh. 3
OTHER SKIN   None 1   SENSIBILITY Normal   1
CONDITIONS   Descr.   Impaired 2
               below 2

MUSCLE POWER   No or light reduction   1
                       Significant reduction   2

Specify:

STATE OF   AMOUNT Ordinary 1   Prominent
TISSUE   Scarce   2   femur
                   Excessive 3   Yes 1   No 2
FIRMNESS Ordinary   1
          Indurated 2
          Flabby   3
OTHER   None   1
CONDITIONS Descr. below 2

OTHER LEG   Normal   1   Specify: ....
            Not normal 2

OTHER FUNCTION REDUCING FACTORS   None   1
                                   Descr. below 2

CIRCULATION at rest   OEDEMA None or minimal 1
                              Excessive   2
COLOUR OF Normal   1   TEMPERATURE Normal 1
SKIN   Cyanotic 2   OF SKIN   Cold   2

OTHER   None   1
CONDIT.   Descr. below 2

PAIN Spontaneous Yes 1   Pain after Yes 1
     pain at rest No 2   exercise   No 2

Local stump Yes 1   Palpable   Yes 1
pain   No 2   neuroma   No 2

Pain in   Yes 1   Other   None   1
hip joint No 2   conditions Descr. below 2

Circumf.

BODY BUILD
Average 1
Light   2
Heavy   3

Weight
kg

Full length

Skeletal end to
soft tissue end

Mark
Position
of fibula

Main descriptions	Assessment of present prosthetic fitting				Use of former prosthesis
Measurements					
Shape					
Skin					
State of tissue					
Circulation					
Pain					
Joint function					
Muscle power					
Other leg					
Other factors					
No objection					
Wait for improvement					
Special precautions					
Surgery needed					
Fitting unsuitable					

SUMMARY AND EVALUATION

COMMENTS

Full-time continuous use
Interruptions necessary daytime
Interruptions necessary for days or longer

UPPSALA UNIVERSITY WALKING SCHOOL
EEN & HOLMGRENS ORTOPEDISKA AB
INTERN. STANDARDS ORGAN. ISO

KNEE DISARTICULATION AND TRANSFEMORAL AMPUTEE

Name

Date of examination .... Examiner ....

Overall situation

AMPUTATION	Diabetes	1	Trauma	3	
DIAGNOSIS	Other vascular		Tumour	4	
	disease	2	Other	5	

| Described side | Right 1 | |
| Bilateral amputees: Use two forms | Left 2 | |

Not fitted before 1   Date of previous
Renewal 2   renewal _____

Reason for present _____
consultation _____

ACTIVITY LEVEL: Average for age 1
Exceptionally active 2
Exceptionally low activity 3 ☐

JOINT FUNCTION IN HIP   Limited range of movement
Record deficit only   Degrees
Normal 1   ☐
Not normal 2   Flexion ☐
Other   None 1   ☐   Extension ☐
conditions Descr. below 2   Abduction ☐
_____   Adduction ☐

SHAPE   Cylindrical 1
_____ Conical 2
Comments _____ Bulbous 3 ☐

SKIN SITUATION Normal 1 ☐ INCISION   OK 1 ☐
IN GENERAL Sores 2   Not healed 2
Fold or adh. 3
OTHER SKIN None 1 ☐ SENSIBILITY Normal 1 ☐
CONDITIONS Descr.   Impaired 2
below 2

MUSCLE POWER   No or light reduction 1
Significant reduction 2 ☐

Specify : _____

STATE OF AMOUNT Ordinary 1 ☐   Prominent
TISSUE   Scarce 2   femur
Excessive 3   Yes 1 No 2 ☐

OTHER LEG   Normal 1 ☐   Specify : _____
Not normal 2

FIRMNESS Ordinary 1 ☐
Indurated 2
Flabby 3
OTHER None 1 ☐
CONDITIONS Descr. below 2

OTHER FUNCTION REDUCING FACTORS   None 1 ☐
Descr. below 2

CIRCULATION at rest   OEDEMA None or minimal 1
Excessive 2 ☐
COLOUR OF Normal 1 ☐ TEMPERATURE Normal 1 ☐
SKIN Cyanotic 2   OF SKIN Cold 2
OTHER None 1 ☐
CONDIT. Descr. below 2

Skeletal end to
soft tissue end ☐☐☐

PAIN Spontaneous Yes 1 ☐   Pain after Yes 1 ☐
pain at rest No 2   exercise No 2
Local stump Yes 1 ☐   Palpable Yes 1 ☐
pain No 2   neuroma No 2
Pain in Yes 1 ☐   Other None 1 ☐
hip joint No 2   conditions Descr. below 2

BODY BUILD

Full length ☐☐☐

Average 1
Light 2
Heavy 3 ☐☐

Weight ☐☐☐
kg

Circumf. ☐☐
☐☐
☐☐
☐☐

COMMENTS
_____
_____
_____
_____
_____
_____
_____
_____
_____
_____
_____
_____
_____
_____

SUMMARY AND EVALUATION			
Main descriptions	Assessment of present prosthetic fitting	Use of former prosthesis	
Measurements			
Shape			
Skin			
State of tissue			
Circulation			
Pain			
Joint function			
Muscle power			
Other leg			
Other factors			
No objection			
Wait for improvement			
Special precautions			
Surgery needed			
Fitting unsuitable			
Full-time continuous use			
Interruptions necessary daytime			
Interruptions necessary for days or longer			

UPPSALA UNIVERSITY WALKING SCHOOL
EEN & HOLMGRENS ORTOPEDISKA AB
INTERN. STANDARDS ORGAN. ISO

54

Role of the Government in the Prosthetic Care of the Amputee

G. ROBERTSON

The role of government

As the role of government in the prosthetic care of the amputee is a particular application of the general role of government, this chapter will consider first that general role and thereafter government's role in the delivery of health care followed by the prosthetic care of the amputee.

Governments are created or elected to serve the people of the country by protecting their rights and by promoting and developing their aspirations and well-being. However, debate centres not on the role of government but on the way governments seek, by their policies, to fulfil their objective by ensuring that their policies are implemented by the responsible authorities using their executive arm, the Civil Services. A number of factors influence governments when they are formulating their policies, three of the most important being public opinion as perceived by them, the strength of their mandate, and the attitude of the people to government policies; this third factor varies from country to country, ranging from the apathetic to vigorous opposition when necessary. But the prime aim of all governments should always be that their policies are and will continue to be generally acceptable to the people. As Thomas Jefferson said, on the American Declaration of Independence, 'To secure these rights, Governments are instituted among men, deriving their just powers from the consent of the governed'. Governments must, therefore, listen to, and more importantly hear, the voice of the governed.

In determining the resource to be applied to particular policies, governments have to decide the priority to accord to each, and it is this need, whether it is the relative priorities between different sectors of government or within one sector, that gives rise to the fiercest argument and debate, even within the government itself.

When these arguments have been won and lost the policies have to be implemented; and most if not all governments find it much easier to prepare and present policies than to ensure their implementation. There are a number of reasons for this:

(a) In many areas, particularly in services such as education, housing and health, governments do not implement their policies on their own but are dependent on other organizations and authorities to do so; and these different authorities may not be so enchanted with the policies as the government, even though some may have a closer relationship to governments than others (e.g. Health Boards in the United Kingdom compared to local authorities).

(b) There may be very real practical difficulties in implementation which were not foreseen when the policies were prepared, particularly if at that time the policy-makers were not in government.

(c) Circumstances may change, leading either to reduced priority for the policy or to a rethink, further consultation and a revised policy.

(d) A particular policy may not have been accorded the necessary priority by the Executive.

With these and other constraints frequently acting against the early implementation of policies, governments must have adequate review and monitoring arrangements aimed at assessing the progress being made in implementing the policy, the reaction of interested parties to the effect of the policy, and the way resources, both manpower and funds, are being applied in terms of cost-effectiveness. Only in this way is government able to detect problems and to take necessary action to resolve them.

Different governments will adopt different styles of governing: there are, for example, interventionist and non-interventionist styles, though often these present to the people a distinction without a difference. The interventionist government will become involved, at times almost to the point of interference, in the direct implementation of policies whether or not they have the competence or it is appropriate for them to do so. The non-interventionist government will attempt to stand back from direct involvement. It will, however, continue to require a check of the implementation of its policies and in particular to ensure that public expenditure is not being misspent. This being so it will become interventionist to the extent that it will almost certainly strive to have sound review and monitoring arrangements, financial management systems, cash limits, budgetary controls, etc. The danger to be avoided here is for policy to be determined purely on financial grounds.

It is important once governments have determined their policies and indicated them clearly to responsible authorities, underlining their declared priorities within the particular policy, that they should then allow the authorities charged with the responsibility of implementing the policies to get on with doing just that, subject, of course, to sensible financial control as referred to above. In other words, it is important for governments to recognize when they should let go and not attempt to become directly involved in the implementation of policies which is the responsibility of other authorities. Failure to do this can all too easily result in the executive arm of government becoming so involved in the detail of implementation that it loses sight of what its main purpose should be, namely to keep the implications of the policy under review, to identify general problems, and to seek ways of clearing these. They should, in effect, be creating the climate in which the policies can most effectively be introduced.

The delivery of health care

Turning now to the government role in the delivery of health care, there will probably be general agreement that the role of all governments is to promote the health and well-being of the people. The ways they seek to do this will undoubtedly vary from country to country, but this aim will be constant.

If the United Kingdom, and more particularly Scotland, is taken as an illustration, the Secretary of State for Scotland has been charged under the health service legislation, since the National Health Service was introduced in 1948:
'to promote in Scotland a comprehensive and integrated health service designed to secure:

(a) improvement in the physical and mental health of the people of Scotland, and

(b) the prevention, diagnosis and treatment of illness and for that purpose to provide or secure the effective provision of services'.
(United Kingdom, National Health Service, 1978).
Later Sections of the Act provide for the appointment of authorities to undertake prescribed functions under the Act. In furtherance of this statutory duty the government has identified its priority groups. This has been done in two documents, first *The Health Service in Scotland, The Way Ahead* (1976), and secondly *Scottish Health Authorities, Priorities for the Eighties* (1980). Paragraph 4.15 of the earlier document, *The Way Ahead,* states that 'services for the physically handicapped have suffered from a shortage of financial resources for many years . . . The aim will be to maintain and possibly improve services of special importance to the physically handicapped, e.g. the prosthetic and orthotic services'. The thrust of both documents is that more emphasis should be given to the movement of resources into the priority fields.

The difficulty that the government has had in bringing about the switch of resources to the priority groups they have identified illustrates the problems governments face in having a declared policy implemented. It is not surprising, in the context of the health service, that those responsible for the acute service will argue strong and hard that the resource in that service is required for that service and cannot be diverted to the long-stay services, however deserving that may be: the argument is that more resource is needed.

The call for more resource as something that will cure all ills is all too common, and very often is not the answer to the particular problem. First of all there must be an examination to assess how effectively existing resources are being deployed and the extent to which there is a wasteful use of resources. If this is done and acted upon, it might well be possible to move resources into the priority area, in this case the services for the disabled, including the prosthetic and orthotic services. This is where the monitoring and review arrangements of government can and should play an important part and do much to move health authorities in the direction of the implementation of declared government policies.

It is appropriate at this point to consider how governments might undertake a review and monitoring function in the delivery of health care; and the considerations would apply equally to the prosthetic service. There would seem to be two main aspects of this function: first, the quality of the health care provided in the different services and, second, how effectively resources are being deployed within the declared policy of the government, particularly where public expenditure is involved.

The prime aim of all involved in the delivery of health care must be as high a quality of service to the patient as is possible. This makes the first aspect of the review function all important. The government will have a general appreciation of the level of care being provided in the different services from correspondence received and the response of those in the field, and will be able to take appropriate action on these. But as government itself will not have the competence to come to meaningful judgements there will be a continuing need for formal arrangements to obtain expert advice and opinion as necessary. Within these formal arrangements governments will no doubt wish to ensure that 'peer reviews' are undertaken as and when necessary to keep particular services up to standard.

So far as the effective deployment of resources is concerned, much of this can and will be done by having sound information retrieval systems and using them wisely to come to judgements on, for example, the cost-effectiveness of comparable units. This, coupled with good day-to-day financial management and budget provisions, if used properly, will identify those units where resources are not being deployed effectively, and will enable government to take remedial action which will in many cases not only cut out waste but also lead to a higher quality service with consequent benefit to the patient. It is, of course, equally important for governments to monitor their own activities to ensure that they too are cost-effective.

Prosthetic care of the amputee

We have thus reached in the United Kingdom — and this is probably the position in many other countries following the International Year of Disabled People in 1981 — the point where increasing emphasis is being given to the needs of disabled people and where government decisions have been taken that more resources should be channelled into this area. But it is important that those directly responsible for the prosthetic care of the amputee should not stand back and accept that such additional resource when it arrives will cure all ills. This will probably not be so, particularly if those concerned are assuming that it will. There is always a need for a self-examination to assess whether the service being provided is as effective and efficient as it might be. The service can often be significantly improved without additional resources. For example, sound use of resources in the training and education of prosthetists and other staff leads to better fitting arrangements and better and quicker rehabilitation of the amputee, with a consequent reduction in total resources required if the patient has a shorter stay in hospital and is saved from frequent returns to the clinic. Most important of all, leaving aside resource implications, is the improvement in patient care and the benefits that accrue to the particular patient. It is the function of government to take the appropriate steps to ensure that those directly responsible for the service pursue this with full vigour. The government role is thus not passive — it certainly should not be — but a positive and active one. The prosthetic service, however, in the submission of this chapter, is clearly an integral part of the health care of the patient, and as such should be undertaken by those charged with responsibility for health care, whoever that might be in different countries, and not directly by government.

The positive and active role of government in this field can perhaps be illustrated by the application of research and development advances. Governments recognize the need for research and development and fund approved projects. But research and development in the prosthetic service, to be in any way meaningful, must lead to better patient care; it is governments who have the power, not always exercised as urgently as it should be, to ensure that research and development advances are introduced into service use without undue delay.

A particular case of interest is CAD/CAM — computer-aided design and manufacture — which was the subject of a special edition of *Prosthetics and Orthotics International.* This shows good international co-operation and heavy government funding, certainly in the United Kingdom. It would be both sad and disappointing if, when this work is proved, there was undue delay in introducing it into the prosthetic service for general use. It would seem very relevant for governments to act promptly on this, as the advances will not only lead to better prosthetic care but also prove much more cost-effective than present procedures. As Murdoch (1985) states in his editorial to the journal, the publication of the details of this work 'will alert Governments and other funding authorities to the state of the art and provoke, one hopes, serious thought to its implications for patient care.'

The Scottish experience

The role and influence of government in determining the appropriate policy to be followed in a particular service is well demonstrated by what might well be called 'The Scottish Experience' so far as the prosthetic service is concerned. On the introduction of the National Health Service in the United Kingdom in 1948 responsibility for the care of the amputee was vested in the then Ministry of Pensions which was responsible for disabled ex-servicemen, but in 1953 this function was transferred to the health ministers (United Kingdom, Ministry of Pensions, 1953). At that time the government, recognizing the circumstances pertaining in Scotland so far as the location of artificial limb centres was concerned, vested the responsibility for the prosthetic services in the health authorities. This decision, which differed from that taken for England and Wales, led to the direct involvement of orthopaedic consultants and other health service staff in the fitting of artificial limbs. Deficiencies and defects in the service were identified by them and pressure built up for changes to be effected. Ministers were quick to realize that this was a Scottish problem, for which a Scottish solution had to be found, and so set up a working party to examine the way the artificial limb service should be developed in Scotland in the future. That working party reported in 1970, and the government of the day, following full consultation with all interested parties on the recommendations of the report, accepted the report in total (Scottish Home and Health Department 1970). At a later stage — and following a change of government — practical and other considerations led to part of the report not being implemented.

The government had thus been responsive to health service opinion, and had acted positively to have the service examined in depth, to obtain all the facts and to assess them. It now had to show the will to ensure that the change was effected. Again, seeing this as a Scottish solution for a Scottish problem and having accepted all the recommendations in the report, it took the lead to ensure the implementation of two of the more important recommendations, first the establishing of a course centre for the training and education of prosthetists and, secondly, the transfer of prosthetists to health service employment: on the first, money was required, and on the second its negotiating powers. Both responsibilities were accepted.

At the time the recommendation that prosthetists should be transferred to health service employment was the one on which attention was mainly focused. But now, a decade or so further on, there is no doubt that the critical recommendation was the establishment of a course centre. The thinking behind the recommendation was that there was a need to bring limb fitters up to a level of competence where they could, with confidence, participate fully as a professional part of the clinic team on all matters relating to the fitting of the artificial limb to the patient: and having brought them to that level they should, by follow-up refresher courses, be maintained at that level and be alive to an understanding of innovations in the field of prosthetic hardware.

The centre was thus aimed at both the basic training of the prosthetist and the postgraduate training. As is now well known, it has in fact gone beyond that and has also become a centre for short courses for all health care staff involved in the prosthetic and orthotic field as well as for the evaluation of new hardware and the dissemination of information.

The prosthetist having been so trained can thus do two things that would have been difficult, through no fault of his own, a decade or so ago: first, help to identify defects and deficiencies in the hardware available for particular patient needs, and by passing this information on to the researchers, for example those in the different companies or at clinical centres, hopefully assist in the forward movement of relevant research; and secondly, by his direct and indirect involvement with a wide training programme, he is able more easily to identify and advise his colleagues on the most appropriate limb for the particular patient.

The result of 'The Scottish Experience' therefore is that the prosthetist is now contributing in a much more effective way to the delivery of care to the amputee, which in turn improves the quality of the work of the clinic team leading to a higher quality of patient care which, at the end of the day, must be the aim of all involved in the service.

The decision by government to intervene directly to resolve a problem and to effect policy changes which significantly affected the way the service has developed should bring a further benefit. The greater all-round competence of the clinic team should lead to a more cost-effective service. As the government in the United Kingdom has ultimate responsibility for health care, its executive arm (that is the Scottish Home and Health Department) must now ensure that these benefits do accrue; this will no doubt be done through sound review and monitoring arrangements, as outlined above, leaving the authorities responsible for health care to discharge their responsibility in the clinical field without undue interference.

Conclusion

This chapter has attempted to set out the general role of government and then move to the more particular areas of health service and the prosthetic service. All the factors relating to the role of government in the general sense apply equally to individual services, in particular the need to keep all policies, with the priorities within them, under regular review with appropriate monitoring arrangements. No government, irrespective of the level of resources available, should settle for mediocrity. Its aim should be the highest possible quality of service in every instance within the resources that it can make available for a particular service; and a higher level, more often than not, can be achieved by a more effective deployment of resources. It is perhaps even more important that all involved in the different services — and in the health service and prosthetic service in particular — must also not settle for mediocrity, but should at all times pursue excellence.

Finally, it is salutary for governments, when fulfilling their role, to remind themselves of the words of Lord Beveridge, whose report led to the United Kingdom's social legislation of the 1940s and in particular to our National Health Service, when he said, 'The object of government in peace and in war is not the glory of the rulers or of races but the happiness of the common man.'

References

Murdoch G. (1985) Editorial. *Prosthetics and Orthotics International* **9**, 2.
Scottish Home and Health Department (1970) *The Future of the Artificial Limb Service in Scotland: report of a working party set up by the Secretary of State for Scotland.* London: HMSO.

Scottish Home and Health Department (1976) *The Health Service in Scotland: the Way Ahead.* London: HMSO.

Scottish Home and Health Department Scottish Health Service Planning Council (1980) *Scottish Health Authorities, Priorities for the Eighties.* London: HMSO.

United Kingdom, Ministry of Pensions (1953) *The Transfer of Functions: Order 1953.* London: HMSO.

United Kingdom National Health Service (1978) *National Health Service (Scotland) Act 1978* (Section 1[1]). London: HMSO.

55

Evaluation in Lower Limb Prosthetics

A.B. WILSON JR

Introduction

The evaluation of individual results of any research and development programme is not an easy task; evaluation of components and techniques in lower limb prosthetics is a positively formidable problem because of the large number of interdependent variables. Nevertheless an unbiased appraisal of new developments emerging from both government and privately supported research and development efforts is needed if these efforts are to be efficient and effective.

Devices and procedures are known that seem to work well when applied by the group that developed them, but which fail to gain widespread acceptance. There are also a number of prototype designs that appeared to be promising in view of trials by the development group, but were never picked up by a manufacturer so that they could be made available generally. A well-run evaluation programme conducted by an organization quite independent of the research and development group would provide manufacturers, educators, and clinicians with the information needed before investing the money and time required to make these devices and techniques available to patients who can benefit from them.

No two developments take the same course in an evaluation programme but certain factors are common and critical to each item being evaluated. An orderly research and development programme obviously would have an evaluation element at each stage of the process. Prototype trial is essentially an evaluation function in itself and does not usually need the formal services of an independent group. However, it is essential that a sufficient number of patients have been treated using the new device to warrant the cost of making a preproduction run of sufficient quantity for a relatively large clinical study, usually 50 or more. Obviously, the device must be evaluated for safety. It is also helpful if quantitative data such as locomotion pattern and velocity are collected and presented at this point.

Clinical evaluation

One method of clinical evaluation that has proven to be effective consists of a network of rehabilitation clinics that apply an experimental device or technique concurrently using a common protocol that has been agreed to by all participants. An organization independent of the development group co-ordinates the work, collects and analyses the data from the participating clinics, and prepares a draft of a comprehensive report, which is reviewed and completed by the participating clinics. For a device or procedure to qualify for a full-scale clinical programme it must meet the following requirements:

1 The device or procedure must be safe for use on patients.

2 There must be available sufficient instructional material to cover the application of the device or procedure.

3 An adequate supply of identical devices must be available.

4 In the case of devices, provisions for maintenance must have been made.

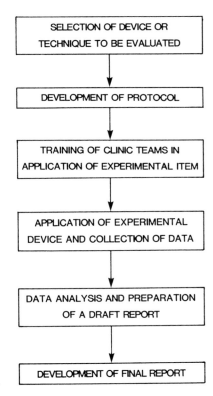

Fig. 55.1 Major steps in a clinical evaluation programme.

The basic steps in a clinical evaluation programme are (Fig. 55.1):

1 Selection of devices. All of the participating clinics must agree that the device or technique is worthy of evaluation.

2 Development of protocol. A draft is prepared by the co-ordinating group, and reviewed and refined by the development group and clinical participants.

3 Training in application of the experimental device or technique. All participating clinic teams are trained at the same time and place by the development group.

4 Data collection. Data are forwarded to the co-ordinating group who maintain close liaison with each of the participating clinics and provide assistance as needed.

5 Data analysis and preparation of draft report. The co-ordinating group pools the data and after analysis prepares a draft report.

6 Development of final report. Representatives of the participating clinics are brought together to review thoroughly the draft report and complete it for publication.

Some important considerations are:

1 The staff of the co-ordinating group should include a prosthetist, a physician, and a therapist who have had clinical experience.

2 The participating clinics should contact the co-ordinating group concerning any problems rather than going directly to the development group. This procedure makes it possible for all of the participating groups to be notified of any changes in procedure that might be worthwhile.

3 It is extremely important that each of the participating clinics receives identical instruction, if good results are to be expected.

This system of evaluation proved to be effective in the United States between 1968 and 1975 when it had an organized research and development programme in prosthetics and orthotics. Some efforts are currently being made to revive it.

A possible improvement

In an effort to be more objective in the evaluation of lower limb prostheses (and, in fact, in most programmes for treatment of locomotion disorders) the author's centre at the University of Virginia has undertaken a study to determine the usefulness of heart beats and vertical acceleration events in measuring changes in energy requirement and activity levels for periods of up to 24 hours, as reported by MacGregor (1980). Programming of an IPM–PCXT to count the events against time is nearly complete, and the technique appears to be promising. The hypothesis of the experiment is that, if the device or treatment is effective, the subject, over the period of a day, will either be more active or use less energy, or some combination of both. If this technique is proven to be practical, it is believed that the number of subjects needed in current clinical evaluation projects can be reduced greatly and that the elapsed time required can be reduced significantly.

Reference

MacGregor J. (1980) Rehabilitation ambulatory monitoring. In *Rehabilitation of the Disabled* (eds Kenedi R. M. & Paul J. P.), pp. 159–172. London: MacMillan Press.

EDUCATION AND TRAINING

56

A Perspective on Prosthetics-Orthotics Education

S. FISHMAN

The problem of developing and implementing an acceptable educational programme for the prosthetist–orthotist is quite complex, since historically people in these fields have not had access to a basic professional training programme. It might be well, therefore, to review the desired responsibilities and functions of the *professional* prosthetist–orthotist.

1   *To serve as a member of the clinic,* along with the physician or surgeon and therapist, *providing consultative advice,* participating in discussions, *and sharing in decisions* regarding prescription, evaluation, and formulation of the prosthetic–orthotic treatment programme.

2   *To provide prosthetic–orthotic service to patients,* which implies all of the necessary intellectual and manual skills (design, measure, cast, fit, align, etc.) required to supply an appliance of excellent quality.

3   *To be aware of and contribute to the progress and growth of the profession* through such means as research and development activities, participating and exercising leadership in professional associations, and recruiting and training new entrants into the field.

In order to fulfil these responsibilities, it becomes quite clear that there are six areas of skill and knowledge which are indispensable:

(a)   Physical sciences including mathematics.
(b)   Biological sciences.
(c)   Psychological sciences.
(d)   Mechanical skills and crafts.
(e)   Communication skills.
(f)   Personal and cultural qualifications.

Before proceeding with any further discussion, several basic assumptions on which the curriculum rests must also be agreed.

1   Graduates will practise their profession using *prefabricated prosthetic–orthotic components.* Therefore, training in the production of such items as prosthetic feet and orthotic joints need not be offered.

2   *The fields of prosthetics and orthotics are not separate and distinct entities.* Rather, there is a considerable (and growing) degree of overlap in the knowledge

and skill required in both areas. Therefore, the educational programme should offer concurrent training in both specialties.

3   The academic level of the educational programme, and *the value and acceptance of the degree or diploma* issued on successful completion of the course of study *must be comparable to that earned by other health professionals* (therapists, counsellors, etc.).

4   *The training should be offered at existing, accredited, and recognized educational institutions on the post-secondary school level.*

Bearing in mind the responsibilities of the prosthetists and orthotists and the four prior assumptions, a reasonable programme of instruction would be as indicated in Table 56.1. Although this proposed course of study is four years in duration, the time can be reduced to three years by eliminating or markedly reducing the communication, liberal arts, and cultural courses. In the author's view this is not advisable, but in any event the other courses are absolutely mandatory.

It is important to note that the last group of courses entitled 'professional specialization' accounts for approximately 60% of the total number of instructional hours. When the additional 10% devoted to 'manual skills and concepts' instruction is added one approaches 70% of the total class contact hours required for the specialized prosthetic–orthotic training. This reflects the considerable amount of time required to develop the necessary prosthetic–orthotic skills. However, even with this substantial time allocation it is necessary to be very selective and to limit the variety and types of prostheses and orthoses fitted and fabricated by the students so as to assure an unquestioned understanding of basic principles and procedures. Specifically, the student learns the practical clinical aspects of this field in four steps:

(a)   Basic shop training in metal, wood and plastic.

(b)   Specialized training in the application of these techniques to prosthetics and orthotics.

(c)   Laboratory courses in the fabrication and fitting of appliances for a variety of patients.

(d)   Clinical internships at certified facilities.

Space will not permit any detailed examination of the content of the specialized prosthetic–orthotic courses; it will suffice to point out that considerable agreement regarding the topics to be covered in these specialized courses has been achieved and documented in four separate well-represented international meetings. The first of these was the United Nations Interregional Seminar on Standards for the Training of Prosthetists held in Holte, Denmark, in 1968 (United Nations 1969); the second was the International Conference on Prosthetics and Orthotics conducted by ISPO in Cairo, Egypt, in 1972 under the sponsorship of the Vocational Rehabilitation Administration, HEW (International Society of Prosthetics and Orthotics 1974); the third was the International Study Week on Prosthetic–Orthotic Education conducted by the University of Strathclyde in Glasgow, Scotland, in 1974 under the sponsorship of the Scottish Home and Health Department (Hughes 1976); and lastly the International Symposium of Prosthetic Orthotic Educators in Toronto, Canada,

Table 56.1 Suggested prosthetic–orthotic curriculum (four years).

	Lecture	Laboratory	Class hours Total
Physical sciences (including mathematics)			
Algebra and trigonometry	45	—	45
Introductory chemistry	45	45	90
Introductory physics	45	60	105
*Mechanics	45	—	45
*Properties of materials	30	—	30
	210	105	315 (8%)
Biological sciences			
Introductory biology	45	60	105
Anatomy and physiology	60	60	120
Orthopaedic and neuromuscular pathology	30	—	30
	135	120	255 (6%)
Psychological sciences			
Introductory psychology	45	45	90
Psychology of the physically handicapped	45	—	45
	90	45	135 (3%)
Communication — personal and cultural			
English composition and speech, social sciences, humanities, liberal arts, and other sciences	570 (approx.)		570 (14%)
Manual skills and concepts			
Mechanical drawing	15	75	90
General metalworking	15	75	90
*Prosthetic and orthotic techniques	30	180	210
	60	330	390 (10%)
Professional specialization			
*Biomechanics	30	—	30
*Above-knee prosthetics	40	200	240
*Below-knee prosthetics	30	150	180
*Lower-limb orthotics	60	90	150
*Upper-limb prosthetics	30	105	135
*Upper-limb orthotics	15	60	75
*Spinal orthotics	30	105	135
*Professional problems in prosthetics and orthotics	30	—	30
*Clincial affiliation (supervised practical experience)	—	1440	1440
	265	2150	2415 (59%)
Total	1330 (33%)	2750 (67%)	4080 (100%)

*Offered in the author's own facility by his own faculty — remaining courses are given by other departments in the University.

obvious differences in details emanating from these various meetings there was unanimous agreement regarding the basic areas of knowledge and skill required by the prosthetist–orthotist — these subjects being essentially those outlined previously. It was further affirmed that an acceptable programme of instruction in prosthetics and orthotics requires a minimum of three years for completion.

In the almost total absence of any formal educational experience or tradition in these fields, it would have been impossible to organize and offer comprehensive long-term educational programmes without an important preliminary step which occurred in the early 1950s. This initial step involved the establishment of short-term, practically oriented, intensive instructional programmes of several weeks' duration for individuals already engaged in prosthetic–orthotic work to upgrade their existing skills. It was only after short-term instructional programmes were well under way that it became possible for a number of institutions to turn their attention to *long-term* training programmes leading to a Bachelor's degree, the first of these being inaugurated at New York University in 1963. At present there appears to be approximately 20 identifiable institutions in the industrial nations offering long-term instruction in prosthetics and orthotics, of which 18 follow the general pattern of instruction described in this paper — seven in the United States, three in Canada, and one each in Scotland, Argentina, Australia, Japan, Norway, Portugal, Spain and Sweden.

Although at first sight 20 institutions offering long-term prosthetic–orthotic instruction may seem to be an impressive number when compared with none in 1950, an analysis of the location of these schools shows that there are large significant regions of the world where there are no schools, indicating that much needs to be done in establishing additional educational institutions. Within the last few years the number of new schools being activated has been negligible, and there is no evidence of any revival of growth. This stagnant situation is one which requires attention on the part of ISPO and other international organizations so that the significant progress to date continues in the years ahead.

Another problem is the continuing paucity of prosthetists–orthotists with appropriate educational qualifications to serve as directors and teachers in various prosthetic–orthotic education programmes throughout the world. The number of potential faculty members with appropriate educational qualifications available to these programmes is negligible.

It should also be noted that, to date, no systematic training in research methodology has been available to the profession, and this undoubtedly explains the minimal involvement of the prosthetist–orthotist in research activities. Prosthetics and orthotics, to an overwhelming degree, has been dependent on the research done by other professions — notably medicine and engineering — certainly not an optimal state of affairs. Intensive detailed instruction in clinical management has also been generally unavailable to the prosthetic–orthotic student, since the time demands for 'basic' education associated with the current levels of training have frequently precluded any serious attention to this more sophisticated instruction. Lastly, the intellectual level and maturity of some of the present undergraduate students makes even moderately sophisticated research and pedagogical and clinical management instruction inappropriate.

It is also important that the prosthetist–orthotist maintains parity in professional growth and status with other colleagues on the treatment team, in particular the physical and occupational therapist. With graduate level education, selected students will be intellectually and emotionally more mature, have more comprehensive educational backgrounds, and will have the opportunity to develop specific competence in *research methods, teaching and/or clinical management*. Lastly, it must be clearly understood that it is not suggested that all practitioners require training at the graduate level — only those preparing for positions of leadership.

The author should like to offer one suggestion regarding a significant simplification in prosthetics–orthotics education, thereby making it more efficient and economical. Most programmes offer substantial instruction in upper limb prosthetics and orthotics, consuming perhaps as much as 30% of the total specialized instructional time on these topics. Although accurate statistics are hard to come by, upper limb prosthetics and orthotics practice (at least in the United States) represents perhaps only 10% of the entire field. Furthermore, a substantial segment of this practice is concentrated in specialized centres emphasizing the care of upper limb disabilities. This results in a situation where the preponderant number of graduates of prosthetics–orthotics schools never have the opportunity to provide these services. This leads to the anomalous situation of investing a goodly segment of training monies in teaching individuals skills that most will not use. It would, therefore, be more sensible to consider upper limb prosthetics and orthotics as a sub-specialty area to be taught *only* to those who have a need for such knowledge, after they have achieved basic competency in lower limb and spinal prosthetics and/or orthotics. The savings would be substantial and the time which would then become free could be better used for more extensive and intensive instruction in the 'bread and butter' aspects of the field.

References

Hughes J. (ed.) (1976) *International Study Week on Prosthetic/Orthotic Education: National Centre for Training and Education in Prosthetics and Orthotics, University of Strathclyde, Glasgow, July 1974.* London: HMSO.

International Society for Prosthetics and Orthotics (1974) *Report of an ISPO International Conference on Prosthetics and Orthotics: Cairo and Alexandria, Egypt, May 1–11 1972.* Cairo: S.O.P. Press.

United Nations (1969) *Report of the United Nations Inter-regional Seminar on Standards for the Training of Prosthetists:* organized by the United Nations and the Government of Denmark with the co-operation of the International Committee on Prosthetics and Orthotics of the International Society for Rehabilitation of the Disabled, Holte, Denmark, 1–19 July 1968. New York: U.N.

57

Education and Training in Prosthetics in the Developing World

W. KAPHINGST & S. HEIM

Introduction

The question of the differences in training requirements for prosthetics and orthotics in Third World countries and in the industrial nations is always worth discussing (International Society for Prosthetics and Orthotics 1985). In exploring this question it is essential to consider the need for orthopaedic treatment in the country involved. This may be:

Substandard technology.
Simplified technology.
Appropriate technology.

'Appropriate' is taken to mean devices adapted in a proper biomechanical and technical sense as well as properly adapted to the local circumstances such as climate and available materials. It can be assumed that no professional takes this concept for granted. However, technologists working in developing countries cannot disregard 'simplified technology' for a number of reasons.

First of all, a few words on the definition of the term 'developing country'. These countries are extremely variable in their economic, social, and technical structure. In some the level of general development is low, while others show a higher level of culture, craftsmanship, and local traditions. It is impossible to make a statement covering all countries. Around the world the definition is linked to the per capita income; countries are subdivided into lowest income countries, 'threshold countries', etc. At the present all these countries share a perceptible common factor in that the orthopaedic care centres in the capital and other large cities are mainly filled with personnel trained in industrial countries and employing techniques acquired abroad. The result is that technically sophisticated orthopaedic treatment is offered, which is not in keeping with the local circumstances. Elsewhere the only technical orthopaedic treatment available is offered by unqualified personnel and is absolutely substandard. This present widespread situation can only be changed by appropriate and extensive training.

With respect to prosthetics, the patients involved exhibit amputations at all levels, just as in the industrial world. Of the lower limb amputations, the commonest is the below-knee followed by knee disarticulation and amputation of the foot. Very often the condition of the stump when presented for prosthetic fitting is unsatisfactory. Contractures of the joints, protruding bony ends and unhealed wounds are all too common. These complications of the stump are mostly due to the fact that amputations are usually carried out by medical officers instead of surgeons. Such circumstances require maximum skills on the part of the prosthetic technologist. Above all, he should be capable of manufacturing the necessary components himself, or at least be able to give instructions for their manufacture. It follows that it is not sufficient to learn to construct a prosthesis; the training and education must be so organized that the professional, when working in the field, is able to translate his acquired knowledge to meet local and very often difficult circumstances. At the other extreme it is certainly not necessary to introduce hydraulic knee joint mechanisms to students in Third World countries or teach them myoelectric principles.

Training system

In the authors' view there is no fundamental difference with respect to training curricula in comparison with other schools. The training in theoretical subjects for the field of prosthetics is composed as follows:

(a) Information on materials including all materials used for the manufacture of prostheses, starting with wood and leather and proceeding to modern synthetics.
(b) Basic mechanical principles: as a prerequisite to biomechanical understanding.
(c) Biomechanics, subdivided in:
  1 Three-dimensional reference lines.
  2 Human locomotion and gait analysis.
  3 Pathological gait.
  4 Socket design and the stump–socket interface.
  5 Prosthetic alignment.
  6 Mechanics and the reciprocal influence of components.
(d) Anatomy and physiology.
(e) Orthopaedic pathology including the anatomy and physiology of amputations and the resultant stumps.
(f) Clinical work with patients. Assessment and check-out.

The last item clearly crosses the borderline between theoretical and practical work. Graphic design is another essential part of theoretical training. Graphic recording, along with analysing, understanding, and finally translating that understanding, is essential in stimulating three-dimensional thinking, which is of major importance, especially among African students. Since a large part of the training is dedicated to practical work, the theoretical part covers approximately 25–28% of the total training time. This often leads to controversy, since the English educational systems, adopted by all English-speaking countries, usually stress theoretical subjects.

The practical part is composed as follows:

(a) Acquiring the basic principles of the manufacture of foot and knee components. This orientation course represents a necessary basis for developing countries. Separate workshops can thus be created to manufacture their own components where there is a lack of prefabricated ones. At the same time basic manual skills are taught. Since repairing the prosthesis is part of the daily routine and no exchangeable components are available, the manufacturing process teaches the technician how to effect repairs.

(b) Bench alignment of BK and AK prostheses is also seen as basic information. During this course students are informed on three or four of the currently available types. A comparison of the alignment of prefabricated and self-made components fails to demonstrate any significant differences in the alignment guidelines.

(c) Discussion of the patients' disability, functional and cultural requirements, and the prescription itself leading to the taking of measurements, cast work, prosthetic alignment, dynamic correction and manufacture is an essential part of practical training. Instruction is confined to those types of prostheses which are adapted to the country and to its structure.

These methods and the contents of both education and training are comparable to those of other schools. The programme is essentially standard practice. The fabrication of simple prostheses such as peg-legs and those used to accommodate a flexed knee do not permit shortening or simplification of the training process, if indeed these simple devices are to be truly functional.

Social and environmental problems of the patients are significant criteria for this type of training. The choice and knowledge of materials play a decisive role with regard to comfort and durability. Parts that are subject to frequent repair are simplified, or, if possible, eliminated. Moreover, techniques are developed and elaborated and taught as part of the curriculum for the manufacture of prostheses in rural workshops where there is a minimum or even absence of powered machinery, low-pressure air suction supplies for laminating work, etc.

What is important for African students, as for all and already stressed several times, is the understanding of the problems. They must be able to recognize problems in order to comprehend and, if possible, solve them.

In conclusion, it is a good thing to list some of the difficulties that affect prosthetic care and the construction of prosthetic appliances and therefore should be reflected in the formation of a training programme.

1 Medical care cannot be compared to European or American standards.

2 Frequently physiotherapy training for the patients is lacking.

3 The patient's social background is very often the decisive factor in accepting or refusing treatment.

4 There are no social workers to take on this aspect of rehabilitation.

This is not a complete list, but it does demonstrate the kind of additional information which should be passed on to the future prosthetic technologist, so that he can assume a professional stature. It must be realized that he will be left to himself after graduation. He will neither find a well-running workshop, nor be supported by *'Meisters'* or older benchworkers. Therefore it is recommended that there should be no simplification of the training requirements for prosthetic technologists in developing countries. On the contrary, they need to develop more specific manual skills and practical knowledge in order to make a good and lasting contribution to our profession.

Reference

International Society for Prosthetics and Orthotics (1985) *Report of a Workshop on Prosthetics and Orthotics in the Developing World with respect to Training and Education and Clinical Services, Moshi, Tanzania, 1984.* Copenhagen: ISPO.

58

The Dundee Experience

G. MURDOCH, D.N. CONDIE, D. GARDNER, E. RAMSAY,
A. SMITH, C.P.U. STEWART, A.J.G. SWANSON &
I.M. TROUP

Introduction

This chapter provides information regarding the Dundee Limb Fitting Centre's 20-year experience in the management of the primary amputee. In addition to that work the group is responsible for the prosthetic care of more than 700 amputees and many more patients requiring a range of other services under the general heading of rehabilitation engineering.

Prior to the inception of the National Health Service in the United Kingdom in 1948, limb fitting was provided by the Ministry of Pensions and later transferred to the then Ministry of Health in 1953. At that time the Scottish Home and Health Department (SHHD) decided that the care of the amputee, including limb fitting, should be devolved to the Health Boards and responsibility for these patients placed with identified orthopaedic surgeons. In the years following, by deliberate and assiduous brain picking through the medium of fellowships, the running of conferences, and the collaboration of the SHHD and the Tayside Health Board, a philosophy of patient management was developed. Tribute must be paid to the influence in particular of Knud Jansen, the founding president of the International Society for Prosthetics and Orthotics: also A. Bennett Wilson Jr, at that time Director of the Committee for Prosthetic Research and Development in the National Academy of Sciences in the United States; to Anthony Staros, at that time Director of the Prosthetic Service in the Veterans Administration in the United States; to Charles Radcliffe of the University of California, Berkeley; to Jim Foort of the University of British Columbia; to Marian Weiss of Kinstantin, Poland; to Dugald McKenzie and Mirek Vitali of Roehampton; and to many others.

Dundee Limb Fitting Centre (DLFC) was opened in September, 1965, and at that time was the only centre in Western Europe offering in-patient care exclusively for the amputee. The number of beds (17) has remained the same but nevertheless considerable development has taken place. Approximately 100 primary amputation cases are treated each year; 86% of these patients suffer from atherosclerosis or vascular problems associated with diabetes. Typically the patients have several handicaps and the rehabilitation provided is designed to meet these circumstances and is based on the concept of the clinic team. Most cases are referred from the general surgical wards and occasionally from medical wards within Tayside, but direct referrals to the service are also made. In either event a comprehensive assessment is undertaken for each patient in the vascular laboratory; these investigations have proved to be critical to the patient's rehabilitation.

All referrals for amputation surgery and arrangements for assessment, surgery and relevant transfer are channelled through the clinical secretary in DLFC. If the vascular surgeon sees no hope of limb salvage by vascular surgery, the patient is seen by one of the two orthopaedic teams involved in the amputation surgery service and the patient is admitted for amputation to a specialist unit where nursing and theatre facilities are available. There are clear advantages in this arrangement as the hospital provides a location for the surgical teams and a high level of nursing care is immediately available. The concentration of surgical expertise has ensured a comprehensive surgical experience for trainees.

Early transfer to DLFC is effected on the second, third or fourth post-operative day. There, the whole clinic team becomes involved at a very early stage. The team consists of doctors, nurses, therapists, prosthetists and bioengineers. All aspects of the total care programme are readily co-ordinated and stump environment can be accurately monitored. Very early prosthetic provison is possible — within five days of prescription and earlier if required. Close co-operation is possible between the prosthetists and therapists, thus optimizing alignment procedures in a controlled situation. At the same time the occupational therapist is able to provide information and training in the use of aids to daily living and links with the Social Work Department in the community in providing adaptations and other aids in time fo the patient's return home. On discharge, follow-up is maintained in the out-patient clinic which provides services for some 700–800 amputees. Three prosthetists are involved in the service and so far as possible prostheses designed by them on the basis of the clinic team's prescription are fabricated in the Centre. In addition to the regular prosthetic clinic a Special Panel Clinic meets at two-monthly intervals to discuss special problems relating to individual patients.

Pre-operative care

Medical care of the patient about to have an amputation can be difficult. It involves the referring clinician who decides that amputation may be necessary, the surgeon who decides it is and determines, after assessment, its level, and the prosthetic clinician who will have the responsibility for continuing care. All too often the prosthetic clinician is presented with an amputee without any previous consultation.

In Dundee a consultative system has been developed which ensures that there is a close liaison between all the professionals involved. The prosthetic clinician is involved in such matters as level decisions and this encourages a close liaison with his surgical colleagues. It also ensures that specific prosthetic implications are considered in decisions about amputation level; for instance the effect of hip flexion. It ensures that optimum results are achieved in such matters as stump length and construction and that prosthetic problems are minimized in future care.

In continuing care the prosthetic clinician is responsible for the recognition of problems such as infection of the stump and delayed or failed healing. Inevitably he must therefore be involved in pre-operative measures to resolve these problems. The opportunity to question procedures leads to close scrutiny of such things as skin preparation prior to surgery, the use of drugs to control pain and infection and general patient management. This close co-operation is the only foundation on which to build continuing amputee care.

Most important of all is the ability to establish patient contact, and a system has been developed which allows the prosthetic clinician directly responsible for patient care to outline in some detail the likely steps in convalescence following amputation. Patient counselling is of extreme importance — the patient who fears the future is immediately at a disadvantage.

Surgery

Between 1971 and 1982 the total number of amputations in England and Wales remained virtually static. A simple break-down of these figures also showed that the ratio of above-knee amputations to below-knee amputations remained at approximately 2:1. In Dundee in 1966, just after the setting up of the Dundee Limb Fitting Centre, the above-knee/below-knee ratio was comparable, viz. just under 2:1. However, an aggressive policy commenced in 1967, of salvaging the knee joint wherever possible, reduced this ratio almost immediately, to 1:1. By 1971 the ratio had been reversed, being 1:1.5, and by 1973 the ratio had become over three below-knee amputations to every one above-knee amputation. Although there was a variation in the ratio in the ensuing years it was never worse than approximately two below-knee amputations for every above-knee. By 1984 not only was a ratio of 3:1 BK/AK being achieved, but in addition local studies showed a success rate in the region of 90% for below-knee amputations. In view of this persistently better BK to AK ratio in Dundee compared with the rest of Scotland, and certainly with England and Wales, it was felt that a prospective study should be set up to confirm these figures and, in so doing, highlight the value of both modern vascular techniques and the concentration of clinical expertise. The study was externally monitored throughout.*

One hundred consecutive patients with major peripheral vascular disease for whom no vascular, or no further vascular, salvage procedures could be performed were admitted prospectively into the study. The mean age of these patients was 73 and the male/female ratio was 59:41. The number suffering from diabetes was 45, which at first sight seemed relatively high. However, the criterion for describing

*Mr Peter McCollum, FRCSI, St James' Hospital, Dublin.

a patient as diabetic was previously established diabetes mellitus or an abnormal glucose tolerance test. Of the 100 patients, 69 presented with gangrene plus rest pain, 19 had gangrene alone and 12 had rest pain alone. Pre-amputation assessment included clinical evaluation and vascular laboratory examination. In the latter, emphasis was placed on two tests, skin blood flow measurement and the thermoscan. The skin blood flow tests were carried out routinely at three sites, two anteriorly 10 cm distal to the tibial tuberosity and 3 cm on either side of the tibial crest, and a third, 15 cm distal to the tibial tuberosity in the midline posteriorly. These results were then superimposed on a thermoscan taken at the same event. The thermoscan, using 15 colour-coded grades of 0.4 °C and related to the skin blood flow, indicated the rapidity of the skin temperature fall-off not only in the long axis of the limb, but also in the mediolateral plane. Because of the precision of this gradient the thermoscan could be used to delineate skew flaps, and indeed on two patients this information was used in planning the operation, thus salvaging the knee.

Table 58.1 Skin blood flow results. Mean skin blood flows (averages) in above- and below-knee groups for diabetics and non-diabetics (ml/100 g/min).

	Diabetics	Non-diabetics
Above-knee group (10) (recommended)	1.0 ± 1.3 ($n = 3$)	1.3 ± 0.9 ($n = 7$)
Above-knee group (9) (not recommended)	8.5 ± 7.6 ($n = 2$)	6.5 ± 3.9 ($n = 7$)
Below-knee group (81)	9.6 ± 5.2 ($n = 40$)	8.4 ± 3.3 ($n = 41$)

Using the skin blood flow results (Table 58.1) and the thermoscan, ten patients were recommended to have an above-knee amputation as their flow fell considerably below the recommended level of 2.5 ml per 100 g per minute using ^{125}I-4-iodo-antipyrine. Nine patients were recommended by the vascular laboratory as being able to have a below-knee amputation but in fact had an above-knee amputation for clinical reasons, such as fixed flexion contracture of the knee. This left a total of 81 patients on whom vascular laboratory analysis had suggested that a below-knee amputation could be carried out and was indeed carried out. It was also noted on evaluation of the skin blood flow results that diabetics had a higher skin blood flow average than non-diabetics.

Results

Of the 100 patients there was an operative mortality of zero. Of the 19 above-knee amputations (including one through-knee amputation), all healed, 18 of them primarily and one after a further revision. Of the 81 below-knee amputations there were six failures, two of which in retrospect were felt to be due to poor surgical technique and one due to severe infection. Of the 75 patients left, seven below-knee stumps failed in the sense that they required a local 'wedge resection'. However, these wedge resections were successful, and in all seven patients a below-knee level was retained giving a total of 75 patients whose end result was a successful below-knee amputation.

In conclusion, of the 100 patients entered into the trial, 19 were selected either by vascular laboratory or by clinical evaluation to have an above-knee amputation which was successful in each case. Eighty-one patients were recommended to have a below-knee amputation, and 75 of these patients had a successful below-knee amputation. This gives a ratio of three below-knee amputations to each above-knee amputation out of 100 consecutive patients and a success rate in the below-knee amputation of 93%. It is recommended therefore that below-knee amputation should be considered seriously in almost all cases of major vascular disease and that by using vascular laboratory techniques such as skin blood flow and thermography a success rate of over 90% can be achieved by surgeons with the appropriate expertise.

Clinical team practice

Post-operative care

The clinician in charge of prosthetic care must be involved from the first post-operative day and, further, his involvement must be within an environment conducive to total integrated care. He must have the support of nursing staff, therapists, prosthetists, engineers and others, all of whom must be familiar with the specific problems to be overcome. Certain conditions require special mention — diabetes, other manifestations of vascular disease, cardiovascular problems and many others. There are also the social implications of limb loss — what is the patient's social status?; how supportive is the family? All these matters require co-ordination, and case conferences are held regularly to achieve this end.

Post-operative care in a specialized unit allows close monitoring of stump care — it allows strict measures to be applied in order to control stump volume. Post-surgical failure such as non-viability, delayed healing and infection can be critically observed and measures can be taken to amend treatment and management as necessary. These activities once again depend on the environment and the professionals involved.

The final stage is when decisions must be made regarding prosthetic fitting. This involves the prosthetist and therapists as well as the medical staff. Once again group consultation is necessary to optimize care. If a decision is made not to embark on prosthetic fitting, efforts must then be directed at wheelchair mobility and maximization of self-care.

Nursing

Dundee Limb Fitting Centre, being a converted house, lends itself to creating a homely atmosphere with its small intimate wards, three of which are four-bedded and one five-bedded. Each ward is furnished with variable-height beds and combined wardrobe–locker units where patients can keep their day clothes. The wearing of personal clothing helps patients regain their identity and individuality and is a most effective way of boosting their morale and confidence. All patients initially use a wheelchair to promote independence and mobility from the day of admission. To secure as normal an environment as possible, all meals are served in the dining room, where patients are encouraged to transfer to dining room chairs and integrate with others.

It is normally the nursing staff who have the first contact with the patient on his arrival at the Centre, two to three days after operation. The relatives usually telephone a short time after the patient's admission. This initial telephone call gives an opportunity to encourage the relatives to visit and it can also help to foster good relationships. At this stage the patient feels very insecure and apprehensive so the nursing staff strive to create a pleasant and relaxed environment and provide support, reassurance and encouragement, and allay fears regarding treatment, domestic circumstances and future capabilities. Such anxieties can have a detrimental effect on the patient's recovery, so timely discussion with, and referral to, the other disciplines is important in averting future difficulties.

Friendly contact with relatives is imperative if their fears about the patient's future, and his return home, are to be allayed. Often relatives require as much reassurance and support as the patient himself. Information gained from this contact must be shared with colleagues as the attitude of the relatives can have a substantial influence on the patient's progress. The handling of such situations requires experienced staff, and the Centre is particularly fortunate as many of the staff have been there for a considerable time. Both the ward sisters have worked at the Centre for a number of years, and, although most of the other members of the nursing staff are part-time they live locally, and over half of them have remained for longer than nine years. Such stability engenders trust and confidence between patients, their relatives and the staff.

The training of new staff, however, is vitally important if the standard of nursing care is to be maintained, and therefore a planned programme of orientation is given to new members over a period of a month. The nursing staff must, of course, be proficient in:
(a) Basic nursing care and in assessing the patient both mentally and physically, but also must have specialized knowledge in
(b) Use of rigid dressings, controlled environment treatment and soft dressings.
(c) Transfers and wheelchair training.
(d) Skin care.

(e) Stump care.

(f) Liaison and communication with other disciplines.

As patients with peripheral vascular disease have a high risk of developing pressure sores, special attention is paid to the skin. Research carried out by Miss Marjorie Wood, the first Senior Nurse at the Centre, showed that 27.1% of all patients admitted to Dundee Limb Fitting Centre after amputation surgery had some degree of skin damage. Following this research Miss Wood started a campaign in the Dundee hospitals to minimize this problem. In consequence, the nursing staff have been well disciplined in the care of the skin, and for this reason patients are seldom admitted with pressure sores from the main referring hospital or develop such a sore during their stay in the Centre. Occasionally, however, patients are admitted with pressure sores after a prolonged illness at home or in other hospitals. It is also important that the nurse affords the same intensity of care and attention to the contralateral leg if deterioration of the remaining foot is to be avoided. Frequent change of position is advocated to prevent decubitus ulceration, but with the help of the physiotherapists and occupational therapists it has been found that the regime of early mobilization is one of the most effective ways of both preventing and healing pressure sores, and of improving the circulation to the contralateral leg.

Stump care is also stressed when training staff. Nurses are made aware of the importance of reducing stump volume in preparation for prosthetic fitting, and of the significance of bandaging the stump correctly and frequently after wound healing. The bandaging regime is taught and supervised on several occasions before the nurses are allowed to perform the task on their own. The nurse not only has to be proficient in the bandaging technique, but must also be able to train and supervise both the patient and his relatives in preparation for the patient's discharge.

Co-operation and communication with the other disciplines cannot be over-emphasized, as all disciplines are interdependent and good relationships are a prime factor in creating the happy and secure environment which is conducive to the patient's progress. As the discipline providing the 24-hour service, the nursing staff have to supervise care of the prosthesis and walking training in the evenings and at weekends, and any significant changes are reported to the therapists on their return.

To provide continuity of service the community nurse visits the Centre once a week for an update on patients almost ready for discharge. In this way preparation for visits by the health visitor, general practitioner and community nurse, if necessary, can be arranged well in advance of the patient's discharge, and a two-way link with the community is established.

Physiotherapy

Physiotherapy treatment of the amputee starts on the day of admission or the morning after. Each morning the patient receives general maintenance exercises and stump exercises aimed at preventing contractures and in preparation for prosthetic use. These exercises are carried out in the wards. Screens are not drawn around the bed for these sessions. These *individual, manually resisted* exercises allow the physiotherapy staff to get an impression of the patient not only regarding strength and range of movement, but also regarding his personality and mental state. There is the opportunity to talk with the patient about his fears and hopes for the future. The nursing staff and the occupational therapist gather other useful background information from the patient's relatives and friends.

From about 10 o'clock onwards, the patients are up and dressed in their day clothes and are encouraged to move around the Unit independently in the wheelchair supplied to them on admission. Both measures help the patient feel more human and less dependent on others. Because of the layout of the Unit, no-one is required to fetch the patient from the ward area. The patients wheel themselves about and tend to congregate in the physiotherapy department of their own choice. There is always something going on there and they watch each other's progress with interest. This is not discouraged as it is felt that the advantages of the patient being immediately available far outweigh any disadvantages of lack of privacy. Privacy can be attained by taking the patient to another quieter area of the Unit. Because the patients are on hand, the duration and frequency of treatment sessions can be adjusted as required.

In the initial stages of walking training the patient is taught to stand and then hop between parallel bars. The fitter patients progress quickly to axillary crutches and are encouraged to go out and about if they are safe in their use. Crutches may also be supplied to some patients for use at home to go to the toilet during the night. This is preferable to having a commode or urinal in their bedroom. Patients are not encouraged to hop with a Zimmer or walker as it encourages a flexed hip posture. The below-knee amputees start walking with the pneumatic post-amputation mobility aid (PPAM) at seven days post-operatively, as they are normally in a rigid dressing at this stage. The through-knee and Syme amputees will start gait training on adapted walking plasters at seven days. The bilateral amputee who already has a satisfactorily fitting prosthesis on one side will be progressed in the same way as the single amputee, standing, hopping and using a PPAM aid. Unfortunately, a suitable early mobilization device for use with the above-knee amputee has yet to be identified.

As time passes, an impression will be gained as to the patient's likely ability to cope with the prosthesis. Although the majority of patients are satisfactorily fitted, there are some whose needs will not be best met by provision of a prosthesis. These patients will be supplied with a suitable wheelchair and be trained to be as independent as possible using this. On average the below-knee amputees receive their first prosthesis 31 days post-operatively and the above-knee amputees 21 days post-operatively. The alignment unit will still be in the prosthesis at this stage. Initial instructions to the patient regarding walking are kept to a few simple sentences and the patient is allowed to walk. Gait problems are dealt with as they arise. The prosthetist makes regular checks on the patient's performance and makes any alignment changes or socket adjustments as necessary. During this period the patient's gait will alter as he gains confidence and adapts to prosthetic wear.

Since the majority of the above-knee amputees are atherosclerotic and elderly, they are initially fitted with a prosthesis with a semi-automatic knee lock as it is preferable for the patient to feel confident enough to venture out of the house than have a knee mechanism which he does not trust to support him. If the patient walks very well with a knee lock from the outset, then the knee unit can be changed on a trial basis to a free knee at an early stage.

Regular checks are made on the stump condition during walking training. If the suture line is not completely healed, the nursing staff are consulted about the most suitable type of dressing to protect this area during limb wear.

Both physiotherapists and nursing staff are involved in teaching the patients how to put on their prosthesis, take it off and wash and care for their stump and prosthesis. Patients are also taught to recognize the number of stump socks required to achieve a good fit, as the stump volume gradually decreases. They soon progress to wearing the limb all day, and the nursing staff maintain the patients' prosthetic training in the evenings and at weekends.

Once the patient is walking independently with the appropriate walking aid and the prosthetist is satisfied with the alignment, the limb is taken to the workshops for removal of the alignment unit and final fabrication. On return of the completed prosthesis the patient will be discouraged from using his wheelchair and will be walking everywhere within the Centre and outside in the grounds. The occupational therapist will report about the size, layout and surroundings of the patient's home which provides guidelines about the level of activity the patient will require to cope at home.

The majority of the amputees are discharged home walking with two canes/ sticks. It is hoped that they will have at least achieved the following goals:
1 Putting on and taking off the limb independently.
2 Walking indoors on carpeted and vinyl surfaces.
3 Ascending and descending a flight of stairs with one banister.
4 Ascending and descending one step without a handrail.
5 Walking on outdoor surfaces, as appropriate to the patient's home, and use of a car.

Occupational therapy

At Dundee Limb Fitting Centre, occupational therapy is carried out with the co-operation of, and in conjunction with, all other disciplines, most especially with physiotherapy and nursing. The occupational therapist is directly concerned with providing advice and instruction to the patient, with the aim of promoting independence in activities of daily living (ADL). Such instruction is geared as appropriate to the different stages of the patient's progress and includes:
(a) Instruction with dressing, this being undertaken only where appropriate.

(b) Instruction as to the most relevant techniques which will allow independent and confident toileting and bathing.

(c) Developing the patient's level of proficiency in transfer, both prior to limb supply and after issue of the limb. The patient is taught how to transfer safely and confidently to and from the bed, to and from a domestic chair, and to and from a car. In the situation where the patient will be resuming use of a car, information pertaining to financial assistance and those vehicle adaptations which are available is supplied.

(d) Also undertaken, as necessary, is assessment and retraining, or instruction in domestic activities.

The occupational therapist is concerned also with the patient's ability with reference to wheelchair independence, manoeuvrability and general mobility, both within the Centre and, if necessary, on discharge. Any special adaptations to be made to the wheelchair may be discussed with the physiotherapist or engineering staff. Should the permanent provision of a wheelchair be required, the size and model of chair provided would be related primarily to the patient's personal needs, but with consideration as to his home circumstances or environment on discharge.

To provide the most suitable and relevant service to patients, it is necessary to know their aspirations and background. Accordingly, discussion with both the patient and, if possible, relatives is very important. This information obtained by the occupational therapist supplements that already received by physiotherapy and nursing staff. Following discussions with the patient, a home visit would be carried out, initially without the patient, but involving a family member or carer, and a representative of the community services. The physical information gained from a home visit concerns walking surfaces, potential hazards and areas likely to require adaptation, and may prove to be useful to the other disciplines in terms of directing training. For example, access may involve negotiating stairs and steps although these may have already been adapted for his particular needs. Additionally, this visit should provide the staff with an impression of the patient's level of self-care when at home. Both factors will provide indications as to the most appropriate community services to contact. This is usually done after conference with the other disciplines within the Centre. A provisional order of aids or adaptations to the home may be made at this point.

A further home visit should be carried out when appropriate. On this occasion the visit should be made with the patient, along with the physiotherapist, and a representative of the community services. This visit allows both the patient and accompanying staff members to estimate the problems which the patient may encounter on discharge. It also allows the community representative an opportunity of meeting the patient, when his capabilities in the company of staff from the Centre may be observed, as opposed to meeting him only after discharge, or in a more artificial hospital environment. This also provides for the patient a familiar face after discharge, when he may otherwise be confronted by community representatives who are unfamiliar.

Communication is a very large part of the role of occupational therapists. It is their responsibility to relay patient's progress to the community services, with the aim of providing the maximum *required* support on discharge, and to supply the Centre with progress reports regarding the provision of aids and the installation of adaptations. Continuity of service is provided by visiting the patient at home one week to ten days after discharge. In this way the occupational therapist can confirm that all requested services have been supplied and, at that stage in the patient's progress, are applicable. Should such a visit prove impractical, the relevant information is relayed to the Centre by the community service via the occupational therapist.

Follow-up has a two-way benefit. On the one hand it allows the therapist to check the patient's level of ability at home and relate any relevant information to the Centre, and on the other the patient is made aware of the Centre's continuing interest in his welfare.

Prosthetic supply

Prior to 1980 the supply of prostheses in Tayside, as in the rest of the United Kingdom, was achieved by virtue of a centrally negotiated contract with a commercial limb fitting company which was responsible for the operation of a workshop located within Dundee Limb Fitting Centre staffed by both prosthetists and prosthetic technicians. In 1980, in partial fulfilment of one of the principal recommendations of the report of a Working Party on the Future of the Artificial Limb Service in Scotland (Scottish Home and Health Department 1970), prosthetists in the employ of a contractor were offered the opportunity of transferring to the National Health Service. Following the acceptance of this proposal a new contract was negotiated with the company which now operates solely in the capacity of a prosthetic fabricator. The original Working Party proposals had envisaged a complete NHS takeover of the entire prosthetic supply process which would have included transfer of the prosthetic technicians along with the prosthetists; this combined transfer did not prove possible (and has still not come about) and the transfer of the prosthetists alone had to be accepted. In spite of initial misgivings regarding this compromise, successful working procedures have been established with the company and its representatives in the Limb Fitting Centre, including, crucially, the opportunity for NHS prosthetists to consult directly with individual technical staff carrying out fabrication.

The second major recommendation of the Working Party relating to the training and education of prosthetists resulted in the creation of the National Centre for Training and Education in Prosthetics and Orthotics within the University of Strathclyde. From the day that the Centre 'opened its doors' in 1973 the Tayside Health Board has supported, both in principle and financially, a policy of sponsoring student prosthetists during their training at the National Centre, and it is recorded with pride that the first two graduates to enter the limb fitting service in Scotland were employed in Dundee in 1978. The present staffing of the Prosthetic Section comprises a principal prosthetist and two prosthetists, who are responsible for an amputee population of 712 patients. The department has been accredited as suitable for the internship training of graduate prosthetists from the National Centre.

The reorganization of the prosthetic service, which derives from the Working Party report, has resulted in a number of important changes in the manner of operation of the service in Dundee. In the bluntest terms it has freed the prosthetists from the inevitable conflict of loyalties which must occur when attempting to reconcile the clinical needs of the patient and the responsibility to uphold the commercial interests of an employer. This particular change in the manner of operation is most clearly demonstrated by reference to current prescription policy. Prior to the transfer of the prosthetists all prostheses supplied in Dundee used components manufactured by a single commercial supplier or one of its associated companies. Since the transfer it has become policy to prescribe and request the supply of a range of different makes of prostheses selected by the team on the basis of clinical considerations alone.

For many years prior to the reorganization an NHS controlled and staffed workshop was operated, enabling the supply of 'temporary' prostheses to below-knee patients virtually on demand. These prostheses, which incorporated a custom PTB socket and a simple re-usable pylon and SACH foot, were used during initial mobilization and to delay placing an order for the first commercially manufactured prostheses while the stump volume stabilized. During the negotiations following the transfer of prosthetists, which included a ban on all future NHS fabrication activities, this experience was exploited to obtain favourable delivery times for all prostheses delivered in Dundee.

Arrangements styled 'projected limb arrival' (PLA) exist for all the Scottish prosthetic centres and allow 20 working days between the placement of an order for a prosthesis and its delivery 'ready for fitting'. An unofficial arrangement in Dundee has enabled this delivery period to be reduced to only five days. An even more favourable arrangement relating to the finishing of prostheses has enabled the period from the completion of the fitting until the delivery of the finished prosthesis to be reduced from the official 20 days to as little as 24 hours when prior notice is given. This arrangement ensures the minimum interruption in the patient's programme of mobilization and is obviously of considerable importance when considering bed occupancy.

Several other innovations are worthy of mention. While not participating on a routine basis in the biweekly ward rounds, prosthetists are immediately available for 'ad hoc' consultation with the rehabilitation consultant at any time during the early post-operative phase when the patient is being assessed with regard to future prosthetic supply. Every amputee in Dundee is personally allocated to an individual prosthetist who will be responsible for all future prosthetic treatment. This apparently obvious arrangement was not possible during the previous commercial regime.

A particularly important practice which has been instituted even before the transfer of the prosthetists is the use of an 'extended fitting period'. This practice, which is only possible because of the existence of in-patient facilities, allows primary amputees the opportunity of wearing their prosthesis in the unfinished form for as long as is necessary to ensure that its fit and function are acceptable. During this period, which is normally about a week, the prosthetist and the physiotherapist will collaborate in resolving any problems with the socket and optimizing the alignment. It is believed that this practice, allied to the intensive measures applied to the control of stump volume, is a principal factor in determining the service life which is typically obtained from first prostheses. Statistics collected during a one-year study demonstrate that on average the first prosthesis is used for 147 days, loss of fit of the socket being the usual cause of withdrawal.

It is necessary when describing prosthetic practices in Dundee to pay tribute to the roles of first Charles Radcliffe and later Jim Foort, who during their visits to Scotland in 1967 and 1969 respectively were responsible for introducing many of the prosthetic techniques which form the backbone of our service today. It is fortunate that this role has formally passed to the National Centre for Training and Education in Prosthetics and Orthotics, which should guarantee the ability to maintain a high standard of prosthetic practice.

The clinical environment at Dundee Limb Fitting Centre with its multi-disciplinary staffing and workshop and laboratory facilities offers an ideal environment for research. In the past this has been exploited to permit a wide range of research activities including electromyographic studies of stump musculature, the evaluation of post-operative management techniques and clinical trials of new prosthetic products. A current study of amputee activity is employing a range of techniques including step counters, and a clinical trial of Rapidform sockets for above-knee patients commissioned by the Bioengineering Centre at Roehampton is being completed. This tradition of research will be continued with the initiation of a project designed to establish a routine prosthetic gait analysis service, utilizing the facilities of the modern gait analysis laboratory.

At this time when the structure of the service in other parts of the United Kingdom is under review, it is important for those in Dundee and in the rest of Scotland to state without any doubt their favourable view of the changes which took place some years ago. These changes have resulted in an improved prosthetic supply and additional benefits which include increased confidence in the ability of the prosthetic service in Scotland to face the challenges which remain to be overcome.

Rehabilitation outcome

Discharge from the Dundee Limb Fitting Centre occurs on average on the 41st day after admission (Table 58.2). 81.8% are sufficiently independent to return home or to be placed in sheltered accommodation. The traditional pylon prosthesis is never used and it has been the practice to fit a definitive limb from the outset. The patients return for prosthetic review six weeks after discharge; they may telephone for an earlier appointment if they feel it is necessary.

Table 58.2 Discharge placement of primary amputees.

Home	79.3%	(range 71.7%–89.5%)	} 81.8%
Residential home for the elderly	2.5%		
Long-term geriatric ward	10.7%		
Acute hospital	3.8%		
Rehabilitation centre	0.3%		
Died in DLFC	3.4%		

The first visit allows the patients the opportunity to tell the staff how they have managed at home. It further ensures that reinforcement of training undertaken at the Centre can occur as renewed contact with nursing, physiotherapy, occupational therapy, prosthetic and medical staff is encouraged. The patient's prosthesis is reviewed and the prosthetic prescription is reconsidered. Prosthetic prescription is further reviewed at the subsequent out-patient visits, usually occurring initially at three- and six-monthly intervals. Procedures for supply of a new prosthesis can be instituted at any of these visits or at other times if considered necessary.

It has been found that patients' walking independence continues to improve after discharge from the Centre. Reviewing 57 primary amputees during the six months after discharge, it was found that the number who required to use two sticks to aid walking reduced from 41.5% at the time of discharge to 27.8% by the six months review period. It can be seen, however, that the amputation resulted in significant loss of total independence. In a comparison of 15 primary below-knee amputees, five primary above-knee amputees and 12 age-related non-amputee peers, it was found that the peers achieved on average 8366 steps a day while the amputees only achieved 2498 steps a day. This indicated that the amputees were much less independent than the peer group.

When the patient achieves an overall stable state a yearly letter is sent asking if they require a review. In this way all the patients are given the opportunity to visit the prosthetic clinic at least once a year.

Patient data have been collected since the inception of the unit. This represents 20 years of practice of amputee care and over 1200 primary amputees. The data include information on age, sex, concurrent disabilities, principal cause of amputation, level of amputation, revision of stump, prosthetic fitting, wheelchair supply and patient survival. The latter is obtained from Register House in Edinburgh and from those records kept in Tayside Health Board offices. The results showed the predominance of men in the primary amputee population. The age of the amputee has been remarkably steady for the period 1966–1981. However, in the year 1984 there appeared to be a rise in the numbers over the age of 60 years (Table 58.3). The cause of amputation showed the significance of vascular disease, but in addition to the amputation aetiology it was found that the patient had two or three other significant pathological problems (Table 58.4).

Table 58.3 Age at amputation.

Mean age	70 years
Constant for years 1966–1981	

Slight increase in 1984 with 73.8% over the age of 60 years compared with 70.1% for previous years

In 1984, using a glucose tolerance test prior to surgery, the incidence of diabetes mellitus was found to be almost 50% in the vascular-related amputee patients. This was confirmed by a fasting blood sugar taken once the stump was soundly healed.

Table 58.4 Aetiology of amputations (1232 cases).

59.8%	PVD	(741 cases)	} 86.7% vascular
26.9%	Diabetes mellitus	(329 cases)	
13.3%	Other	(162 cases)	

It can be seen that over the 20 years there has been a predominance of below-knee amputations (Table 58.5). In 1984, 68.4% were amputated at below-knee and 29.8% above-knee, there being no Syme amputation and only one through-knee amputation. It can be observed that over the years there has been a dramatic reversal of the above-knee/below-knee ratio in favour of the below-knee level (Fig. 58.1). The surgery failed however in 20% of cases, usually at below-knee level, but by the use of the wedge resection technique in 12% only 8% overall required an amputation to a higher level (Table 58.6). Prostheses were supplied to 87.1% of the patients (Table 58.7). Some patients were considered unsuitable for fitting with an artificial limb and were supplied with a wheelchair for home use, a few having both limb and wheelchair.

Table 58.5 Amputation levels — 1966–1984, all diagnoses.

30.8%	AK
58%	BK
4%	Syme
6.2%	Through-knee
1%	TH/HQ

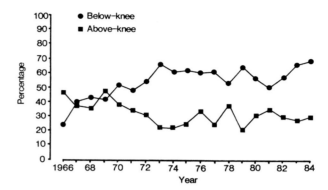

Fig. 58.1 Amputation level —
all diagnoses, 1966–1984.

Table 58.6 Secondary surgery.

Overall 20.4%	
PVD 13.2%	Wedge resections 12.3% (same level).
DM 6.6%	
	Higher amputation 8.1%
Other 0.6%	

Table 58.7 Supply of prostheses.

87.1% of patients supplied with prostheses (range 75–96.1%)

12.1% of patients not supplied (0.8% not recorded)

A contralateral amputation at a later date was necessary in over 180 cases. Below-knee amputation was again the amputation of choice (Table 58.8). The resultant second amputation produced 45.8% double below-knee amputees (Table 58.9), and again the majority were vascular-related amputations (Table 58.10). At the second amputation, surgery failed in nearly 30% of cases but with the use of the wedge resection only 11% required a reamputation to a higher level. Following

Table 58.8 Secondary amputation levels.

32.4%	AK
61.5%	BK
2.3%	Syme
1.1%	Through-knee
2.8%	Foot

Table 58.9 Final level of bilateral amputations.

Overall	27.7% double AK
	45.8% double BK
	17.5% AK/BK
	9% other

Overall the amputation on the contralateral leg was at BK level

Table 58.10 Double amputees on file — cause of second amputation.

61.9%	PVD	
35.4%	DM	} 97.4% vascular
1.1%	Trauma	
1.6%	Other	

Table 58.11 Double amputees on file.

Disposal	
68.3%	Fitted with prosthesis
29.1%	Not fitted
2.6%	Missing

Table 58.12 Double amputees on file — discharge placement.

78.2%	Home	
2.7%	Residential home for the elderly	} 80.9% independent (148 cases)
7.7%	Geriatric waiting list	
6.0%	Acute hospital	
4.9%	Died in DLFC	
0.5%	Transfer to rehabilitation hospital	

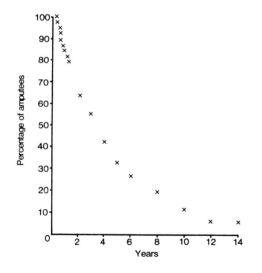

Fig. 58.2 Amputee survival data 1965–1981. Percentage of study surviving against time in years.

Table 58.13 Amputee survival information.

Life expectancy of all vascular patients		3 years 1 month
	AK	2 years 11 months
	BK	3 years 3 months
Life expectancy for age peers (70 years old)		10 years

the second amputation 68.3% were fitted with prostheses (Table 58.11). Despite the second amputation 80.9% were fit enough either to return home or to sheltered accommodation (Table 58.12).

The life expectancy of the Dundee vascular amputee proved to be three years one month. Some 80% of the amputees were still alive two years after amputation, 40% were alive at four years and 10% by ten years (Table 58.13). This life expectancy contrasts markedly with the life expectancy of ten years for a 70-year-old person (Fig. 58.2).

The data collection has allowed the Centre to audit its progress in each successive year. This has ensured that changes can be observed and analysed and alterations made in the clinical practice if deemed appropriate. In this way the Dundee Limb Fitting Centre has ensured a sustained level of interest and confidence in the clinical activities. In particular, the belief in the clinic team has been strengthened and the group is confident that comprehensive assessment, goal setting, careful attention to the technical detail by all members of the clinic team, continuous monitoring of the team's activities and the courage to reset goals when required are all essential to good clinical practice.

Reference

Scottish Home and Health Department (1970) The future of the Artificial Limb Service in Scotland: report of a working party set up by the Secretary of State for Scotland. London: HMSO.

Index

COMPLETED